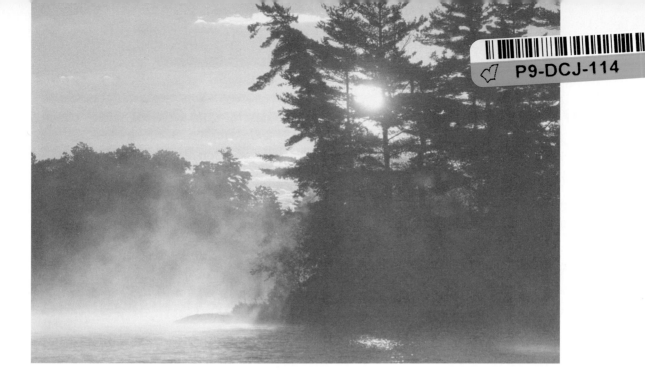

# ETHICAL &
# LEGAL ISSUES

*in Canadian Nursing*

## THIRD EDITION

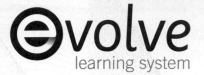
learning system

Evolve provides online access to free learning resources and activities designed specifically for the textbook you are using in your class. The resources will provide you with information that enhances the material covered in the book and much more.

Visit the Web address lised below to start your learning evolution today!

# http://evolve.elsevier.com/Canada/Keatings/ethical/

*Evolve® Student Learning Resources for Keatings,* **Ethical and Legal Issues in Canadian Nursing, 3rd Edition,** *offer the following features:*

## Student Resources

- **Review Questions** test your reading comprehension for each chapter.

- **Critical Thinking Scenarios** provide additional scenarios to the cases presented throughout the textbook.

- **Case Scenarios from the CNA** *Code of Ethics* help you to understand the Code and how it applies to nursing practice.

- **WebLinks** let you link to Web sites carefully chosen to supplement the content of the textbook.

- A **Glossary** comprehensively lists all of the key terms found in the textbook.

ELSEVIER

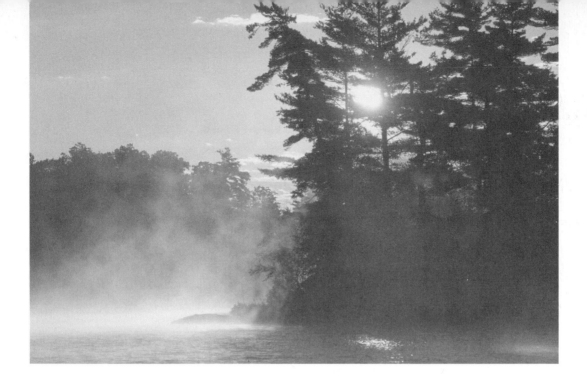

# ETHICAL &
# LEGAL ISSUES

## *in Canadian Nursing*

### THIRD EDITION

Margaret Keatings, RN, MHSc

O'Neil Smith, BA, LLB (of the Ontario Bar)

**MOSBY**
ELSEVIER

**Copyright © 2010 Elsevier Canada, a division of Reed Elsevier Canada, Ltd.**

NOTICE

Knowledge and best practice in this field are constantly changing. As new research and expertise broaden our knowledge, changes in practice, treatment, and drug therapy may become necessary or appropriate. Readers are advised to check the most current information provided (i) on procedures featured or (ii) by the manufacturer of each product to be administered, to verify the recommended dose or formula, the method and duration of administration, and contraindications. It is the responsibility of the practitioner, relying on his or her own experience and knowledge of the patient, to make diagnoses, to determine dosages and the best treatment for each individual patient, and to take all appropriate safety precautions. To the fullest extent of the law, neither the publisher nor the authors assume any liability for any injury and/or damage to persons or property arising out of or related to any use of the material contained in this book.

The Publisher

**Library and Archives Canada Cataloguing in Publication**
Keatings, Margaret
    Ethical & legal issues in Canadian nursing / Margaret Keatings,
O'Neil B. Smith — 3rd ed.
Includes index.
ISBN 978-1-897422-09-0
    1. Nursing ethics—Canada.  2. Nursing—Law and legislation—Canada.
I. Smith, O'Neil B. (O'Neil Brian), 1962–  II. Title.  III. Title: Ethical
and legal issues in Canadian nursing.
RT85.K43 2009        174.2        C2008-907275-8

VICE PRESIDENT, PUBLISHING: Ann Millar
MANAGING DEVELOPMENTAL EDITOR: Tammy Scherer
MANAGING PRODUCTION EDITOR: Roberta A. Spinosa-Millman
COPY EDITOR: Cathy Witlox
COVER, INTERIOR DESIGN: George Kirkpatrick
TYPESETTING AND ASSEMBLY: Jansom
PRINTING AND BINDING: Transcontinental

Elsevier Canada
905 King Street West, 4th Floor
Toronto, ON, Canada M6K 3G9
Phone: 1-866-896-3331
Fax: 1-866-359-9534

Printed in Canada

1 2 3 4 5      13 12 11 10 09

# Contents

**Chapter 6**     **Consent to Treatment  155**

**Chapter 7**    **The Nurse's Legal Accountabilities: Professional Competence, Misconduct, Malpractice, and Nursing Documentation  188**

**Chapter 11**    **Caregiver Rights 348**

In appreciation of the love and support I receive from my father Patrick, sister Linda, niece Kathleen, godson Erik, and in loving memory of my mother Jean and brother Frank.

MARGARET KEATINGS

To Claudia, Ksenia and Stephanie with all my love.

O'NEIL SMITH

# Preface

SINCE THE FIRST EDITION of this book was published in 1994, the role of ethics in the day-to-day practice of nurses has grown significantly. With the introduction of ethical theory into the curriculum, nurses are becoming more aware of what constitutes ethical issues in health care, acquiring greater knowledge about ethical theory and principles, and gaining competence in addressing ethical challenges. As a result, as health care team members, they are becoming confident participants in the important dialogue surrounding individual issues and in reaching a consensus on the best course of action or approach in a difficult situation. At the same time, the ethical issues facing nurses and the interprofessional team have grown in both complexity and prevalence. Ethics and the law are becoming increasingly intertwined as new legislation is introduced to ensure ethical standards are met. In other words, previously common or best practices are now being regulated (e.g., the regulations for consent to treatment, which were formerly embedded in common law and standards of practice). Further, as ethics and the law become integrated into the core curriculum of all health care professions, nurses are embracing new roles, such as that of the clinical ethicist—an expert resource, for the health care team and families of patients or clients, who supports and facilitates ethical decision making.

As with the previous two editions, *Ethical and Legal Issues in Canadian Nursing* is by no means a comprehensive or exhaustive text. Chapters are arranged to facilitate both class discussion and individual study. Point-form learning objectives guide the reader through the material; each chapter summary reiterates and reinforces the key points. In this edition, additional case scenarios have been introduced to focus discussion of the issues raised and to encourage class participation. Case scenarios at the end of each chapter encourage critical thinking, discussion, and debate among students or practitioners and their colleagues. Following the case scenarios are questions for discussion, which are intended to integrate the chapter's key concepts. Narratives that further exemplify central themes are woven throughout selected chapters. Relevant current Canadian case law has been updated, and additional references provide readers with sources for further investigation into the legal issues facing the nursing profession.

This edition includes Evolve® online resources to accompany the text, for both students and instructors, which can be found at http://evolve.elsevier.com/Canada/Keatings/ethical. These include additional case scenarios, Weblinks, review questions, critical thinking scenarios that further explore chapter themes, a test bank, and PowerPoint® presentation slides.

In this edition, chapters have been extensively rearranged. Chapter 1 expands on previous editions and provides a more extensive introduction to ethics and the law. Chapter 2 delves into ethical theory and thought, and includes new material related to care and narrative ethics. Chapter 3 is a new chapter that examines the resources available to support nurses when dealing with ethical challenges, and concludes with a discussion of the values expounded in the CNA's *Code of Ethics for Registered Nurses* (2008). It includes case scenario examples that illustrate each value, found at http://evolve.elsevier.com/Canada/Keatings/ethical. Chapter 4 introduces the fundamentals of the Canadian legal system, as well as the differences between the common law and civil law traditions. Chapter 5 reviews the provincial regulatory systems that govern the nursing profession. Chapter 6 focuses on respectful and ethical strategies for obtaining informed consent to treatment, and considers patients' rights and the nurse's role. Nursing documentation has been integrated into Chapter 7, which examines the nurse's legal accountabilities (i.e., professional competence, misconduct, and malpractice), in which proper documentation is critical. The complex chapter "Ethical and Legal Issues at the Extremes of the Life Continuum," included in previous editions, has been separated into two chapters (Chapters 8 and 9) to enable updated discussions of the challenges and regulations related to the end of life and evolving and advancing technology. Chapter 10 contains an expanded focus on the rights of the patient, including patient safety, a key priority in Canadian health care and for accreditation bodies, and increasing cultural diversity, which introduces significant challenges in a system and culture with beliefs and values that may differ from those of new immigrants to Canada. Chapter 11 contains an added focus on the right to health and safety in the workplace: Individual nurses and leaders alike must pay attention to the critical issues associated with ensuring a healthy, safe, and violence-free work environment. A new final chapter, Chapter 12, has been introduced to discuss the ethical and legal complexities related to health care team interaction; the importance of patient- and family-centred care, leadership, and organizations; and approaches to processes such as recruitment.

Our goal throughout this book is to explain current ethical and legal concepts in Canadian nursing in as lucid a style as possible. To this end, tables and figures are included to illustrate pertinent concepts. Boxes highlight information of interest, such as the key points of historical codes of ethics or the health beliefs and practices of various cultural groups. Key terms are indicated in bold type and are further defined and explained in the Glossary, which has been expanded for this edition.

Throughout the book, we refer to the "patient" or "client." The term *patient* is used primarily to refer to those being cared for in an environment such as a hospital or an acute-care or long-term care setting (e.g., the seriously ill, accident victims), whereas the term *client* refers more to those being cared for in their own home or in a community setting (e.g., people accessing wellness programs or baby-care clinics).

We continue to regard *Ethical and Legal Issues in Canadian Nursing* as a work in progress. Many of the issues discussed continue to be debated in Parliament, provincial legislatures, the courts, and health care institutions. We welcome suggestions, criticism, and comments from readers in our continuing effort to improve this work.

The third edition of *Ethical and Legal Issues in Canadian Nursing* states the law as it stood in August, 2008. While every attempt has been made to ensure the accuracy of the information given, the authors and publisher emphasize that they are not engaged in providing medical, legal, or other professional advice. Those desiring such advice are encouraged to seek the assistance of appropriate professionals.

## Acknowledgements

The challenge of preparing a third edition of this book was no less difficult than writing the first two editions. During preparation of the manuscript, we relied upon the help, support, and encouragement of people too numerous to mention.

We wish to thank Ann Millar, Martina van de Velde, Tammy Scherer, Roberta Spinosa-Millman, Jane Clark, and especially Cathy Witlox at Elsevier Canada for their patience and understanding. We also acknowledge and thank those who reviewed the manuscript and provided helpful comments, constructive criticism, and suggestions for improvements:

Craig Duncan, Laurentian University
Marie Edwards, University of Manitoba
Carol Fine, Ryerson University
Jean Hughes, Dalhousie University
Rosemary MacDonald, University of Prince Edward Island
Joanne O'Brecht, Seneca College
Beth Perry, Athabasca University
Elizabeth Peter, University of Toronto
Linda Mary Scott, Centennial College
Riek van den Berg, University of Ottawa/The Ottawa Hospital
Wendy Wagner, Vancouver Island University

We wish to thank those nurses who shared their stories with us so that the case scenarios would more accurately reflect real practice situations. In particular, Margaret would like to acknowledge not only her own family members and friends but also the patients and families she has met over the years, whose experiences in the health care system inspired many of the text's case scenarios and added a new dimension to her appreciation of what constitutes ethical nursing practice.

Margaret would also like to acknowledge the support, guidance, and input she received from many of her colleagues at the Hospital for Sick Children and Hamilton Health Sciences. Their insights, stories, and ideas have enabled a deeper comprehension of the complex ethical and legal challenges faced in nursing and health care today.

Finally, we wish to thank our families and friends for their patience and understanding during the many hours spent away from them during the preparation of this third edition. Their sacrifice has not gone unnoticed, and their immense support has made this difficult work a good deal easier.

Margaret Keatings, RN, MHSc
O'Neil Smith, BA, LLB
January, 2009

# Chapter 1

## Introduction to Nursing Law and Ethics

**Learning Objectives**

The purpose of this chapter is to enable you to understand:

- Why nurses must be familiar with the law and ethics
- The knowledge nurses require to practise according to ethical and legal standards
- The role of professionals in serving the public interest
- How and why the field of ethics has grown over recent years
- The challenges nurses face when dealing with complex legal and ethical issues
- Key ethical and legal issues that arise in the practice of nursing

## Introduction

A CENTURY AGO, BEFORE THE nursing profession was regulated and before the technology available today was in place, nurses had no need to concern themselves with the legalities of their practice. Although there probably existed issues of negligence and malpractice, they were rarely considered because there was absolute faith in the medical system. However, even in early nursing schools, the study of ethics was deemed fundamental to the training of nurses. The major challenges faced at that time related primarily to:

- Behaving appropriately in the new health care environment (primarily hospitals at that time)
- Recognizing one's own faults, biases, and personality traits (e.g., tendency toward anger, impatience, ambition)
- Understanding the repercussions of misconduct, disloyalty, insubordination, and so on

Consider the following ethical issues identified in a textbook on nursing ethics first published in 1916 (Aikens, 1926):

Loyalty to the physician is one of the duties demanded of every nurse, not only because the physician is her superior officer, but chiefly because the confidence of the patient in his physician is one of the important elements in the management of his illness, and nothing should be said or done that would weaken this faith or create doubts as to the character or ability or methods of the physician on whom he is depending. (p. 25)

Aikens continues:

To learn to do the thing ordered punctually, when she is busy, when her own judgment opposes it or when she feels it to be unnecessary; to refrain from arguing the case when she feels she has a strong side to present; to make no grumbling comments about the order; to grasp the thought that the thing ordered is to be done even if it be inconvenient and so difficult as to be well-nigh impossible—these are qualities to be coveted and cultivated in every nurse. To make for herself a reputation for being faithful and dependable is possible for every nurse. (p. 66)

Much has changed over the past century. Today, nurses are expected to think critically, to offer evidence-informed solutions, and to respectfully challenge physicians or other health care professionals when they have concerns about the treatment plans of patients. Nursing has evolved into an autonomous profession, distinct from medicine, resulting in increasingly complex ethical challenges for nurses within the context of a more sophisticated and collaborative health care team.

Like other professionals, nurses operate within a set of professional standards as well as a framework of legal and ethical rules and guidelines. These are aimed at ensuring the consistency, quality, competence, and safety of health services, while preserving respect for individual rights and human dignity. As part of their professional role, nurses make and act on decisions that relate to both independent practice and collaborative relationships with other professionals; patients, clients, and their families; government agencies; and others. For all of these decisions and actions, the nursing professional must answer to individual clients or patients, their families, fellow health care team members, regulatory bodies, employers, their communities, the profession, and society in general. These multiple accountabilities may often be in conflict, posing challenges for nurses. Nurses, therefore, require a sound knowledge base, including familiarity with the law, ethics, ethical theory, and the workings of Canada's legal system; practical skills and reasoning skills; and a willingness both to take risks and to be accountable.

## Nursing, the Law, and Ethics

### Introduction

Members of professional groups have an obligation to serve the public interest and the common good because their roles, missions, and ethical foundations focus not only on the individuals they serve but on society as a whole. Professionals have this authority, and they accept this responsibility, because of their unique body of knowledge, skills, and expertise. Society has traditionally depended on professionals as custodians of such fields of knowledge as health, law, and education. They are placed in a position of respect and are accordingly given the power to engage in decisions that influence and shape public policy, law, and societal norms. As technology advances and the issues society faces become more complex, existing professions are becoming more specialized and new professions are emerging (Jennings, Callahan, & Wolf, 1987).

In recent years, the field of ethics in health care has gained greater prominence because of the increasing complexity and volume of ethical dilemmas, a result of the growing sophistication of science and technology. Consider the rapidly evolving field of genetics. We are capable of predicting congenital abnormalities and future illnesses at the embryonic stage of life. In this climate, questions arise: Is it right to do this? What precisely are we capable of doing? And if we proceed, what are we to do with the knowledge and information we gain? Advances in technology, too, have made it possible for us to affect various life processes in ways that pose moral and legal questions for health professionals, patients, and society alike. A growing awareness of patients' rights and a greater emphasis on respect for individual autonomy have consequently led to the establishment of advocacy groups representing the interests of various patient constituencies.

Nurses, in particular, have been challenged by an increasing number of ethical and legal concerns. As they confront each new issue, it is easy for them to be confused by the often conflicting interplay of ethics and law. Moreover, nurses must deal with these conflicts while providing quality, ethical care to patients within the context of a health care system strained by limited funds and resources. More than any other health professional, they are in sustained contact with patients in the home, in the community, and in the institutional setting. Nurses fulfill the important task of supporting patients and their families, as well as intervening or advocating on behalf of those patients when necessary. Their role involves building professional and trusting relationships with people throughout the life continuum. All of this must be achieved within the requirements of ethical rules and the law.

To aid them in the difficult decisions they make, nurses must have knowledge of ethics. Chapter 2 explores theories, principles, and decisional frameworks that guide nurses' ethical choices. This material is not exhaustive but is intended only to provide nurses with a foundation in ethics. In Chapter 3, these theories will be applied to the Canadian Nurses Association's *Code of Ethics for Registered Nurses*. This will begin the process of lifelong professional learning in ethics and provide a framework for the specific ethical themes discussed in later chapters.

## The Need to Know the Law

The situations nurses face as health professionals may involve clear institutional rules and procedures or straightforward legal rules and statutes. Yet, many situations are more complicated and require nurses to decide, from many possible alternative courses of action, the morally correct thing to do. At times, nurses may face situations in which what they believe to be the most ethically and legally correct course of action may not be supported by law, or in which they are clear on the right action but are unable to act upon it. An example of an ethical solution that is opposed by law can be found in the challenging and emotional debate surrounding euthanasia. One might believe that the most compassionate approach is desirable when death is inevitable; however, the **Criminal Code of Canada** clearly makes it an offence for a person to assist another person in taking his or her own life (*Criminal Code*, 1985).

Society holds nurses to high standards of professional, moral, and ethical competence, but it also affords them certain rights and privileges. The law strives to keep these competing interests in constant balance. It regulates the education and licensing of nurses; the conditions of their employment; their collective bargaining rights; their rights, duties, and responsibilities toward patients, physicians, other health care professionals, the public, and each other; and a host of other matters. Furthermore, the legal system provides a forum for resolving disputes and conflicts, which inevitably arise when these divergent interests clash.

Thus, for example, under occupational health and safety legislation in force in some provinces, a nurse who is being made to work in conditions that are unsafe or even dangerous has recourse against his or her employer. Likewise, a patient who has suffered injury or harm as a result of the negligence of a nurse may commence a civil suit in the courts for damages against that nurse and the health care facility.

In recent years, more attention has been paid to patient safety. There is a growing focus on the role of systems versus the individual when harm occurs. The culture is evolving into one of blamelessness and understanding in which nurses are obliged to disclose any harm that may have occurred to patients and their families. There is also more recognition that nurses' work environments must be healthy and that health care employers must ensure a work culture that is ethical, safe, and supportive. The ultimate aim is to provide an environment with a low tolerance for disrespect, especially between nurses and within the health care team.

As Canadian society becomes culturally more diverse, there is correspondingly more diversity among patients as well as within the interprofessional team. Diversity in other forms (e.g., same-sex parents, people with physical or psychological challenges) is becoming increasingly evident and understood as well. Nurses therefore need a greater understanding, empathy, and respect for these differences and for differences in values and beliefs.

There are many other reasons why nurses should familiarize themselves with the law and have a basic understanding of Canada's legal system. First, the Canadian Nurses Association's *Code of Ethics for Registered Nurses*[1] (Canadian Nurses Association [CNA], 2008), which is discussed in Chapter 3, and each provincial regulatory body have certain requirements with respect to nurses' level of professional knowledge and skill. Failure to meet these requirements, or undertaking the practice of nursing without adequate education, leaves the nurse open to disciplinary action from his or her provincial professional governing body and, if the conduct is serious enough, the courts, by way of either criminal prosecution (in cases in which the conduct involves a breach of criminal law), or a lawsuit (in which the nurse is sued for negligence due to the breach of an accepted standard of nursing care). Chapter 4 outlines the principles of Canada's legal system in order to provide nurses with a basic understanding of what often seems an obscure and confusing institution. The roles of legislatures and executive branches of government are briefly discussed, as are some of the legal concepts and principles applicable to nursing law. These provide a framework for the chapters that follow. Chapter 5 describes the structure, role, and workings of various provincial professional regulatory bodies and institutions. Against this background, nurses can begin to appreciate how their profession is regulated and, in particular, how the concept of self-government is integrated into this regulatory structure and into professional codes of ethics.

Second, nurses have access to drugs that are heavily regulated by legislation and hospital procedures governing their use, prescription, dispensation, and handling (see, for example, the *Drug and Pharmacies Regulation Act*, 1990). In addition, in some provinces, nurse practitioners (NPs) have the authority to prescribe medication in certain situations (see, for example, Nova Scotia's *Registered Nurses' Regulations*, N.S. Reg. 155/2001, section 28(1), and Nova Scotia College of Nurses' *Authorized Practice Schedule, Schedule of Drugs and Drug Interventions for Primary Health Care Nurse Practitioners*, available on the college's Web site). An understanding of the legal system, and of the law and rules surrounding negligence, underscores the importance of following such procedures and regulations when administering any medication. Not only civil, but also criminal, consequences can flow from a breach of such laws. Chapter 7 deals with issues of negligence and standards of care in the nursing profession.

---

1. Visit http://www.cna-aiic.ca/CNA/practice/ethics/code/default_e.aspx to obtain a copy of the Code.

It describes how nurses' conduct and professionalism in carrying out their duties are measured in relation to the law and current ethical standards. Chapter 7 also explores the legal, ethical, and practical aspects of proper documentation. Ensuring a high standard of documentation is important in maintaining effective communication, which is key to professional nursing practice. The nurse's assessment and progress notes monitor, on a continuing basis, the course of a patient's treatment and the effect of interventions. Inadequate documentation or the failure to review client information and history has a negative influence on the quality of care. Given that multiple caregivers may be involved, it is impossible to achieve effective communication and continuity of care without accurate documentation.

Third, the rights of patients influence the everyday actions and decisions made by nurses. These actions and decisions may involve going beyond the usual consensual barriers. For instance, a patient who needs an injection may readily consent by holding out an arm to the nurse who administers it. However, if a patient is unable to consent to a procedure owing to physical or mental incapacity, including impairment by illness or the effects of medication, the nurse bears the onus of ensuring that any action taken or treatment administered is in the patient's best interests and is consistent with that patient's wishes. It is often difficult to determine whether the patient is truly capable of giving consent. However, failure to do so leaves the nurse open to the risk of a civil suit for damages from the nonconsenting patient or the next of kin. There are also challenges with respect to the consent of children and the sincerity of substitute decision makers. Most provinces and territories have enacted legislation that clearly defines the parameters of consent, the patient's capacity, the manner of giving consent, express versus implied consent, and so forth. This legislation is discussed in detail in Chapter 6. Furthermore, health professionals are legally obligated to ensure that the patient understands the nature of the illness, the need for treatment, and all the attendant risks and benefits of such treatment if that patient is to give as fully informed a consent as the law requires. Issues of consent to treatment and the many subissues arising from this area are also addressed in Chapter 6.

Chapter 8 discusses the challenging legal and ethical issues associated with the end of life. Current subjects such as euthanasia, assisted suicide, and organ donation will be explored. These topics have gained public prominence in recent years and hold profound implications for nurses. The fear of death has led to an emphasis on finding ways to extend life at all costs. Yet, there is a heavy price when extending someone's life also diminishes the quality and dignity that give life its meaning. As means of dealing with death and the dying process change, nurses are challenged to find new ways to preserve patients' human values, autonomy, and dignity.

Recent, extraordinary advances in medical technology have made it possible both to manipulate the reproductive process at one end of the life continuum and, at the other, to extend life in cases in which death would once have been certain. Chapter 9 explores complex technologies such as those related to reproductive and genetic science. Technologies now exist that not only attempt to overcome infertility but have the capacity to identify genetic anomalies much earlier and to control the characteristics of the children produced. This overwhelming power to manipulate the creation of life has the potential to reshape our society and to redefine future generations.

Often, these situations arise before laws can be made to deal with them. The law, therefore, is not an exhaustive source of guidance and direction in such matters and is sometimes slow to adapt legal solutions for them. Through knowledge of our legal system, the nurse will see that the law is also, not infrequently, out of step with current societal values. Law is usually perceived as a "black and white" proposition, while ethical situations—such as euthanasia and physician-assisted suicide, as mentioned earlier—are vastly more complicated by shades of grey. Today, the single biggest challenge facing lawmakers and the legal system is the attempt to come to terms with the grey areas and to provide more realistic and practical guidelines for dealing with ethical problems. Law often evolves from ethical principles and common sense. For example, the law now recognizes that a person's consent is essential before a health care professional initiates any physical contact. This stems from the principle of autonomy in that a person has the ethical right to ultimately control what will be done to his or her body and person. There is also now an increasing awareness that the law must respect individual privacy and the security of health records.

A further reason for understanding the law as it applies to nursing is that nurses have access to confidential information about individual patients. They have both legal and ethical obligations to keep all such information confidential and not to divulge it without the patient's consent. When that consent cannot be obtained, they may reveal only as much as is absolutely necessary in the interests of the patient and only to persons whose participation in the patient's treatment is necessary (i.e., the "circle of care"). There may be cases in which nurses are required to disclose such information in court in the form of testimony, or in which it is essential to prevent harm to the patient or others. Most provinces have enacted privacy legislation governing health records that clearly delineates the responsibilities of the custodians of such records, the use that may be made of confidential patient information, who may consent to its release, and to whom such information can be disclosed. This legislation is discussed in Chapters 4 and 7. Knowledge of the workings of the law, the rules of evidence, ethics, and the judicial system provides a framework when determining whether to disclose sensitive and confidential information about a particular patient. Ill or injured patients are in a vulnerable state and are not always able to protect their rights as citizens. To ensure that the interests of their patients or clients are represented, nurses must understand the rights of their clients as well as their own professional obligations to protect or respect these rights. These issues are explored in Chapter 10.

If nurses have obligations to their clients, they also have rights regarding what they can expect as professionals. Like all other Canadians, under the *Charter of Rights and Freedoms*, nurses have the right to privacy and respect, and to freedom of expression—the right to think, say, write, or otherwise act in accordance with their beliefs. However, these rights must be considered in the context of nurses' responsibilities as professionals and of their obligations to patients and clients. Chapter 11 focuses on the balance between these rights and obligations.

## Why Should Nurses Study Ethics?

Nurses function within a health care team and collaborate with many other health care professionals. Today, nurses practise in many different contexts beyond the traditional health care settings: in the community or the home; in continuing care or rehabilitation; in business or industry; in adult and pediatric long-term care facilities; and in many other areas such as government. In some situations, nurses may interact with other professionals who do not share the same perspective about or understanding of nursing or health care in general. Each member of the team may have a different perspective on an ethical issue, or some may share a similar position. However, similarities—as well as differences—must be clarified. Without discussion and clarification, on occasion others may interpret decisions made and actions taken by members of the team as wrong. If the reasons, values, and perspectives behind these decisions and actions are explained, however, they may more readily be understood and respected, if not accepted, by others. There is a growing focus on the nurse within the context of interprofessional practice, and this will be discussed in Chapter 12.

Most importantly, nurses must study ethics because morality (i.e., doing good) is at the heart of traditional theoretical perspectives of nursing practice. Many nursing theorists consider "care" not only a key dimension of nursing practice but the very core of it (Benner, 1990; see also Leininger, 1988a; Leininger, 1988b; and Watson, 1988). Recent ethical theorists view care as both a therapeutic interaction and a moral imperative (Roach, 1992). To that end, nurses are viewed as "moral agents" charged with nurturing the humanity of those for whom they care (Cloyes, 2002).

Within health care, choices are often not easy: it may be difficult to determine, from among many alternatives, which is best. Consider, for example, a situation in which the medical team is aggressively treating a terminally ill patient in an Intensive Care Unit. Some nurses involved with the person's care may consider this approach wrong because they believe that it will only diminish the quality of the patient's remaining life and result in a painful death. If the medical team involved were to clarify its position—say, at a team conference—the nurses and other team members might discover that the physicians' decisions were based on a belief in the sanctity of life and the view that their collective role is to preserve life at all costs. Possibly, on an earlier occasion, the patient asked a doctor to try anything that might save his life. Or, perhaps, the physician has other knowledge about the patient's story, such as a particular religious or cultural perspective he observes that requires every effort be taken to sustain life. Perhaps there was an advance directive stating this, or perhaps the family was awaiting a beloved relative's arrival from out of town so that final goodbyes could be said. Though the views of some nurses or team members may not change, they may come to a better understanding of the reasons behind the physicians' actions. Such discussion would reduce the moral conflict and distress experienced by some nurses and ensure better relationships among those on the interprofessional team.

It is imperative that patients or clients, families, physicians, nurses, and other team members discuss such issues together and attempt to reach consensus on a course of action. Since many ethical quandaries do not have clear-cut answers, collaboration and effective communication, as well as a respect for one another's values and beliefs, can enhance the resolution process. The communication that is necessary to clarify and justify our moral actions and choices to our professional colleagues is improved through a shared language grounded in a solid foundation of ethical theory. This shared language also involves the interplay of law relative to such difficult dilemmas as withdrawal of treatment and the use of advance directives in making treatment decisions for incapacitated patients.

The study of ethics provides nurses with some tools to be better able to manage and contribute to such discussions. Knowledge of abstract philosophical theories and terminologies does not always provide solutions to ethical problems; however, such knowledge can serve to help us better understand the moral context and the values and beliefs of ourselves and others.

Nurses face ethical choices every day in practice. These may deal with the areas of pain control, patient comfort, restraints, patient choice, and family involvement in care. The issues do not always make headlines. Ethics is involved when nurses decide how to allocate time and nursing care to patients; whose needs are to be met first; and how to show respect to patients, families, each other, and the interprofessional team.

Nurses are involved not only in the ethical context of the individual nurse–patient or nurse–client relationship; they are also affected by—and are in a position to influence—policy, the wider context of health care, and the health care system.

For example, advances in the areas of organ transplantation and reproductive technology force questions about how we allocate these scarce resources and, indeed, whether we should be using this technology at all. The growth of the consumer movement, the proliferation of special interest groups, and the occupational issues that arise from collective bargaining and unionization all influence the context of health care and hence nurses' ethical choices. The effect of financial restraints on the nurse–client ratio poses additional challenges relative to how nurses allocate their time and services. Further, the role of the nurse is expanding: nurses are being given more autonomy and, with that, more authority and responsibility.

## Moral Justification

Persons involved in the field of ethics draw upon ethical theories and principles not only to select an ethical approach to an issue but also to justify and defend their positions to others. Points of view, especially in controversial areas, are open to criticism and debate and require justification, an argued defence of one's perspective. Theories and principles of ethics can clarify relationships between reasons and conclusions. Points of view are justified through reasoned arguments and evidence, and are subject to criticism and counterexamples. Arguments can be disguised by rhetoric, irrelevancies, redundancies, and connections with other arguments, and can mislead those not comfortable with ethical language and theory (Beauchamp & Walters, 2003). As moral problems in the health care environment increase in frequency and intensity, it becomes increasingly important for nurses to have knowledge of ethical theory and some skill in justifying and defending their positions to others.

## Everyday Ethical Issues Faced by Nurses

Nurses have the opportunity to defend and protect patient rights, to promote compassionate care, and to enhance the dignity and autonomy of their patients or clients. They are often required to choose from among a number of good or "least wrong" alternatives and to assess and defend the choices made or actions taken; however, they may not even be aware of the ethical nature of their choices. Since options are not always clear, how does one decide what the right thing to do is? In order to address ethical challenges, nurses first need to be aware that these challenges exist and be able to identify them as ethical in nature.

Within the context of a health care system strained by limited funds and resources, every day, nurses face a challenge in providing high-quality and ethical care to patients. The following scenarios are not uncommon.

An infant in a pediatric centre has been diagnosed with a malignant cerebral tumour. The infant is comatose, nonresponsive, and on life-support systems. There is nothing the team can do to halt the progress of this terminal disease. They believe it would be in the child's best interest to discontinue life support and to allow the child to die a natural death. The parents disagree and want all measures taken to save their child's life.

Who decides the best interests of this child? Do patients or families have the right to expensive, futile health care? How do the nurses support the parents through this crisis and the loss of their child? How do they ensure quality care for this child throughout the dying process?

Joe, a 20-year-old man diagnosed with schizophrenia at the age of 16, is admitted to the psychiatric unit of a community hospital. He is agitated and expresses a wish to "end all this pain." He refuses all medications to deal with his symptoms. He wants to go home.

What rights does Joe have in this situation? Is there meaning behind Joe's wish to "end all this pain," or is this merely a symptom of his disease process?

A man with end-stage cancer of the liver is receiving palliative care at home. His wife and children, with some support from home care and community nurses, are his primary caregivers. As his condition deteriorates, his symptoms become more difficult to manage. Drained, the family questions whether he might be better off in a hospital. The patient, however, has always stated his preference is to die at home.

How does the community nurse manage the conflicting interests of this patient and his family? What is society's role in ensuring adequate resources to address the needs of a dying patient at home?

continued on following page >>

A 40-year-old single man is recovering from surgery to his lower back. Though he is still in pain and continues to have difficulty with mobility, the hospital needs the bed, and he has reached his expected length of stay. The hospital nurse discusses his transition to the community with the home care case managers, who determine that he does not qualify for homemaker support, even though he does not have family or friends at home to help him.

How do these nurses ensure this man a safe transition to his home? How do they deal with the rules that limit needed resources in the community?

An occupational health nurse in an industrial setting is managing the case of a worker who was injured at work. He has recovered and is functionally able to return to his former work. Management is eager to have him return as soon as possible. However, the worker confides to the nurse that his front-line manager constantly harasses him and his co-workers; he believes that it was this stressful environment that led to his accident in the first place. He asks the nurse to keep this information confidential, as he fears repercussions.

How does the nurse balance the responsibility to ensure this worker's safe return to work—and concern for the safety of other workers in this hostile environment—with the obligation to honour the worker's request for confidentiality?

An older adult in a geriatric unit is confused and agitated. The use of physical restraints is considered.

How do nurses caring for this patient balance the risks and benefits of this option while respecting the patient's wishes?

It is the middle of an evening shift on a busy medical unit. A patient is dying; family and friends are not around.

Should nurses let this patient die alone?

A child is dying. The parents, clearly distressed, have been with the child for weeks and are seriously sleep deprived. The father, who has grown increasingly agitated, goes to the nursing station to request additional pain medication for his child. When 10 minutes pass with no response, he becomes enraged and yells at the team, using profanity, aggressive language, and other threatening behaviours.

How does the nursing team balance the needs of the parents and the child with the rights of the nurses and staff to a safe work environment? How could the situation have been prevented?

John has recently begun working as a nurse in a small hospital in a rural community. He moved there with his partner, who was recently appointed as a manager in a nearby mine. Since he started a few months earlier, John has found it difficult to engage with other staff members. They routinely fail to help him if he is busy and have never invited him to join them on a break. Already feeling marginalized, he overhears three of the nurses discussing his personal relationship and speculating on why a man would ever become a nurse.

What is happening here? What options does John have to address this uncomfortable situation?

These are only a few examples of the types of complex and challenging situations faced by nurses on a daily basis. It is not uncommon for nurses to be confronted with a number of these ethical issues and questions simultaneously. A better understanding of ethical theory, greater awareness of the ethical issues, increased knowledge and skill to address them, and appropriate system supports may limit or better address these challenges.

Now, take some time to reflect on the above scenarios. What choices would you make? What are your reasons for making them? Is your rationale consistent from one scenario to the next, or does your approach vary depending on the situation or your past experience? Are you able to defend your approach to your colleagues?

After you review the theoretical perspectives discussed in Chapter 2, return to these scenarios. Was your approach to these problems consistent with any of Chapter 2's theories? Did your views change as you read through the chapter? Did these perspectives provide you with arguments to assist in defending your position? Are you better able to identify the ethical issues in these scenarios? Do the theories help you decide on a course of action?

## Summary

Clearly, the impact of the law and ethics on the nursing profession is widespread and significant. An understanding of the law's structures, terminology, and mechanisms is essential to the nurse's ability to operate within society's expectations and standards; similarly, a familiarity with and a willingness to be guided by the values and ethical standards of the nursing profession is essential to practising within a system with high standards of patient care. The authors have tried to lay the basis for such an understanding in the chapters that follow.

This chapter conveyed the reasons nurses must be familiar with the law and ethics and have the knowledge to practise according to these standards. Professionals have a significant role in serving the interests of the public and must be sure they have their trust. As we have seen from the scenarios above, the complexity of ethical issues has grown alongside the increasing reliance upon ethics in guiding and supporting decisions. It is clear that ethics and law intersect on many levels, and a strong understanding of both is essential to exemplary nursing practice.

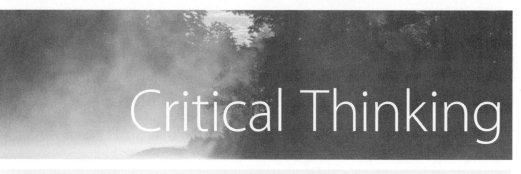

Critical Thinking

## Discussion Points

These questions are intended to encourage self-reflection.

1. Why did you decide to enter the nursing profession?
2. What personal values do you share with the nursing profession?
3. Have you or a family member had a memorable experience with the health care system? What did you most appreciate about this experience? What did you least like about it?
4. In your opinion, what are the most significant legal issues that nurses may face? What significant ethical issues might a nurse face?
5. If you were a patient or client today, what would you expect from the nurses caring for you? If a member of your family were a patient or client today, what would you expect? As a nurse or a nursing student, do you meet these expectations with your own patients or clients?

## References

### Statutes

*Criminal Code*, R.S.C. 1985, c. C-46 (Canada), s. 241; R.S., 1985, c. 27 (1st Supp.), s. 7.
*Drug and Pharmacies Regulation Act*, R.S.O. 1990, c. H.4 (Ontario).

### Regulations

Nova Scotia's *Registered nurses' regulations*, N.S. Reg. 155/2001 (Nova Scotia).

### Regulatory Body Policies

Nova Scotia College of Nurses (2008). *Authorized practice schedule, schedule of drugs and drug interventions for primary health care nurse practitioners*. Retrieved July, 2008 from http://www.crnns.ca/documents/AuthorizedPracticesScheduleofDrugsPHCNPsJuly2008.pdf

### Texts and Articles

Aikens, C. A. (1926). *Studies in ethics for nurses* (2nd ed.). Philadelphia, PA: W.B. Saunders Company.
Beauchamp, T. L., & Walters, L. (2003). *Contemporary issues in bioethics* (6th ed.). Belmont, CA: Wadsworth Publishing Company.

Benner, P. (1990). The moral dimensions of caring. In J. S. Stevenson & T. Tripp-Reimer (Eds.), *Knowledge about care and caring: State of the art and future developments* (pp. 5–17). Kansas City, MO: American Academy of Nursing.

Canadian Nurses Association. (2008). *Code of ethics for registered nurses*. Ottawa, ON: Author.

Cloyes, K. G. (2002). Agonizing care: Care ethics, agonistic feminism and a political theory of care. *Nursing Inquiry, 9*(3), 203–214.

Jennings, B., Callahan, D., & Wolf, S. M. (1987, February). The professions: Public interest and common good. *Hastings Center Report* (special supplement), 3–4.

Leininger, M. M. (1988a). Care: The essence of nursing and health. In M. M. Leininger (Ed.), *Care: The essence of nursing* (pp. 3–15). Detroit, MI: Wayne State University Press.

Leininger, M. M. (1988b). *Caring: An essential human need*. Detroit, MI: Wayne State University Press.

Roach, M. S. (1992). *The human act of caring: A blueprint for the health professions*. Ottawa, ON: Canadian Hospital Association.

Watson, M. J. (1988). New dimensions of human caring theory. *Nursing Science Quarterly, 1*(4), 175–81.

Chapter 2

# Ethical Theoretical Perspectives

**Learning Objectives**

The purpose of this chapter is to enable you to understand:

- The moral complexity of the practice environment and the role of the nurse as a moral agent
- The challenging ethical choices nurses make
- The influence of values on ethical decision making
- The relevance of a solid understanding of ethical theory and principles to the practice of nursing
- The basics of historical and contemporary ethical theory and principles and their application to nursing
- The evolution of present-day ethical thinking in nursing
- The application of ethical theory and principles to nursing practice

## Introduction

NURSES ENJOY A POSITION of extraordinary responsibility in Canadian society. Their actions, both independent and collaborative, affect the well-being of Canadians. Whether nurses are influencing the quality of a person's death, protecting the vulnerable, such as children and older adults, promoting the health of the community, or advocating for policy or legislation that affects either the profession itself or Canadians as a whole, they have been awarded the trust of individuals, communities, and society at large, who view them as moral agents. That is, society assumes nurses will choose to do what is right. Because of the responsibility they have been given, nurses must be able to understand, clarify, and justify their choices and actions to others: patients, clients, colleagues, the profession, employers, the justice system, and society. To do this effectively, nurses must study ethics and develop the skills and tools to support their positions.

Every day, nurses make complex choices within the context of a challenging health care environment. They may not always be aware, however, that the issues and challenges they face and their subsequent choices are ethical in nature. When nurses are aware of the ethical challenges they face, how do they then choose a course of action from several alternatives when the relative merit of these choices may be unclear? How do they make choices that ensure an optimal level of care? How do they know that the decisions they make and actions they take are the right ones? How are ethical dilemmas and violations identified? When are ethical violations the result of poor communication, inadequate system support and resources, or substandard patient care processes? Within this complex health care environment, how can nurses be supported in their relationships with patients, clients, family members, and the community? This chapter will demonstrate how a solid understanding of ethical theory and principles can facilitate or guide the process of making and defending ethical choices.

Reflect on the ethical challenges in the following scenario.

### Margaret's Story

Margaret is a novice nurse working an evening shift in a busy medical unit. She has just returned from break and realizes that the unit is in utter chaos. One of her patients, an older gentleman with congestive heart failure, has had a cardiac arrest. The arrest team is attempting resuscitation. Meanwhile, she hears screaming and discovers other members of the staff restraining his wife, who is attempting to go into her husband's room. Margaret tries to calm her and explains what is happening to her husband. She describes the chaos in the room and how difficult it would be for her to observe the activities of the team. The wife insists that she wants to be in the room and promises to stay focused on her husband regardless of what the team is doing. Margaret is very uncomfortable. She knows that family members are not permitted to be in attendance during emergency situations. She enters the room, explains the situation, and asks the team to reconsider this "rule" in these circumstances.

continued on following page >>

Immediately, the senior nurse participating in the resuscitation attempts responds that the wife would find it too disturbing. The medical team refuses as well, saying they would be uncomfortable with the wife observing their actions. Margaret leaves to explain this to the wife, who says, "He is my husband, not yours. I want to be with him if he dies."

This story raises a number of issues and challenges, which include:

• The nurse's professional relationship to the patient and family
• The well-being of the patient
• The rights of the team caring for the patient
• The rights of the spouse and family
• The nurse's role as a representative of the interests of the patient

This chapter will focus on the key theories and principles that guide ethical decision making and actions. Before proceeding with your review of these theories and principles, spend some time reflecting on your responses to the situation. What do you think are the key ethical issues and challenges? As various ethical theories and principles are discussed in this chapter, we will revisit Margaret's story and consider how these may have guided her actions. At the end of this chapter, the complete story of what Margaret actually did will be shared.

## An Introduction to Ethical Theory

A number of factors influence our thinking about what is right and wrong. These factors may include the norms and beliefs of society, the context of the particular situation, previous experiences with similar situations, the potential outcomes or consequences of actions, the relationship of the individuals involved, and professional and individual values and beliefs.

Over the centuries, many philosophers have tried to uncover the foundations of morality in an attempt to understand the key moral principles that guide our decisions regarding right and wrong. Believing that decisions about morality transcend our emotions, philosophers of the past developed theories and identified principles grounded in a "reasoned" or "rational" approach to ethical decision making. **Rationality** is related to the notion of thinking and reasoning. It is associated with comprehension, intelligence, or inference, particularly when an inference or a conclusion results from a thought process. Rationality is also linked to explanation, understanding, or justification, particularly if it provides a ground or a motive. "Irrational," therefore, is defined as that which is not endowed with such reason or understanding (Landauer & Rowlands, 2001).

In recent decades, thinking has evolved beyond these "rational" views to acknowledge the influence of emotion, caring, and relationships. Early ethical theories were developed by men, who did not at the time consider women's input relevant; however, recent theories established by both men and women take into account the feminine perspective. Emerging theories also consider the role of nursing and the growing complexity of ethical challenges in health care. To better appreciate contemporary perspectives, one must understand the evolution of ethical theory, so in this chapter, some of the well-known historical and present-day views will be discussed, as will their application to nursing today.

As mentioned, in the discipline of philosophy, making decisions about what is right and wrong traditionally involved a reasoning process. Opinions without arguments or reasons to support them were discouraged. Although these rationalistic approaches devalued the role of emotion and instinct, as will be seen later in this chapter, our emotional responses are considered by some contemporary thinkers to be important guides to moral behaviour.

Before proceeding with descriptions of the theories developed to aid us in ethical decision making, let us discuss some key definitions.

**Ethics**, the philosophical study of morality, is the systematic exploration of what is morally right and morally wrong. The study of ethics enables us to recognize and evaluate the variables that influence our moral decisions, our obligations, our character, our sense of responsibility, our sense of social justice, and the nature of the good life (Grassian, 1981). **Ethical theory** is the study of the nature and justification of general ethical principles that can be applied to moral problems (Beauchamp & Walters, 2003). It attempts to provide a more rigorous and systematic approach to how we make decisions about what is right and wrong. The field of **biomedical ethics** explores ethical questions and moral issues associated with health care. **Nursing ethics** focuses on the moral questions within the sphere of nursing practice, the nurse–patient or nurse–client relationship, the moral character of nurses, and the nurse as a moral agent.

Morality is the tradition of beliefs and norms within a culture or society about right and wrong human conduct. It is guided by explicit codes of conduct and rules governing behaviour. A well-known example is the "golden rule": Do unto others as you would have them do unto you. As children grow up, they are taught the moral rules of their culture and society, along with other mores and social norms (Beauchamp & Walters, 2003). Since Canada is a pluralistic society, the notion of respecting differences and understanding the influence of culture in ethics is vital, so Chapter 12 includes a comprehensive section on diversity and multicultural ethics.

There are two approaches to the study of morality: nonnormative and normative. *Nonnormative* approaches to ethics involve analyzing morality without taking a moral position, whereas *normative* ethics approaches focus on the question of what is right and what is wrong (Beauchamp & Walters, 2003).

Nonnormative studies include the fields of descriptive ethics and metaethics. **Descriptive ethics** encompasses factual descriptions and explanations of moral behaviours and beliefs. By looking at a wide range of moral beliefs and behaviours, this field of study attempts to explain how moral attitudes, codes, and beliefs differ from person to person and across societies and cultures. **Metaethics** analyzes the meanings of key terms such as *right*, *obligation*, *good*, and *virtue*, and attempts to distinguish between what is moral and what is not—for example, the difference between a moral rule and a social rule. Further, metaethics analyzes the structure or logic of moral reasoning and justification and explores the nature of morality and the meanings and interrelationships of the fundamental concepts of moral language (Grassian, 1981). For example, in metaethics, answers to the following questions are pursued:

- How is a moral principle different from a nonmoral one?
- What do we mean when we say an act is right?
- What does it mean to have "free will" or to be "morally responsible"? (Grassian, 1981)

In normative ethics, attempts are made to identify the basic principles and **virtues** that guide morality and to provide coherent, systematic, and justifiable answers to moral questions (Grassian, 1981). Through the development of ethical theory, normative ethics provides a system of moral principles or virtues and focuses on the reasons or arguments that guide decisions about what is right and what is wrong (Grassian, 1981).

**Applied ethics** is the field of ethics in which these theories and principles are applied to actual moral problems, for example, in health care (Beauchamp & Walters, 2003).

**Ethical dilemmas** arise when the best course of action is unclear, when strong moral reasons support each position (i.e., when good reasons for mutually exclusive alternatives can be cited) (Beauchamp & Walters, 2003), and when we must choose between the most right and the least wrong. The first step to resolving ethical dilemmas is simply obtaining all of the facts and information concerning the areas of moral controversy (Beauchamp & Walters, 2003), which requires the cooperation of all involved. It is therefore important for members of the interprofessional health care team, the patient, and the family to work together to address difficult ethical issues, and for members of the interprofessional team to be able to communicate about ethical issues with each other, as well as with patients and families. Ethical issues related to interprofessional teams and patient- and family-centred care will also be addressed in Chapter 12.

**Moral distress** results when we are not able to face these issues and deal effectively with them. It occurs when we believe that a particular course of action is right but we are not permitted or able to act or to influence the decision (Rushton, 2008). Moral distress may contribute to feelings of guilt, discomfort, and dissatisfaction in not being able to do what we think is best. This can cause long-term consequences, especially when supports are not in place to aid the nurse in these circumstances. Some of these supports and resources are described in Chapter 3.

Ethical theories provide a framework of **principles** and guidelines to help identify ethical issues and reconcile problems or conflicts. While the solutions to these problems may not always be clear, these theories help in guiding ethical discussions. Thus, it is important that nurses have a deep understanding of normative ethics and the many theories and principles available to guide ethical reflection and discussion. Although these theories and principles may not be able, in every circumstance, to help resolve an ethical conflict, they nevertheless serve as a template or guide to assist nurses in justifying their moral position to others.

## Values

Before describing the more common ethical theories that are available to guide care and ethical decision making, it is important to clarify the influence of values, not only on ethical theory but on the norms, rules, and laws of our society. A **value** is an ideal that has significant meaning or importance to an individual, a group, or a society. For example, Canadian society values individual freedom, health, fairness, honesty, and integrity. Evidence of these values is found in Canada's laws, the *Canadian Charter of Rights and Freedoms*, and individual and collective actions and behaviours. The structure of the Canadian health care system demonstrates that Canadians value equality, individual rights, health and well-being, quality of life, and human dignity. This is evident in the principle of universality contained in the *Canada Health Act*—that is, the attempt to provide equal access to health care to all Canadians, regardless of where they live and their socioeconomic status.

Since Canada comprises a mosaic of cultural and religious perspectives, nurses care for patients and families whose basic value systems—and hence beliefs, rituals, and customs—may differ from their own. Therefore, an understanding of the concept of values helps to ensure respect for differences. For example, a particular group or society may have cultural values or beliefs that influence the treatment of the body after death and the rituals and behaviours associated with death and dying. Let us consider some of the values within the Buddhist tradition. Within this culture there exists the notion of *karuna*—compassion, which includes the need for families to continue to ensure comfort, support, and love for as long as there is life. Once a person is dying, Buddhists will chant, believing this helps the spirit of the dying person to be led away by the higher being (Ives-Baine, 2007). How might the nurse ensure this significant ritual is respected, whether in the home or in an institutional setting? Nurses who understand such values can clarify their role and enrich their relationships with patients, clients, and families.

Dealing with values and rituals that are different from our own can be challenging if these differences are not understood. It is also important, though, for us to understand and respect our own values; for when our behaviours are not congruent with them, internal conflicts can arise.

The Canadian Nurses Association's *Code of Ethics for Registered Nurses* (described in Chapter 3) is based on the values that are deemed important for the profession of nursing. An understanding of the values of the nursing profession then will assist nurses in comprehending and applying the Code, which articulates value statements, or principles, to guide the ethical behaviour of nurses and the profession (CNA, 2008).

### Influence of Values on Ethical Decision Making

Values influence our own individual beliefs, our views of others, and our opinions in such areas as literature, art, objectives, and ideals. Our behaviours, rituals, symbols, structures, rules, and laws represent the collective values and beliefs of our society. Nurses' values may have an effect on their responses to ethical issues, their decisions, and the care they provide to patients and clients. Because Canadian nurses work with and care for patients who represent a broad spectrum of cultural and religious perspectives, they must strive to clarify their own values and learn to respect and understand those of others.

Values within a culture may shift over time. For example, in recent years, Canadian society has become more focused on the meaning and quality of life rather than on prolonging life at all costs. This is evident in debates over euthanasia and assisted suicide. Palliative care health practices reinforce this growing concern for quality and dignity in the dying process. Respect for individual rights and freedoms, more prevalent in Western societies, is a modern concept that has emerged only over the past couple of centuries. Values around individual rights have led to legislation regarding consent to treatment, confidentiality, and so forth.

Values emerge through our associations with others—family, friends, classmates, teachers, colleagues—life experiences, religious beliefs, and the environment we live in. In recent times, the media have also had a strong influence on value development. Gender is also said to affect the development of values in individuals and groups (Gilligan, 1988), significant when considering the nursing profession, which continues to be dominated by women, although this is changing, as is the gender profile of medicine, previously dominated by men. Nurses have historically interacted with physicians. As disciplines in health care have evolved, however, nurses now interact with a broader interprofessional team, which may include other regulated health professionals such as dieticians, physiotherapists, pharmacists, and so on, depending on the setting. For example, in long-term care settings, recreational therapists are key members of the team, as are child-life professionals in the pediatric setting. The respective values of nurses, doctors, and other health care professionals may influence the perspectives that each brings to ethical issues and dilemmas. As the importance of teams in health care grows, so too does the necessity to understand and respect the contribution each member makes to ethical discussion.

Professional values build on and expand on personal values, and emerge as nurses are socialized into the profession. Sometimes they will experience a struggle between their personal beliefs and professional responsibilities. As health professionals, nurses face life-and-death situations, joy, pain, inequity, and sorrow that may alter their perspectives and reframe and reprioritize their values.

Value conflicts arise in situations in which our actions or others' are at odds with our beliefs. Conflict is evident when professionals disagree about how a particular ethical situation (e.g., withdrawal of treatment, abortion, euthanasia, patient restraint) should be managed. Our duty as professionals and as members of a health care team requires that we understand and respect the values of other members of that team. Since conflict in values can result in moral distress, it is imperative that we understand our own values, articulate and clarify them to one another, and establish processes whereby this can be done.

## Value Clarification

Value clarification is an ongoing process through which individuals come to understand the values they hold and the relative importance of each of these values. To facilitate understanding among the interprofessional team, patients, clients, and their families requires open discussion, active listening, and mutual respect. The process is enhanced if we use the same language and terminology in relation to ethical issues. A focus on specific situations, stories, or narratives helps nurses to identify values, evaluate responses to specific situations, and hence come to understand the various perspectives.

Frequently, workload demands in the health care field restrict the opportunity for these important discussions. However, making the time for such dialogue is a worthwhile investment. The rewards include improved communication and collaboration among professionals, a reduction in moral distress, and subsequent improvement in patient care as ethical problems are addressed and action plans identified.

## Relativism

Prior to reviewing some of the best-known ethical theories, we would like to note that not all thinkers and philosophers agree on a single, correct, and objective framework for morality (Grassian, 1981; Beauchamp & Walters, 2003). Some consider individual and group responses to morality to be relative to the norms and values of that particular culture or society, or to the situation presenting itself. This view is labelled **cultural** or **normative relativism**.

Relativists consider morality to be more a matter of cultural differences and taste, an arbitrary notion of what one believes or feels, and not based on some deeper set of objectively justifiable principles (Grassian, 1981; Beauchamp & Walters, 2003). Proponents of relativism believe that moral beliefs and principles relate only to individual cultures or persons, and that the values of one person or one culture do not govern the conduct of others. What is morally right and morally wrong, they believe, varies from place to place. There are no absolute or universal moral standards that can apply to all persons at all times (Beauchamp & Walters, 2003). Concepts of rightness and wrongness are, therefore, meaningless apart from the specific contexts in which they arise. Relativists note that what is deemed worthy of moral approval or disapproval in one society differs from standards in other societies, even though all possess a moral conscience or general sense of right and wrong. A moral standard is a historical product, sanctioned by custom over time, and moral beliefs of individuals vary according to historical, environmental, and familial differences. The particular actions, motives, and rules that are praised or blamed vary greatly from culture to culture (Beauchamp & Walters, 2003); therefore, according to relativists, there are no universal norms.

Opponents to this view argue that despite apparent differences in conclusions, there is a "universal structure of human nature, or at least a universal set of human needs which leads to the adoption of similar or even identical principles in all cultures" (Beauchamp & Walters, 2003). Individuals or groups may disagree about the ethics of a particular situation or practice, but this does not mean that they hold different moral standards or principles (Beauchamp & Walters, 2003). Presenting a view different from that of relativists, universalists assert that conflicts between moral beliefs across cultures are not basic or fundamental; rather, they believe disagreements over critical facts or concepts are usually the underlying source of moral diversity. A society may agree on ideals of individual liberty and general happiness yet disagree on when society has the right to make people happy in spite of themselves. They may agree on principles but disagree on their range of application. For example, consider the historical practice of older Inuit who wished to choose the time and place of their death. This practice was based on the belief that one's status in the afterlife reflected that person's condition at the end of life on earth (Eskimo Old Age, n.d.). Therefore, from the Inuit perspective, it was better to die when one's mental and physical capabilities were more or less intact.

## Normative Ethical Theories

As mentioned earlier, ethical theories that are intended to provide frameworks and rules to guide decisions about what is right and wrong are called normative. They provide a system of principles by which to determine what ought and ought not to be done. Two traditional categories of ethical theory are teleology (derived from the Greek *teleos*, "end") and deontology (derived from the Greek *deontor*, "duty") (Beauchamp & Walters, 2003). *Deontological* theories make explicit the duties and principles that should guide our actions, whereas *teleological* theories focus on the ends or outcomes and consequences of decisions and action. Teleologists look ahead to the consequences of action; deontologists look back at the nature of the act itself, evaluating it in terms of the duties and obligations one has, either by virtue of being a human being or by the morality of the specific person and his or her social relationships (Grassian, 1981).

The following discussion is not intended to be an exhaustive presentation of all ethical theories but a review of some better-known theoretical perspectives, theories that provide a historical foundation and those that offer relevance to nursing practice today. Each theory will be used to reflect on Margaret's story.

### Teleological Theories

The most well-known teleological theory that considers ends, outcomes, and the consequences of decisions and actions is utilitarianism, which is explored below.

#### UTILITARIAN THEORY

Those who espouse **utilitarianism** believe that the ethical choice is the one with the best consequences, outcomes, or results. They believe that an "action or practice is right (when compared to any alternative action or practice) if it leads to the greatest possible balance of good consequences or to the least possible balance of bad consequences in the world as a whole" (Beauchamp & Walters, 2003). In utilitarian theories, there are no absolute principles, moral codes, duties, or rules; rather, there is the assumption that good can be quantified and that we can calculate the relative good or harm that would result from our actions

(Beauchamp & Walters, 2003). One acts best by choosing the route that provides the greatest good and the least harm for the greatest number of people. Essentially, the consequences of an act consist of the sum total of differences that act will make in the world.

Utilitarian theories provide us with evaluative standards for assessing and ordering consequences. One may choose to evaluate the moral value of an act based on outcomes that may be related to happiness, welfare, pleasure, pain, risk, or costs and benefits. (This is explored below in the chapter, when the theory of value is discussed.) The consequences of an act are measured in their totality. For example, in a situation in which withdrawal of treatment is being considered, the consequences of this action would be evaluated not only in relation to the patient but also to the family, the health professionals involved, and society as a whole. Both immediate and long-term consequences would be considered.

*Mill's Utilitarianism*
Utilitarianism, one of the best-known normative theories, was formulated by the philosopher John Stuart Mill (1806–1873), based on the earlier work of Jeremy Bentham (1748–1832) (Mill, 1948). The theory articulated by Mill is founded on the principle of **utility**, which he described as the greatest happiness for the greatest number of people. Mill's utilitarianism has both a normative and psychological foundation: normative in the principle of utility, and psychological in Mill's views of human nature. Vital to the validity of his theory was his belief that most people desire unity and harmony with one another and essentially wish to benefit others (Mill, 1948). These basic goals—to benefit others and to control harm—ensure, Mill believed, a commitment from all rational beings to strive to do their best. Mill viewed a moral framework as a means not only to fulfill individuals' needs but also to facilitate the achievement of broad social goals (Mill, 1948).

From a normative perspective, Mill argued that the principle of utility is grounded in the pursuit of pleasure and the avoidance of pain, which he believed to be the main goals of life. In fact, actions, he argued, have even greater moral significance when they have a greater effect on the pleasure or pain of others (Mill, 1948). Mill believed that actions are right when they promote happiness, wrong when they produce the opposite. In choosing among alternatives, he believed an act to be right if and only if its utility (benefit or value) is higher than the utility of any other act the person could have done instead (Mill, 1948). Because of our desire for unity and harmony with others, we should intend our actions to produce the greatest happiness for the greatest number. Mill argued that we could reasonably predict and evaluate what actions would produce the most happiness and, therefore, the best consequences, by relying on our common sense, our habits, and our past experiences.

*A Theory of Value*
A utilitarian theory or the notion of utility depends on the theory of value or intrinsic good: There needs to be an identifiable good or value in order to evaluate the outcome or consequence of right actions. Debate among utilitarians focuses on what result has the greatest utility or value—the ultimate intrinsic good. Many differences in views relate to

the distinction between what is instrumentally good (good because of its consequences) and intrinsically good (good in and of itself).

Bentham and Mill fall within the category of hedonistic utilitarians in that they saw utility in terms of pleasure or happiness. They argued that the ultimate intrinsic good is happiness and that all other goods are instrumental toward this end. Happiness, to Mill, was not merely "pleasurable excitement" but a "realistic appraisal of the pleasurable moments afforded in life, whether they take the form of tranquility or passion" (Beauchamp & Walters, 2003). He argued that pleasure and freedom from pain can be measured and compared. Thus, the moral value of an action is determined by adding the total happiness produced and subtracting the pain involved (Beauchamp & Walters, 2003).

Utilitarians do not always agree on these goals and values, whose goals count, or why. Pluralistic utilitarians, for example, believe that no single goal or state constitutes good. They accept many values—such as friendship, love, devotion, welfare, health, beauty, and moral qualities such as fairness—as having intrinsic worth. They consider this total range of intrinsic values, not pleasure alone, to be important products of a good action, and believe the greatest aggregate good is achieved when these multiple intrinsic goods are considered in the analysis of right and wrong actions (Beauchamp & Walters, 2003).

*Act and Rule Utilitarianism*

There are two approaches to utilitarian theory: one considers particular acts in relation to particular circumstances; the other formulates rules of conduct that determine what is right and wrong in general. In *act utilitarianism*, each act is judged on its consequences ("What good and evil consequences will result directly from this action in this circumstance?") (Beauchamp & Walters, 2003). In *rule utilitarianism*, the utility of general patterns of behaviour is considered, rather than that of specific actions ("What good and evil consequences will result generally from this sort of action?") (Beauchamp & Walters, 2003). A rule is correct provided that more utility would be produced by people following it rather than any other rule that would apply to the situation or act. (Some argue that this approach is similar to Kant's notion of universality, which is discussed next.)

In practice, then, a person might list the alternative actions available, consider the possible consequences or outcomes of each act, and then quantify the consequences in relation to what is considered the "good" consequence or outcome. The right alternative or rule would be the one that produced the greatest good or the least harm for the greatest number of people.

Rule utilitarians hold that rules have a central position in morality and cannot be compromised by the demands of a particular situation. The effectiveness of a rule is judged by determining that its observance would, in theory, maximize social utility (Beauchamp & Walters, 2003) better than any possible substitute rule and better than no rule. Theoretically, utilitarian rules are firm and protective of all classes of individuals, independent of factors of social convenience and momentary need (Beauchamp & Walters, 2003).

Critics of rule utilitarianism question how one resolves conflict among moral rules in particular circumstances or situations. They argue that ranking of rules is almost impossible;

therefore, in circumstances of conflict, the principle of utility decides, and the theory is reduced to act utilitarianism (Beauchamp & Walters, 2003). Rule utilitarians argue that every moral theory has practical limitations in cases of conflict, when the right choice is not clear, but that in the majority of circumstances, the rules make sense.

*Criticism of Utilitarianism*

Critics of utilitarianism argue that it is impossible and impractical to use this theory in determining what one ought to do in daily life. They suggest that the model is relatively useless for purposes of objectively quantifying widely different interests in order to determine where maximal value—and therefore right action—lies (Beauchamp & Walters, 2003). Further, given the focus on pleasure as the desired end, critics have concerns that individuals with morally unacceptable preferences would use these in their calculations. In response, supporters suggest most people are not perverse; if they were, then their actions would result in great unhappiness in society, thus demonstrating the validity of the theory (Beauchamp & Walters, 2003). They also argue that we must rely on common sense and our past experiences in quantifying consequences and that we need be only reasonably predictive, recognizing that it is not possible to always be error-free.

Other critics suggest that "good" cannot be measured and comparatively weighed. In response, utilitarians argue that we make crude, rough-and-ready comparisons of values every day, that what is important is to be morally conscientious and serious in our analysis (Beauchamp & Walters, 2003).

One of the more serious judgements against utilitarianism is that it can lead to injustice. Critics argue that the greatest value for the greatest number may bring harm to a minority, thus failing to consider issues of *distributive justice* (Beauchamp & Walters, 2003). Utilitarians respond that considerations regarding justice and social utility are part of the calculations considered in the short- and long-term evaluations of the rightness of a particular act or rule under utilitarian theory. Rule utilitarians deny that single cost–benefit determinations ought to be accepted and believe that general rules of justice should constrain the use of cost–benefit analysis in all cases and ensure that standards of distributive justice are adhered to (Beauchamp & Walters, 2003).

### Relevance to Margaret's Story

Utilitarians would certainly be concerned with the short- and long-term consequences of whatever decision Margaret arrives at. If the wife is allowed into the patient's rooms during the team's resuscitation efforts, team members might be distracted while they should be focused on saving the life of her husband. Some may feel uncomfortable with the wife's presence, and their actions may be inhibited or otherwise influenced. Such distractions might affect the outcome. The patient may die. This might lead to the wife feeling guilty or perhaps angry at the team, blaming them for her husband's death. Preventing her from being present, however,

continued on following page >>

might negatively affect her short- and long-term grieving process because she would have been denied the opportunity to be with her husband when he died.

On the other hand, if she is allowed to be present, perhaps she would not react to the team's activities and would instead take the opportunity to sit quietly with her husband. Perhaps her presence would positively influence the outcome, and resuscitation efforts would be successful. If not, then at least being with her husband when he died might make the bereavement process easier.

Margaret might wish to allow the wife to enter the room, but as a novice nurse, she might be concerned about consequences to her if she were to override the wishes of the team.

These are the types of outcomes a utilitarian would consider. Using the theory, discuss the case in more detail and think about what you would do if you were Margaret.

## Deontological Theory

In deontological theory, rules are established to determine what is right or wrong based on one's obligations and duties, the foundation of which is the unchanging or absolute principles derived from universally shared values. Contrary to teleological theory, including utilitarianism, deontologists believe that standards for moral behaviour exist independently of means or ends (Beauchamp & Walters, 2003). Consequences, they argue, are irrelevant to moral evaluation. An act or rule is right if it satisfies the demands of some overriding principle or principles of duty. Further, they argue, our duties to each other are complex and vary according to our relationships in society, as are the duties and obligations a parent has to a child or the responsibilities physicians and nurses have to patients (Beauchamp & Walters, 2003).

Deontologists attempt to identify the foundation of moral standards in order to make clear the duties and obligations required of moral agents. There are various deontological perspectives on the foundation of duty—for example, the will of God, reason, intuition, universality, or the social contract (Beauchamp & Walters, 2003).

As with utilitarianism, there are two types of deontological theory: act and rule. The *act deontologist* believes that an individual in any situation should grasp immediately what ought to be done without the need to rely on rules. Act deontologists emphasize the particular and changing features of the moral experience and value the intuitive response to situations or circumstances (Beauchamp & Walters, 2003).

*Rule deontologists* promote that acts are right or wrong relative to their "conformity or nonconformity to one or more principles or rules" (Beauchamp & Walters, 2003). Further, there are two types of rule deontologists: pluralistic, who believe that there are many principles to guide moral conduct, and monistic, who hold that there is one fundamental principle that provides "the source from which other more specific moral rules can be derived"—one such example is the golden rule ("Do unto others…") (Beauchamp & Walters, 2003).

Rule deontologists argue that rules facilitate decision making. Further, they suggest that act theories present problems for cooperation and trust, and reduce morality to "rules of thumb." Moral rules, they say, should be binding (Beauchamp & Walters, 2003).

Philosopher Immanuel Kant (1724–1804) formulated the best-known rule-oriented deontological theory, discussed below.

KANTIAN ETHICS

Central to Kant's philosophy is the concept that morality could be explained as "the ultimate commandment of reason, or imperative, from which all duties and obligations derive." This *categorical imperative*, which he set out in his book *Groundwork of the Metaphysics of Morals* (Kant, 1785), denotes an absolute rule or requirement for behaviour that exists in all circumstances. He believed that humanity was special, that the rational person should not need guidance in determining right from wrong, and that this should be clear to every decent human being (Grassian, 1981). The challenge, he believed, was for people to maintain the self-control to do what was right. He set out to establish a comprehensive theory of the nature of morality in order to explain how morality was both possible and rational (Grassian, 1981).

Kant rejected the utilitarian notion that the maximization of human desire was the basis for morality. People, he said, do not derive their dignity or worth from desiring happiness. Morality, he insisted, must be based on the values of rationality and freedom. He argued that one could not be acting morally while justifying one's actions by an appeal to human desires (Grassian, 1981). Further, a focus on the principle of utility, he believed, would lead to grave injustices, there being no assurance that the distribution of happiness would be fair. Kant placed great emphasis on justice and individual liberty (Grassian, 1981).

Kant developed two distinct theories of morality—a theory of moral obligation and a theory of moral value. The theory of moral obligation focused on how we decide an act is right, whereas the theory of moral value considered how we decide when a person is morally good or has a good character (Grassian, 1981).

*Kant's Theory of Moral Obligation*

Kant's theory of moral obligation focuses on how those principles and rules that guide duty should be determined.

Kant tried to establish the foundation for the validity of moral rules in pure reason, not in intuition, conscience, or utility. Morality, he argued, should provide a rational and universal framework of principles and moral rules that constrain and guide everyone, regardless of personal goals and interests (Beauchamp & Walters, 2003). The moral worth of an individual's action depends only on the moral acceptability of the rule upon which that person is acting. He believed that a person's act has moral worth only when performed with the intention of goodwill and in accordance with universally valid moral principles (Beauchamp & Walters, 2003).

Kant believed that valid moral and ethical principles are based on an abstract, a priori foundation that is independent of empirical reality. He argued that morality is objectively and universally binding; it is absolute, not flexible. If an act or behaviour is morally right, then it is right in all circumstances and is not dependent on the outcome or consequences of that act (Albert, Denise, & Peterfreund, 1975). For example, if telling the truth is the morally correct thing to do, then one must always tell the truth, regardless of the context of the situation or the consequences.

Kant believed that we are able to isolate these a priori, or absolute, elements that ground morality through reasoning. He claimed that the universal basis of morality lies in an individual's rational nature rather than in human desires and inclinations (Albert et al., 1975). (Later in this chapter, alternative ways of thinking about rationality will be explored.)

Kant identified one supreme principle that a law of morality must follow and called this the **categorical imperative**; categorical, in that Kant admits to no exceptions to the rule that is absolutely binding, and imperative, in that it gives instructions about how one must act (Albert et al., 1975). Kant set out some guidelines, or maxims, for determining rules of conduct based on the categorical imperative. He stated that an act is morally right if and only if its maxim is universalizable.

The categorical imperative, independent of our goals or desires, is fundamental to Kant's theory of how to identify the rules or principles that guide our actions and moral decisions. Kant expresses the categorical imperative, or moral law, in two significant formulations:

- "I am never to act otherwise than so that I could also will that my maxim should become a universal law. We must be able to will that the maxim of our action should become a universal law. . . . Since you would not want others to behave in the way you propose to behave, you should not behave in that way." (Albert et al., 1975)

In this formulation, Kant suggests that we must determine the implications of universalizing the rules that guide our actions. For example, would we be able to establish a rule that lying is morally correct? What would happen if everyone lied? Whom would we be able to trust? If it were universally acceptable to lie, then no one would believe anyone, contradicting then the assumption of truth. Could we establish a rule that only doctors may decide on treatment options for patients? What would a society be like if we were denied the freedom to make decisions about our own health care? What if it were permissible to cross an intersection on a red light? A rule must undergo such scrutiny. According to Kant, if it can be applied universally, then it is what we "ought" to do. If not, then it is morally wrong.

- "So act as to treat humanity whether in thine own person or in that of any other, in every case as an end withal, never as means only." (Albert et al., 1975)

This formulation requires us to treat each human being or person as an end, never as a means to any other end. This is based on Kant's view that the existence of humanity has in itself absolute worth. Therefore, all human beings should be respected (Grassian, 1981). For example, Kant would argue that we have a duty to tell the truth, since persons ought to be respected and not used as a means to some other desired end (such as keeping the truth from someone to protect our own interests). Even if lying were to produce some desired outcome for the person being lied to, the act would still be disrespectful. However, Kant did not say that, as persons, we would never be used as means—for example, for some instrumental good. But if we are used as an instrument toward some other good, we must also be regarded as ends in ourselves. Hence, for example, the notion of informed consent: Kant would probably agree that it is morally acceptable to use persons for research or organ donation but only if the right to self-determination is respected.

To summarize, according to Kant, a rule, principle, or maxim is a fundamental, object-ive moral law grounded in pure, practical reasoning, upon which all purely rational moral agents would act.

## Kant's Theory of Moral Value

How do we determine whether a person is morally good or has a good character? According to Kant, it is insufficient to look only at actions and the consequences of those actions without also looking at the person's motives and intentions. Actions alone do not give the complete picture of one's moral character, since a bad person may do the right thing for the wrong reasons. The only moral motive, a sign of good character, is the motive of con-scientiousness (acting out of duty). A morally good person is one with goodwill—that is, one who acts out of duty (Grassian, 1981). For example, a person tells the truth because of the duty to tell the truth regardless of the consequences.

Fundamental to Kant's theory of moral value is the notion of freedom and rational-ity. Kant considered individuals to be rational, moral agents who have the right to make their own choices unless those choices interfere with the freedom of others. He believed that morality presupposed the existence of free will and that we have the choice to act from goodwill or not (Grassian, 1981). An action, behaviour, or decision that is chosen in accordance with one's duty or goodwill is therefore right. If an act and one's motivation to do that act is right, then it is intrinsically good; that is, it is good in and of itself. If an act is intrinsically good, then it has moral value (Albert et al., 1975).

Kant placed great emphasis on the performance of one's duty for its own sake. While it is possible to engage in right actions for many reasons—for example, fear or self-interest—Kant considered such actions morally praiseworthy only if they are performed out of duty (Grassian, 1981). Thus, to be moral, an individual must demonstrate goodwill or good intention by doing what he or she ought to do, rather than acting from inclination or self-interest (Albert et al., 1975).

Some actions based on inclination or self-interest may be worthy of praise; they may also happen to be in accordance with duty. But these do not have "moral" value (Albert et al., 1975). For example, a rich benefactor may donate a million dollars to a health care agency in order to have the agency renamed in his honour. This act might be praise-worthy but not in accordance with duty, so it would not have the same moral value. According to Kant, an individual recently unemployed who continues to contribute weekly to his church would be acting out of a sense of duty, and, hence, his actions have moral worth or value. Actions with true moral worth, when they are evaluated, stand alone, independent of other motives. Thus, an act performed out of duty has moral worth because of the principle guiding that act; the worth does not spring from the act's results or outcomes.

Kant emphasized duty as the prominent feature of moral consciousness. Duty accords with moral law, the essential characteristic of which is universality (Albert et al., 1975).

*Criticism of Kant*

There are a number of criticisms of Kant's theory, particularly related to its application in everyday practice. For example, how is duty to be determined when two or more duties are in conflict? What happens if, in order to protect someone from harm, we have to lie or withhold the truth? Consider a situation in which someone provides protection to a woman who is being abused by her husband, and the husband arrives asking about her whereabouts. Kant's theory seems to demand that both relevant duties be fulfilled: the duty to tell the truth and the duty to protect the woman from harm. Kant does not provide a means to deal with this type of situation; he indicates only that we must be true to both duties (Beauchamp & Walters, 2003).

Critics also argue that the categorical imperative is ultimately reduced to a determination of consequences. That is, in looking at the universal application of an action, one is actually looking at the overall consequences of that act. If the universal performance of a certain type of action is undesirable overall, then it is wrong (Beauchamp & Walters, 2003). In response, Kantians argue that consequences are not totally disregarded, but the features of making something right are not dependent on any outcome alone (Beauchamp & Walters, 2003).

## THE DEONTOLOGY OF W.D. ROSS

W. D. Ross, a British philosopher of the early twentieth century, developed a pluralistic, rule-oriented deontological theory that attempts to resolve the problem of conflict of duties. Ross identified **prima facie duties**, those duties that one must always act upon unless they conflict with those of equal or stronger obligation (Beauchamp & Walters, 2003). The stronger duty is determined by an examination of the respective weights of the competing prima facie duties. Ross accepts that prima facie duties are not absolute since they can be overridden. Instead, he argues they have greater moral significance than mere rules of thumb (Beauchamp & Walters, 2003).

When one is faced with a number of alternatives, the "right" choice or action is the one consistent with all the rules. If a number of alternatives are consistent with the rules, then the choice is one of preference. When each choice is consistent with one rule but in conflict with another, then one attempts to appeal to the higher rule to resolve the conflict. For example, sanctity of life would have priority over the rule of veracity or truth telling.

In response to criticisms that it is not always possible to evaluate the respective weights of principles in conflict, Ross reduced his argument to a claim that no moral system is free of conflicts and exceptions (Beauchamp & Walters, 2003).

Would a deontological approach assist Margaret in making the right choice? How? What ethical principles apply to this scenario? Which ones have greater priority?

### Relevance to Margaret's Story

From a deontological perspective, Margaret has a duty to her patient and to his family—in this scenario, his wife. She also has a duty to her team, who expressed their concern about bringing the wife into the room. Is it possible for Margaret to use the categorical imperative to identify the rules or principles that would guide her action in this situation? Are we able to establish a maxim or rule that can be generalized to similar situations? Is it possible to establish a universal law that families may choose to be present during emergency interventions whenever they wish? On the other hand, can we establish that it is always the health care team who decides who may and may not be present? How would we want to be treated if we were the family member?

Continue to reflect on this situation from a deontologist's perspective. How does this theory assist your thinking in this case relative to teleological or utilitarian ethical theory?

## Ethical Principles

Derived from moral theory, ethical principles serve as rules to guide moral conduct and to assist us in taking consistent positions on specific and related issues (Beauchamp & Walters, 2003). Principles provide a framework for ethical decision making that is often used by health care professionals and is a popular approach in health care ethics. Ethical principles are expressed in many professional codes of ethics, which are discussed in Chapter 3.

The use of ethical principles as a guide for ethical decision making in health care was introduced by Beauchamp and Childress in 1983 in *Principles of Biomedical Ethics*, which has since undergone three revisions (see Beauchamp & Childress, 2001). The important principles commonly applied to ethical challenges in health care include sanctity of life, autonomy, nonmaleficence, beneficence, justice, fidelity, and veracity. Ethical principles are considered prima facie; that is, their application may be relative to another principle that may have more weight or priority in a given situation. For example, consider the scenario in which a community client reveals to a nurse that he frequently fantasizes about children. He states he has never acted on these fantasies and certainly has never been convicted of an offence. Recently, she has heard that he just started employment as a janitor in one of the local primary schools. Clearly, this nurse is facing two principles in opposition to each other: confidentiality versus protecting the children from potential harm. Moral reflection and deliberation would assist this nurse in deciding the best course of action based on the principle that has the most weight in this circumstance.

Some individuals may consider particular principles to be a priori or binding, as are Kant's categorical imperatives. For example, some people advocate sanctity of life in all forms and at all costs, while others believe that quality of life may override sanctity of life in some circumstances.

## Autonomy

The principle of **autonomy** (*autos*, from Greek meaning "self"; *nomos*, from Greek meaning "rule") asserts that a capable and competent individual is free to determine, and to act in accordance with, a self-chosen plan (Beauchamp & Childress, 2001). Autonomy, founded on respect for persons, is based on the notion that human beings have worth and moral dignity not possessed by other creatures. To respect persons is to recognize them, without condition, as worthy moral agents who should not be treated as mere means to any other end (Beauchamp & Childress, 2001). Thus, persons should be able to decide their own destiny and should be allowed to make their own evaluations, choices, and actions, so long as these do not harm nor interfere with the liberty or freedom of others (Beauchamp & Walters, 2003). Respect for autonomy also means granting individuals the right to privacy and confidentiality. Confidentiality is important in the health care environment, in which patients and clients must trust health professionals with private information in order to receive safe and competent care. Patients have the right to expect that such information will remain confidential unless there is a risk to self or others, or unless disclosure is required by law.

This principle supports the Kantian view that individuals be respected as ends in and of themselves, and never as means to some other end. As discussed earlier in this chapter, this view is based in Kant's belief that humanity itself has absolute worth. Therefore, all human beings should be respected (Beauchamp & Childress, 2001).

This principle is also consistent with Mill's utilitarian ethics, which states that autonomy maximizes the benefits of all concerned, and that social and political control over individual action is legitimate only if it is necessary to prevent harm to others (Beauchamp & Childress, 2001).

The legal doctrine of **informed consent** is based on respect for the principle of autonomy and an individual's right to the information required to make decisions about one's own health care. Failure to provide a patient with adequate information limits that person's autonomy and interferes with his or her rights. (The elements of informed consent are discussed in Chapter 6.) The concept of the autonomous individual gives rise to the duty of respecting a person's values and choices. Autonomy assumes the person is competent; has the ability to decide rationally, rather than impulsively; and has the ability to act upon those decisions and choices (Beauchamp & Childress, 2001). Autonomy also assumes voluntariness, which means having the freedom to make choices.

In order to be autonomous, a person must be free of external control and be able to take action to control his or her own affairs (Beauchamp & Childress, 2001). Even if it is believed that clients' evaluations or decisions are wrong or potentially harmful to them, as long as acting on them poses no threat of serious harm to others, then the principle of autonomy demands they be respected. On occasion, autonomy conflicts with other principles, such as beneficence—for example, when a patient refuses treatment that the nurse and health care team firmly believe is in the patient's best interest. As nurses know, illness puts limits on individual autonomy. The hospital environment further limits the patient's control. The views of the health care team may be readily apparent to the patient, leading to subtle forms of coercion in relation to choices the patient must make. Patients may experience anxiety and stress, and even be overwhelmed by uncertainty with regard to their future and prognosis. As a moral agent, the nurse has a duty to support the patient through this process, ensure that he or she has the information required to make choices, and give him or her time to reflect on these choices to determine the best course of action.

Some philosophers believe autonomy to be the primary moral principle, which takes precedence over all other moral considerations (Beauchamp & Childress, 2001). The challenge, particularly for health care professionals, is to ensure that clients have the ability to act autonomously; that is, they are making decisions with a full understanding of the facts, issues, and consequences of that decision. Some persons are unable to act autonomously owing to immaturity, incapacity, lack of information, or coercion. A person of diminished autonomy is highly dependent on others and, to some degree, is unable to choose a plan on the basis of controlled deliberations. Young children and the mentally ill may fall into this category of individuals whose rights may need to be protected by others. One must be careful, however, in assuming that the mentally ill and children always have diminished capacity to make decisions on their own behalf. Consider the 15-year-old patient who was diagnosed at age 8 with leukemia. Having experienced a series of treatments and their complications for some time, this patient would likely be capable of making a decision regarding further interventions. Contrast this with a 15-year-old adolescent who has never been in a hospital and is not willing to undergo surgery for a ruptured appendix. As well, people receiving treatment for mental illness may have the capacity to make decisions and also to make an advance directive regarding their care if they become ill.

As autonomy is a prima facie principle, it may at times conflict with another principle of higher moral weight in a particular circumstance. For example, a patient with a terminal illness who is in constant pain may, after careful deliberation, freely decide that assisted suicide is his preferred option. Even if his decision has the support of his family and friends, in this circumstance, the principle of **sanctity of life** continues to have more weight in Canadian society than the principle of autonomy.

Another important principle derived from the principle of autonomy is the principle of **veracity**, the duty to tell the truth. Veracity, or truth telling, is central to ensuring and maintaining trust within the nurse–patient or nurse–client relationship. An individual's right to the truth is linked to respect for persons, inherent in the principle of autonomy. Patients have the right to expect that the nurses caring for them will provide honest responses to their questions and communicate truthfully to them about the nature of their condition and the care they receive.

Conflicts associated with our obligation to the principle of veracity arise when the truth may result in harm. For example, consider a patient who is dying of a terminal disease. How should caregivers respond to questions associated with the outcome of a particular treatment when the likelihood of success is poor but they still wish to communicate some sense of hope? How does one balance the need to share relevant information with a client while sharing that information in a respectful and benevolent manner? How and when to communicate bad news, for example, is a critical ethical issue. One cannot appeal to the principle of veracity as justification for revealing bad news to a patient without considering the timing and manner of communication and the need for follow-up care and support.

Truth telling is fundamental to the establishment and maintenance of trusting relationships. Vital to the relationship between nurses and patients is the nurse's ability to care, to provide comfort, and to maintain honest and truthful communication while continuing to convey a sense of hope and purpose.

## Nonmaleficence

The principle of **nonmaleficence** is associated with the Latin maxim *primum non nocere*: "above all (or first), do no harm." This is expressed in many professional codes of ethics and in the Hippocratic oath: "I will use treatment to help the sick according to my ability and judgement, but I will never use it to injure or wrong them." This principle obliges members of society to act in such a way as to prevent or remove harm (Beauchamp & Childress, 2001).

In nursing, professional practice standards express the competencies that nurses must have to ensure the provision of safe patient care. Some actions of nurses may produce temporary harm (e.g., the administration of medication by injection, restraining patients, painful procedures such as dressings or intravenous insertion). This temporary harm is justified if it is a means to producing a good and if the principle of autonomy is respected.

There are four hierarchical elements related to nonmaleficence (Beauchamp & Childress, 2001), ranked according to standard of obligation. The first three represent adherence to the principle of nonmaleficence, whereas the fourth, the highest standard, relates to the principle of beneficence, described next:

1.  One ought not to inflict evil or harm.
2.  One ought to prevent evil or harm.
3.  One ought to remove evil or harm.
4.  One ought to do or promote good (Beauchamp, 1982).

## Beneficence

The principle of **beneficence** sets a higher standard than nonmaleficence in that it holds that one must make a positive move to produce some good or benefit for another. It asserts an obligation to come to the assistance of those in need and to help others to further their important and legitimate interests (Beauchamp & Childress, 2001). Many thinkers argue that the ideal is to be beneficent but that we are not morally obliged to take positive action to benefit others. Indeed, the law in Canada, except in Quebec, does not require us to assist others, for example, in emergencies. This differs from "good Samaritan" laws in force in some European countries. In France, individuals can face criminal charges for failing to provide assistance in emergencies; in Quebec, a person who fails to render assistance can be sued by the injured person for such failure.

As professionals, nurses have the duty to act in such a manner that not only protects patients from harm but also produces some good or benefit. Failure to do this may violate professional duties and obligations.

At times, the principle of beneficence may conflict with that of autonomy—for example, when a particular intervention is likely to benefit a patient, yet the patient refuses consent. This is often a source of distress for health care professionals. However, ensuring that patients are provided with the information, support, and time to make decisions that are truly in their best interests can help overcome this situation.

### THE INFLUENCE OF PATERNALISTIC OR MATERNALISTIC ATTITUDES

Traditionally, but much less so in recent years, health care professionals have acted in a paternalistic way ("Father or Mother knows best") toward patients in an effort to protect them from the potentially harmful consequences of their choices. That is, out of a desire to be beneficent, physicians and nurses have at times allowed their sense of what they think is best to gain ascendancy over important ethical principles (autonomy, truth telling).

In the past, this approach had the potential to restrict the liberty of individuals. Treatment may have been given or withheld without the client's consent; the justification for such action was either the prevention of some harm clients might have done to themselves or the production of some benefit they might not otherwise have secured (Beauchamp & Childress, 2001). Some health professionals went so far as to withhold information from patients with a terminal illness in order to protect them from the "pain" of knowing their death was imminent. (Of course, even today, patients may choose to have information withheld from them in such circumstances.) Others would fail to disclose all of the side effects or consequences of major surgery in order to secure consent. Paternalism is considered justified in Canadian society today in certain situations, including the following:

- Involuntary committal to a mental health facility
- The prevention of suicide
- Resuscitation without consent
- Denial of unusual, untested, and possibly dangerous treatment requested by the patient or family
- Requirements to use bike helmets and seat belts
- Immunization against disease

## Fidelity

The principle of **fidelity** is the foundation of the nurse–patient relationship. This rule is about nurses' being loyal, keeping promises, and telling the truth (veracity) to those entrusted to their care (Beauchamp & Childress, 2001). Fidelity comes into play when nurses uphold their commitment to provide adequate pain control; to provide quality care, comfort, and support when needed; to represent the interests of their clients; and to tell the truth. This principle is challenged when nurses are placed in situations in which being loyal to a patient may compromise their own ethical principles, as when a terminally ill patient requests assistance to die when pain cannot be controlled and life has lost its dignity. Even if the nurse understands the patient's physical and emotional pain, and agrees that this action would demonstrate care and compassion, he or she is restricted by law (and perhaps by the nurse's own beliefs) from helping the patient in this circumstance.

## Justice

The principle of **justice** is based on the notion of fairness. In particular, theories of justice focus on how we treat individuals and groups within society, how we distribute benefits (e.g., health care) and burdens (e.g., taxes) in an equitable way, and how we compensate those who have been unfairly burdened or harmed. In health care, justice is fundamental to issues associated with the allocation of resources and rationing in times of scarcity or diminishing resources. There are two forms of justice relevant to health care: distributive justice and compensatory justice.

**Distributive justice** is the proper distribution of both social benefits and burdens across society (Beauchamp & Childress, 2001). Unfortunately, most perspectives on justice describe the concept theoretically but fail to provide effective tools to determine equality or proportion, leaving the meaning of "proper distribution" open to interpretation. Decisions regarding the equitable distribution of resources may be based on one of several considerations (Beauchamp & Childress, 2001):

- To each person an equal share
- To each person according to individual need
- To each person according to that person's rights
- To each person according to individual effort
- To each person according to societal contribution
- To each person according to merit

Determining how to distribute resources equitably is a challenge when resources are scarce, as they increasingly are in health care. Nurses are involved with such questions as to how financial resources are distributed, which programs are funded, how staff is allocated, how patient assignments are organized, who gets the rare organ for transplantation, and many others. Recently, major restructuring in a number of Canadian hospitals has led to the introduction of different models of care that include various levels or categories of care providers. These models add a new dimension to resource allocation from a nursing perspective in that there is a further requirement to evaluate the care needs of patients and to determine the type of provider competent to provide that care.

*Rationing* is a method of allocating scarce resources to those who will most benefit. A well-known example of rationing in health care is in the area of organ donation. Even if Canada's federal and provincial governments provided all the health care dollars necessary to perform all the transplants needed, donor organs are still scarce. Thus, transplant programs must determine how this limited resource will be distributed. Should an organ be given to the person who has waited the longest, to the person with the best chance for survival, to the sickest, to the one with the greatest need, or to the person who "deserves" it the most (e.g., the one needing a liver transplant who has never consumed alcohol, or the one needing a lung transplant who has never smoked)?

Macro resource allocation decisions are made at the policy level. Administrators or legislators decide which programs will be funded. For example, should the number of cardiac surgical procedures performed annually be increased, or should a program of prevention be invested in? Individual nurses face micro resource allocation decisions daily. Which patient gets admitted to the one remaining Intensive Care bed? How much home care should be provided to a dying patient? How should time be allocated among the eight home care patients that have to be visited today? If, because of staff shortages, the care needed today can't be administered, what should be eliminated?

*Compensatory justice* involves providing compensation or payment for harm that has been done to an individual or group. Compensation is commonly provided to individuals or groups as a result of a successful suit for negligence or malpractice. For example, federal and provincial governments compensated victims who contracted HIV and hepatitis C through blood transfusions.

### Relevance to Margaret's Story

A number of ethical principles are relevant to this story. The principle of autonomy would suggest that it is the patient's right to decide who may or may not be present with him. In these circumstances, however, the patient is not capable of making such a decision. One would assume, though, that his wife is his substitute decision maker and therefore able to make decisions for him based on an advance directive or his best interests. The principle of beneficence, which requires health care professionals to act to benefit others, too, might require that Margaret allow the wife to be with her husband to provide him comfort. Also, if he were to die, the experience of being present at the time of his death may facilitate a better bereavement process for her. But based on the principle of nonmaleficence, the team might argue that there is the possibility of harm to both the patient (if the team is distracted) and the wife (if she becomes upset by the resuscitation process). Beyond this situation, the principle of justice would require that the hospital review its policy to ensure fairness to all patients and families.

Continue the discussion in light of these principles and compare their relevance with that of the previous theories. Discuss, too, the value of a policy or guideline regarding family presence during emergencies.

## Feminist and Feminine Perspectives on Ethics

In recent years, emerging feminine and feminist perspectives on ethics have offered alternatives to traditional ethical theories. As discussed, deontological and teleological or utilitarian theories of morality place a strong emphasis on rationality and notions of justice. Feminine and feminist perspectives are critical of these theories, all developed by men, as they are based on male perspectives, standards, biases, and experiences (Baier, 1985). If, as Carol Gilligan's 1988 study of moral development argues, the moral development of women differs from that of men, then these approaches can be problematic for women. Gilligan challenges the notion that there is one superior way to think about moral problems—that is, in terms of abstract and general notions of duty, justice, and rights. Given the patriarchal power structures within health care, and the fact that nursing continues to be dominated by women, alternative models to guide moral action have merit in health care, where the challenges involve not only complex care but complex human relationships that are influenced by the milieu of politics and power.

Feminine and feminist theorists resist traditional rationalistic ethics, believing that ethical analysis must make sense and be applicable in the real world (Sherwin, 1992). Feminist thinkers believe there is more to ethics than abstract reasoning: there is the context of the situation, the nature of the relationships involved, and the unique interests of all the individuals involved.

These thinkers argue that traditional ethics searches for a "systematic approach to evaluate the standards or justifications" of morality and that the interest is in "determining which rules ideally should be followed" (Sherwin, 1992). Such rules, they suggest, may not fit the moral experience and intuitions of many women and fail to address the unique perspective of the individual (Sherwin, 1992). The different experiences of women, feminists argue, may be ignored or downplayed in traditional theories. Further, from their perspective, the emphasis on reason and justice offers little help in explaining women's moral duties to children, the ill, or other vulnerable people who have traditionally been cared for by women, rather than men.

The term *feminist ethics* refers to a wide range of feminist-related moral issues. The goal of feminist ethics is to create a plan or ideology that will end the social and political oppression of women. Feminists believe there is a unique female perspective of the world that can be shaped into an important and relevant theory (Reich, 1995).

## Feminist Theory

To provide a context for a discussion of feminine and feminist approaches to ethics, it is important to describe significant feminist perspectives. Two premises are accepted as essential to feminist thinking (L. Shanner, personal communication, March 28, 1995):

- Female and male experiences, bodies, and socialization are not identical.
- Male perspectives are (currently and historically) dominant, and female perspectives are often marginalized, muted, or simply unrecognized.

A feminist is described as anyone who acts to give voice to these different female perspectives, attempts to balance or integrate male and female thinking, or who promotes feminine over masculine views. Feminist work considers gender and sex to be important analytic categories and seeks to understand their operation in the world. The major focus is on the effort to change the distribution and use of power and to stop the oppression of women (Wolf, 1996). While all feminists agree that women are oppressed and that oppression is wrong, various sects of feminists characterize oppression differently and offer different approaches to overcoming it.

### LIBERAL FEMINISM

This branch of feminism is concerned with the equality of women and the equitable distribution of wealth, position, and power. Though not critical of the traditional roles of woman as wife and mother, liberal feminists are concerned about the social, political, and economic forces that channel women into these roles. Liberal feminists affirm individual choice and urge equal rights for women and the reform of systems to ensure their inclusion (Reich, 1995). The liberal tradition emphasizes rights and freedoms, and seeks to replace a patriarchal protection of male freedoms and limitations with equal rights for women. For example, since men can father children well into their later years, a liberal feminist might argue that women should have right of access to postmenopausal infertility treatment (L. Shanner, personal communication, March 28, 1995).

The liberal feminist agenda, then, is to influence the social and political forces that will overcome oppression and provide women with the same rights and opportunities as men. Some strategies include providing greater educational opportunities for women, ensuring women have access to male-dominated professions (such as medicine and engineering), and implementing legislation that ensures equality for women (Valentine, 1994).

From the liberal feminist perspective, the notion of the autonomous-agent model might be acceptable, but both women and men should be able to act as free, rational agents unless their actions constrain the equal rights of others. The concern of the liberal feminist is that women's freedoms are unfairly constrained.

### SOCIAL FEMINISM

Social feminists examine the cultural institutions that contribute to the oppression of women and the relationship between the private sphere of the home and the public domain of productive work. They focus primarily on the role of economic oppression in women's lives (Reich, 1995). Of major concern are poverty, the challenges of single parenthood, and the influence of the social determinants of health on women and children. They argue that equity will not be attained until changes are made to structures such as the patriarchal family, motherhood, housework, and consumerism since these structures influence the distribution of power, wealth, and privilege. Further, they believe that the social and political structures must change so that women's responsibilities within the home, and traditionally female professions such as nursing, are valued to the same extent as those of men (Valentine, 1994).

To help distinguish between social feminism and liberal feminism, consider the different responses of the two groups to the suggestion of in vitro fertilization (IVF)—for example, the freezing of ova—for fertile women in their 20s to allow them to finish their education, launch careers, and have children later in life with reduced risks of birth defects. A social feminist would respond that the educational and business institutions are not structured in ways that allow women to work and have families at the healthiest time in their life cycle, and so the institutions should be restructured. The liberal feminist is more likely to assert the right of women to having both (Dawson & Singer, 1988).

RADICAL FEMINISM

Radical feminists view women-centred perspectives and institutions as the only or primary ones, thus inverting, not just challenging, current patriarchy. They argue that women's oppression is the crucial problem and challenge the concepts and frameworks of traditional philosophical and scientific inquiry. This perspective, in turn, challenges the patriarchal underpinnings of society, since radical feminists seek to analyze and value women's experiences from the perspective of female rather than male standards and biases (Valentine, 1994).

The focus of radical feminism is the development of women-defined thought, culture, and systems; in order for these to evolve, gender discrimination and sexual stereotyping need to be eliminated. Though the childbearing role of women and values such as nurturance are considered important, radical feminists also see them as the historical basis of oppression of women. There is a greater (not universal) tendency in radical feminism to blame men for oppressing women, not merely to acknowledge that structures in a society are problematic (L. Shanner, personal communication, March 28, 1995). An implicit, or explicit, recommendation is that men should be removed from their position of dominance and replaced by women. Thus, the liberal feminist goal of economic and political equality with men is perceived as aiming too low (L. Shanner, personal communication, March 28, 1995).

While the role of childbearing and child rearing in oppression may be a concern within all forms of feminism, for the radical feminist the role of pregnancy is central. All feminists tend to want women, not men, to control the means of reproduction and to have at least an equal voice in reproductive policies. They may argue that women's voices should dominate since women are more greatly affected by pregnancy and reproductive interventions than men are. The liberal feminist wants greater reproductive liberty and thus is more likely to want minimal restrictions on surrogacy, egg selling, and other means of reproductive choice. The social feminist not only wants to change the institutions that limit women's choices so that women can thrive whether or not they choose to have families, but also challenges the values we place on reproduction and family life. (Thus, social feminists may wish to reject some practices, such as surrogacy or egg selling, as exploitative of women and children.) The radical feminist is more likely to characterize a reproductive intervention as a plot to control the bodies of women (L. Shanner, personal communication, March 28, 1995).

Although these three perspectives embrace a broad range of feminist thought and practice, all share the following themes:

• Recognition of the oppression of women
• Support for equal rights and opportunities for women
• An orientation to initiating change (Adamson, Briskin, & McPhail, 1988)

Feminist theory is complex, as are the ethical perspectives it raises. Nurses can benefit through increased awareness of, and interest in, the ethical views that feminist theory offers.

## Feminist Ethics

Feminist approaches to bioethics have historically attempted to expose the ways in which medical practices contribute to the oppression of women. Challenging the paradigms of bioethics, feminists reject liberal assumptions about the autonomy of individuals (Reich, 1995). Humans, they argue, are fundamentally relational, and this in itself is morally significant (Reich, 1995). Of key interest to feminists in the area of bioethics are the debates over abortion, surrogate motherhood, maternal–fetal relations, use of fetal tissue, and medical conditions affecting women that have hitherto been ignored.

In feminist ethics, the oppression of women, the issue of utmost moral concern, "is seen to be morally and politically unacceptable" (Sherwin, 1992). Feminist ethics, therefore, is committed to "eliminating the subordination of women." (Sherwin, 1992). Within the context of feminist ethical thinking, the predominant question asked is "What does this mean for women?" The focus is on changing the status quo, empowering women, and eliminating oppression (Sherwin, 1992). Without such changes, feminists believe a truly ethical reality is not possible.

### Relevance to Margaret's Story

A feminist reflecting on this story would be concerned about the interests of the patient's wife. A feminist might ask questions related to whether rules or policies excluding this woman from her husband's bedside were established primarily by men who, they would be concerned, might make up the hospital hierarchy. The question might also be asked whether if the situation were reversed and the husband wanted to be present, his wishes would be respected. Reflect on whether you think feminist ethics would assist Margaret with her dilemma.

## Feminine Ethics

Feminine ethics as recognized by Carol Gilligan, a feminist thinker, has emerged as a focal point in philosophy. Gilligan (1988) suggests that women and men make ethical choices based on different sets of values, perceptions, and concerns. Feminine views give greater significance to the nature of the relationships within a particular ethical context without the political nature of feministic thinking. Gilligan argues that when faced with a moral issue, women use an empathetic form of reasoning (Reich, 1995) and tend to seek out innovative solutions that will ensure that the needs of all parties are met, whereas men tend to seek the dominant rule, even when someone's interests are sacrificed (Sherwin, 1992). An example might be the various approaches to visiting-hour rules in hospitals. One could treat all visitors the same, imposing strict time limits, or recognize the special needs of individual patients and families, allowing a more open, client-directed approach.

Those with a feminine view of ethics argue that traditional theories are overly concerned with rational and objective thinking. In contrast, the feminine view places greater emphasis on values, feelings, and desires. There is more significance to being present, listening, taking feelings seriously, searching for meaning, and seeing the person and the world from a more holistic perspective (Lind, Wilburn, & Pate, 1986). In contrast to Kantian thinking, in which emotion is seen to have no role in morality, emotion and intuition are viewed as key indicators of right action. Consider the work of Patricia Benner, who observes the expert nurse's ability to detect the changing condition of a patient without apparent changes in physiological status. She places value on nurse's intuition, which she suggests developed through experience in detecting the worries and concerns of patients and families. Brenner proposes that within any complex social interaction, emotions are central to perception and rationality, and can signal preference, danger, attraction, and so on. Within any situation or context, emotions have significance; they influence responses such as compassion and fear and provide insights into the meaning of human interactions and relationships (Benner, 1990, 2000). When we reflect on these experiences and understand our responses and reactions to situations and events, we may gain insight into our moral selves (Malmsten, 2000). In summary, feminine thinkers assert that more than one dimension needs to be considered to understand the moral issues and principles that prevail. The study of feminine ethics is, therefore, essential to understanding and clarifying ethics as it relates to the complex practice and values of nursing and the context and relationships within which care is given.

## An Ethic of Care

Feminine thinkers who accept Gilligan's assertion that women think differently from men propose an "ethic of care" (Reich, 1995). Critical of the dominance of principles and of the historical preference in traditional theories for abstract rules that reinforce a deductive reasoning process, they argue instead for an inductive process in which the starting point is the individual's circumstances or personal story. This approach, they suggest, more accurately depicts real life and ensures that all dimensions of the situation are addressed (Wolf, 1996). Reasoning from abstract rules and principles governed by requirements for universality and impartiality, they argue, overlooks the importance of partiality, context, and relationships. An ethic of care is instead relational, contextual, and empathetic, as opposed to the abstract, universalized, and principled approach of an ethic of justice (Wolf, 1996). An ethic of care is therefore suggested as a new approach to ethical thinking that values feelings, emotions, empathy, and care—all important components of our ethical responses. Further, it recognizes the demands of relationships and the particular situations we face.

Using the experience of women as the foundation of a model of ethical theory, an ethic of care encourages spontaneous caring for others as appropriate to each unique circumstance and experience. Feminine ethical decision making is based on the desire to respond to the unique needs of each person. The focus is on caring rather than on justice or principled approaches. Further, it recognizes the nature of complex relationships and the challenges people face in life. For example, rather than treating all people alike in the name of fairness, it is recognized that some people need and want to be treated differently. Out of interest and concern for each individual's personal context, a focus on caring requires an examination of all of the dynamics of a particular situation. From this perspective, nurses enter another's world in order to see things as that person sees them (Crowley, 1989). Thus, nurses can better understand the values, beliefs, and experiences of their patients or clients. The ethical issues are understood from the experience of entering another's world, being aware of the morally relevant features and responsibilities of the relationships involved, and the context of the situation (Sherwin, 1992). These are all elements of family and patient-centered care, which will be discussed in Chapter 12.

In care ethics, the emphasis is on the process of self-understanding, whereby one offers explanations, or justifications, for choices. The sharing of unique perspectives facilitates a greater understanding of the dynamics of a situation and therefore provides greater insights to guide our choices. This approach enhances the nurse's relationship with the patient and is recommended as a means of understanding and respecting the various views and life experiences of all members of the health care team (Baker & Diekelmann, 1994).

Not all feminine thinkers agree that caring should supplant all principles; some worry that it is a "compassion trap" that will keep women in their traditional roles (Reich, 1995). Some radical feminists have concerns about an emphasis on caring, which they view as a gender trait and a survival skill of a historically oppressed group (Sherwin, 1992). Too much emphasis on the welfare of others, they believe, can drain the resources and energy of women. These feminists do not reject the relevance of caring but instead attempt to identify criteria for determining when it is relevant and when it is not. Social feminists would agree that feelings play a role in ethical decision making but that these need to be balanced with social justice (Sherwin, 1992).

Some suggest that caring, which women take more into consideration because of their traditional role within the family, is the only moral consideration (Sherwin, 1992; Noddings, 1992). This view has been criticized because it suggests the exclusion of women who do not have children and men from the possibility of such caring and nurturing (Condon, 1992). Noddings (1992) argues that an ethic of care is a quest for new virtues based on traditional women's practices and that the traditional female role as nurturer can be shaped into an ethic of care.

## Caring and Relational Ethics in Nursing

Theories in nursing have focused on understanding and clarifying the concept of care. Consider the following quote from well-known nursing theorist Jean Watson (1988):

> At a new level in nursing's caring–healing consciousness, regardless of one's theoretical inclinations, there is the continual need to search and to acknowledge that the traditional models of health–illness and science are inadequate for the lived world of patients and the lived caring–healing processes nurses experience in transpersonal caring moments.

Watson argues that caring avoids reducing persons to the moral status of object and introduces new caring–healing possibilities. Caring ensures the preservation of human dignity and relationship equality within the context of illness and suffering. As a moral ideal, caring is not only a standard that demonstrates commitment to patients but is an end in and of itself. Essentially, it is both the process and goal of nursing (Watson, 1985).

Given the importance of the notion of care and caring in the nursing profession, it is not surprising that care-based approaches are highly relevant to nursing ethics. They emphasize the moral imperative of reducing human suffering as well as the relational aspect of nursing and the nurse–patient relationship (Peter & Gallop, 1994). These approaches are seen as more meaningful alternatives to principles-based approaches. The moral experience of the nurses cannot be limited to principles alone. Rather than serving as tools to facilitate ethical decisions, principles can become a pretence to defend one's own biases and to pass them off as absolutes. Some thinkers note that moral conflicts arise precisely because moral rules and principles cannot be applied to every situation clearly and without contradiction, and that this demonstrates the limitations of this type of reasoning. Furthermore, the role of the nurse as a moral agent may be compromised if a focus on rules leads the nurse to become more detached from the situation—and the person—and become more of a "distant observer," rather than understanding the situation within the context of the caring relationship (Parker, 1990).

Consider the stories of critical care nurses who become distressed when caring for patients receiving aggressive treatment that causes pain and suffering while offering only a slim chance of survival. It may be that the family supports aggressive treatment or that the patient at an earlier time completed an advance directive that agrees with such measures. However, in the reality of the moment, and the present experience of the patient, the nurse may, because of the caring relationship, intuitively believe that the patient's views are now quite different. A focus on principles such as autonomy and quality of life alone in this circumstance would not alleviate the moral distress of the nurse. If only principles are used to justify care, without any connection to the nurse–patient relationship or the human experience, the nurse may become disengaged.

Care ethics organizes social and moral theory around care and the connections that bring us in touch with others through the nurse–patient relationship (Parker, 1990). Care is seen as a relational response to a fundamental human need, central to nursing practice, not only as a therapeutic interaction but as a moral imperative. As the deliverers of care, nurses then become moral agents. Care is also seen as a means of being ethical, therefore a normative moral concept of that which is good (Benner, 1990, 2000). As moral agents, then, nurses "nurture the humanity of those for whom they care" and demonstrate caring attributes of compassion, competence, confidence, commitment, conscience, communication, concern, and courage (Cloyes, 2002).

Essential to an ethical nurse–patient relationship is trust (Peter & Morgan, 2001). Trust is significant in that, frequently, the nurse is in the position of power, especially when caring for those who are most vulnerable. To trust is to make oneself or let oneself be more vulnerable to the power of others, to be confident that one will be cared for and protected from harm

(Baier, 1985). Trust is especially relevant to challenges related to the need for basic care. For example, a patient who loses the ability to control bodily functions essentially hands his or her body over to someone else, the nurse. This patient is totally dependent on the nurse and the nurse's capacity to meet or facilitate the patient's physical, social, and emotional needs.

Some theorists propose that it is difficult to separate the ethic of care from the notion of the "good nurse." Two positions are put forth: Some see caring or relational ethics as a distinct approach to ethics; others see it as the way virtues are acted out within specific relationships (Izumi et al., 2006; Watson, 1992). The characteristics of the nurse are relevant to his or her status as a moral agent. *Virtue ethics* considers the character traits of the person or the moral agent, and views virtue as a socially valuable character trait. In virtue ethics, the normative standard is the good person who will want to do what is good in all circumstances (Pellegrino, 1995). For example, a nurse may provide care that follows policy or protocol, but unless the nurse, because of his or her virtuous character, is also motivated to care about the person, the therapeutic intervention would not be considered caring and ethical (Izumi et al., 2006). Without the commitment to care and to do what is best for that patient in that circumstance, the nurse simply completes a task. It is suggested that there are four qualities that support a caring relationship: being a good person, presenting as a good person, being interested in the other person (patient) as a person, and caring for the other person (patient) (Izumi et al., 2006).

Consider the nurse observed in a rehabilitation setting caring for four older patients who are recovering from orthopedic surgery:

The nurse is attentive to protocol, well organized, and focused on the task at hand. She addresses the men individually as "Papa," likely because of their senior status. She is particularly concerned about one of the men, who is diabetic and is not eating well. Dutifully, she checks his blood sugar and finds that it is very low. She scolds him for not eating and suggests that he drink a glass of orange juice loaded with sugar. He refuses. In frustration with his "noncompliant behaviour," the nurse leaves the room to call the physician. A visitor, also a nurse and the daughter of one of the other patients, has become acquainted with the other patients in her father's room. They are highly competent men with prestigious backgrounds, though vulnerable because of their health issues. She has noted their responses to various caregivers and seen the men bristle when they are addressed as "Papa." She is aware that the patient with diabetes is a businessman who is sad because his partner is taking advantage of his convalescence to visit her family in the Philippines.

The visiting daughter approaches him, listens to him express his frustration about how he is being treated, and then kindly counsels him to drink the orange juice, which he does. He is well aware of how to manage his diabetes and knows the importance of raising his blood sugar level. Is this nurse who is caring for the patient in this setting functioning as a moral agent within the framework of a caring nurse–patient relationship? Does she know the patients she is caring for? Are they receiving ethical and respectful care?

SYNTHESIS OF JUSTICE AND CARING

Those who have a "care versus justice" position on ethics view care and justice as different and divergent approaches to ethics and morality (Cloyes, 2002). Critics of justice-based ethics focus on its "rigidity, inflexibility and failure to account for the caring relationship a nurse develops with a patient" (Olsen, 1992, p. 1023). Critics of caring ethics worry about "its potential for differential regard of patients" (Olsen, 1992, p. 1023).

Though many maintain that care is the superior approach, others argue for the integration of care and justice (Cloyes, 2002; Noddings, 1992; Gilligan, 1995). They argue that models based solely on care have limitations in that without moral obligation to principles such as justice, caring relationships can be exploitative or unfairly partial (Peter & Morgan, 2001). Believing that "the heart and the mind need not be adversaries in moral reflection" and that justice and caring are not mutually exclusive (Olsen, 1992), they promote a combination of an ethic of care and an orientation toward principles that would address injustice while maintaining a more connected sense of social relationships. In fact, research indicates that this is how many nurses frame their ethical reasoning. Researchers studying the guiding ethical framework of nurses have found that both a caring orientation and a justice orientation were frequently present as part of their reflection on moral issues (Millette, 1994). Nurses are often found to be committed to both the principles of patient rights and autonomy and their duty to the patient while at the same time obligated to the caring relationship with the person. The relationship with a patient informs the nurse's moral responses (Cooper, 1991) as engagement facilitates recognition of what autonomy, justice, and so on mean for that person at that time.

### Relevance to Margaret's Story

Caring-oriented thinkers would try to understand the context of the situation with which Margaret is faced. They would be interested in the nature of the relationship Margaret has with the patient and his wife. How long has she cared for him? Does she know their story, understand their values? These thinkers would note and take seriously the wife's reactions and Margaret's responses to the situation. From a relational perspective, they might highlight the long and loving relationship between the patient and his wife and the high likelihood he would not survive. Do we not all want to be with those we love when we die? Can we not appreciate the longer-term consequences of the wife's not being with her husband in his final moments and its implications on her grieving? They would ask what Margaret's inclination is at the time and if she is responding as a caring moral agent wanting to do what is right.

## Uncovering Ethics Through the Story—A Narrative Approach to Ethics

Storytelling has a long tradition in our history. It is how many children learn to understand the world, the nature of relationships, what is right and wrong, how to behave. The experience of nursing is rich in stories that are deep with emotion, sadness, joy, confusion, guilt, stories that make nurses proud, stories in which they wish there was more they could have done. Nurses share these stories with each other every day. Some stories remain in their memory for years.

*Narrative ethics* encourages the sharing of these stories with the goal of gaining a clearer understanding of the ethical issues and challenges embedded in them, which is attained through questioning, challenging, and information-seeking. Reflecting on and discussing narratives with others uncovers the moral dimensions of the experience and enables learning that becomes entrenched in memory more so than that of theory alone (Benner, 1994, 1996; Parker, 1990).

Sharing an experience through narrative also uncovers the respective values and perspectives of the team members. Stories can be shared from a personal or a universal view. Each person or profession may see the situation through a different lens. All of what is seen has meaning, and through the conversation, each team member will become aware of what is important both to him- or herself and to others. One's understanding of the situation will sometimes even be altered. In this way, learning occurs as the team reviews what happened, what can be gained from the experience, and how this experience will influence future practices and behaviour. Storytelling, hence, offers the opportunity to identify both excellence and how things could have been better (Benner, 1994).

Benner has identified the dominant ethical themes that emerge in many of the stories nurses share: those "of care, responsiveness to the other, and responsibility" (Benner, 1996, p. 233). These themes align with an ethic of care, which can be appreciated through the sharing of stories of real experiences. Learning occurs as themes are revealed and one is able to recognize the important ethical issues that arise in various circumstances. For example, in certain situations, it becomes evident that patients, due to their illness and vulnerable state, may not be able to make decisions or act on their own behalf. In these cases, their rights and best interests must be protected. However, since all situations are different, and since the nature of relationships varies, the nurse's approach may alter based on these variations. As different perspectives are shared, it should become clear what the right action is in each situation. And as numerous stories emerge and are shared over time, it will become evident that not all rules apply in all situations—each circumstance is unique.

**Narratives** are different from case studies. Case studies are often used to illustrate ethical theory or principles. Narratives are real situations and encourage an inductive process in which one is able to examine the notions of morality that are embedded in the story. This process reveals the extent to which nurses come to know the patient and family in highly stressful and vulnerable circumstances:

This engaged knowledge of the patient and family can yield wisdom and attuned caring because knowing the patient calls the nurse to respond to the person as other, worthy of care and with no expectation of reciprocity. . . . In naturally occurring narratives, new issues and innovations are introduced as the situation demands, rather than reducing the situation to the preconceived ethical issue. (Benner, 1996, p. 235)

The story provides the background for understanding the ethical components and allows principles to be understood in the context of everyday practice and relationships, making them more meaningful and understandable.

Narrative accounts of practice help nurses in recognizing needs and patterns. This understanding aids the nurse in responding to the concerns, needs, preferences, and tendencies of patients and families. Stories reveal what is good and what is important in relationships, and provide a clearer picture of the context, the nature of the relationships, and the defining elements of the situation. They help to further one's understanding of the patient and others (Benner, 1996).

Through the sharing of stories, the moral engagement of the nurse advances (Benner, 1996). Stories of practice uncover moral concerns and notions of good. As the storyteller reports feelings, thoughts, and experiential knowledge, the actual ethical dimensions can be identified and examined: "We need to listen to our stories of practice to examine distinctions of worth, competing goods, and the relational ethics of care, responsiveness, and responsibility" (Benner, 1994, p. 410).

Leaders in all contexts play a significant role in enabling these stories to be heard. Through the learning resulting from the discourse, the stories advance the moral agency of the nurse and the moral culture of the environment.

### Relevance to Margaret's Story

In Margaret's circumstance, she needed to make a quick decision and take immediate action. She would not have been able to take the time to reflect on the story and share it with others. However, after the fact, sharing the story of the situation and the consequences of whatever action Margaret did take would reveal the moral issues and help the team reach a common understanding of the needs of the patient and his wife and the role nurses play in enabling the best outcomes for patients and families.

Regardless of what choice Margaret made, sharing the story and discussing the consequences of her action would give the team a clearer view of what did happen, what should have happened, and how practice can be improved through this learning experience.

It is important to understand Margaret's perspective as she shares her story. Is she confident that she made the right choice? Why or why not? Does she feel that she made a significant difference for her patient and his wife or not? Did she have the opportunity to debrief with the cardiac arrest team? What were their perspectives? What was the reaction of the patient's wife? Looking back, would Margaret have changed the way she handled the situation? Please consider these questions as you reflect further on Margaret's story.

What action did Margaret actually take? Margaret was profoundly influenced by the comment the wife of her patient made: "He is my husband, not yours. I want to be with him if he dies." Being aware of and understanding the strong bond between the patient and his wife,

continued on following page >>

Margaret was concerned about the wife's well-being if he were die. At the same time, she was worried about the arrest team's response if she were to bring the wife into the room. Margaret was aware of their concerns that family presence might interfere with the resuscitation attempt. However, she had a strong conviction that the right thing to do was to allow the wife to be with her husband and was convinced that the patient's wife would not interfere with any actions of the team. Margaret thought, too, that this would be in the best interest of the patient, who might be aware of his wife's presence. She also believed that, if the patient died, the wife would be better able to accept his loss if she had been present. Margaret was brave enough to announce this decision to the team and accept all responsibility for the consequences of her decision. The patient's wife, escorted by Margaret, came into the room, sat by her husband, and whispered words of comfort and love into his ear as she caressed and comforted him. She paid absolutely no attention to the team. She was at peace with him as he died.

Throughout this chapter, we have explored the complex moral issues raised in this story. There are also legal components to consider. The most obvious one is the right of the patient's wife to be in the room while her husband is being treated. Since the husband was not able to express his wishes, the wife would usually be the person to provide whatever consent to treatment that is required. In fact, many provincial consent-to-treatment statutes state that an incapable patient's spouse (if there is one) is the first to be consulted when a treatment decision is to be made. Consent to treatment is discussed in more detail in Chapter 6.

An extension of the right to be consulted in making a treatment decision is the right of the wife to be near her husband. While there is no clear-cut law that provides for this, common sense dictates that, if the presence of the spouse in the place of treatment would not clearly impair the ability of the health care team to provide effective care and treatment, he or she should be permitted to remain with the patient. In this case, the wife stayed quietly by her husband's head and did not in any way impede the health care team's activities. From an ethical perspective, her dignity and the husband's right to have his spouse with him were respected.

If a spouse's behaviour is seriously disruptive, however, a competing consideration of ensuring the proper standard of care comes into play. Margaret and the health care team might have faced a very difficult choice if the wife's behaviour had been disruptive and seriously impeded the team's activities. Health care professionals have an obligation to provide competent care to the patient. The hospital also has an obligation to ensure that the workplace is safe for its employees. Thus, this story illustrates the interplay between ethics and law and how the two intersect, and provides a good introduction to the legal theory presented in Chapter 4.

You may have surmised that the nurse in this true story is Margaret Keatings, the co-author of this book. This event was transformational for Margaret; the profound effect it had on her influenced her decision to explore ethics in greater detail.

## Summary

In this chapter, traditional theories, principles, codes, and decision frameworks that can guide ethical decision making were introduced. In recent decades, as the field of ethics has grown, the role of the nurse has become more complex. As ethical challenges have emerged in health care, the profession of nursing has responded with perspectives that consider both caring and relationships. The material covered in this chapter is intended to provide nurses with a foundation in ethics that will launch the beginning of a lifelong learning process.

Nurses' commitment and allegiance to the individuals they serve may at times conflict with the interests of society and the common good, and this conflict may emerge in many everyday, practical decisions that nurses face. Such decisions may relate to standards of care, to quality of life, and, indeed, to the very ethic of caring within the nursing profession and the health care system.

Technology has altered the boundaries between living and dying. The irony is that major advances in health care delivery have brought caregivers not a sense of greater control but, rather, increased feelings of powerlessness. This has become a predominant theme in discussions among health care providers. We can extend life, but at what cost? We can influence the creation of life, but should we?

Nurses not only must stay focused on the everyday issues they face but be in a position to influence issues such as poverty, inequity, and the changing role of society. At the same time, nursing leaders must ensure a safe environment for nurses and the patients and clients they serve.

Nurses need a knowledge of ethics and of the various approaches to understanding morality in order to be able to recognize ethical issues, communicate with others about them, make good choices, and evaluate how to provide not only the best but also the most ethical nursing care. This understanding is essential to ensuring the moral agency of the nurse and to advance the important caring relationships nurses have with their patients and clients.

# Critical Thinking

## Discussion Points

1. Are any of the approaches described in this chapter used when discussing ethical issues in your practice environment?
2. What are the limitations of these theories in applied practice?
3. Compare and contrast utilitarian and deontological approaches. Although feminists are critical of these traditional approaches, do they share any similarities with feminism?
4. Is there a theory that is most consistent with your values? How?
5. What trends in health care and nursing reinforce the value of a rigorous ethical reasoning process?
6. Do you think it is possible to develop an ethical theory that will assist in resolving the major ethical issues faced in health care and nursing?
7. Does using a theory to resolve an issue necessarily lead to consensus on the solution? Why or why not?
8. What approaches best guide your nursing practice?
9. What narratives can you share with your colleagues to effect a common understanding of some challenging issues?
10. How can the theories you have been introduced to in this chapter affect your future nursing practice? Will they assist you in ethical reflection?

## Narratives for Ethical Reflection

The following scenarios are presented to provide you with the opportunity to evaluate the various ethical perspectives outlined in this chapter, to facilitate self-reflection, and to be the focus of team discussion.

Maria is the charge nurse on evening shift in an Intensive Care Unit in a major city hospital. It is a busy night: Frank, a 27-year-old male, is dying, having sustained major head injuries in a motor vehicle accident. Another patient, who received a lung transplant earlier in the day, has just gone into cardiac arrest. Meanwhile, the nurses are preparing for an admission from Emergency, and because it is dinnertime, they are relieving one another.

Members of Frank's family have just arrived from out of town and wish to see him. On this unit, two visitors at a time are permitted for 10 minutes of every hour. That maximum has already been met, yet two brothers and two sisters are still waiting. Frank's relief nurse is involved in preparing for the new admission. She informs the family of the rules, stating that it is "just too busy" to have visitors at this time. The family complains to Maria, who sympathizes, especially since she believes Frank will not survive the shift. When approached by Maria, the relief nurse cites unit policy and suggests that her priority is helping the new patient, who, unlike Frank, still has a chance. How can she do her job effectively if Frank's family is in the way?

What are the moral dimensions of this story? On what grounds would the hospital have based its visiting policy? Are these grounds justified? What position would you take in this circumstance? What are the relevant ethical considerations for deciding a course of action?

Joanne is a public health nurse in a rural community in northern Alberta who is caring for a new mother and her two-week-old daughter. Joanne finds the mother, Cathy, more stressed than most new mothers she has worked with. During a recent visit, Joanne observes that Cathy has been crying. Since nurse and client have developed a good therapeutic relationship, Cathy soon reveals the source of her distress.

Cathy and her husband had experienced some difficulties about a year earlier. At that time, she took a vacation with a woman friend. While away, she had sexual relations with a man who lives somewhere in the United States. She has no idea how to contact him, and he knows nothing about her whereabouts. After Cathy returned from vacation, the situation with her husband improved, and she decided not to reveal her indiscretion. She strongly suspects the baby is not her husband's and asks Joanne to keep her confidence.

A few weeks later, Cathy's husband asks Joanne to explain why their daughter has red hair. He can't think of anyone on either side of the family with hair that colour.

What are the moral dimensions of this story? What position would you take in this circumstance? What are the relevant ethical considerations for deciding a course of action?

John is 16 years old. Two years ago, he was diagnosed with a sarcoma (bone cancer) in his right foot. At that time, he received aggressive chemotherapy and had his foot amputated. He has done well since, though he has been unable to participate in the contact sports he loves. Now the cancer has recurred in John's right tibia. The planned treatment involves an above-the-knee amputation and more chemotherapy.

Since John's first round of chemotherapy, treatment approaches and outcomes have improved dramatically. However, John refuses this treatment. He does not believe his doctor's

continued on following page >>

optimistic projections and states he cannot go through chemotherapy again, nor does he want to lose his leg. He maintains his refusal even when informed of its consequences and the pain he will experience without the surgery.

John's parents are very distressed. They ask if he can be forced to accept the treatment.

What are the moral dimensions of this story? What position would you take in this circumstance? What are the relevant ethical considerations for deciding a course of action?

Jolanta is a 40-year-old single woman who works as an accountant with a major consulting firm. She lives in Halifax, though she sometimes travels in her job. Jolanta has two brothers who moved to Vancouver some years ago.

Jolanta's mother died about a year ago; her 82-year-old father continues to live alone in the family home. He has done well but recently was admitted to hospital with pneumonia. He is recovering, and the hospital team would like to discharge him with home care. The home care resources are limited, so they inform Jolanta that her father will need 24-hour assistance from her for at least two to three weeks. She has already taken her vacation for the year, and this is audit time for her clients.

What are the moral dimensions of this story? What position would you take in this circumstance? What are the relevant ethical considerations for deciding a course of action?

## References

### Texts and Articles

Adamson, N., Briskin, L., & McPhail, M. (1988). *Feminists organizing for change: The contemporary women's movement in Canada* (p. 9). Toronto, ON: Oxford University Press.

Albert, E., Denise, T., & Peterfreund, S. (1975). *Great traditions in ethics* (pp. 210–212). New York: Van Nostrand.

Baier A. (1985). What do women want in a moral theory? *Nous, 19,* 53–65.

Baker, C., & Diekelmann, N. (1994). Connecting conversations of caring: Recalling the narrative to clinical practice. *Nursing Outlook, 42,* 65–70.

Beauchamp, T. L. (1982). *Contemporary issues in bioethics* (2nd ed.) Belmont, CA: Wadsworth Publishing Company.

Beauchamp, T. L., & Childress, J. F. (2001). *Principles of biomedical ethics* (4th ed.). New York: Oxford University Press.

Beauchamp, T. L., & Walters L. (2003). *Contemporary issues in bioethics* (6th ed.). Belmont, CA: Wadsworth–Thompson Learning.

Benner, P. (1990). The moral dimensions of caring. In J. S. Stevenson & T. Tripp-Reimer (Eds.), *Knowledge about care and caring: State of the art and future developments* (pp. 5–17). Kansas City, MO: American Academy of Nursing.

Benner, P. (1994). Discovering challenges to ethical theory in experience-based narratives of nurses' everyday ethical comportment. In J. F. Monagle & D. C. Thomasma (Eds.), *Health care ethics: Critical issues* (pp. 401–411). Gaithersburg, MD: Aspen Publishers.

Benner, P. (1996). The primacy of caring and the role of experience, narrative, and community in clinical and ethical expertise. In P. Benner, C. A. Tanner, & C. A. Chesla (Eds.), *Expertise in nursing practice: Caring, clinical judgment, and ethics* (pp. 232–237). New York: Springer Publishing Company.

Benner, P. (2000). The roles of embodiment, emotion and life world for rationality and agency in nursing practice. *Nursing Philosophy, 1*(1), 5–19.

Canadian Nurses Association. (2008). *Code of ethics for registered nurses.* Ottawa, ON: Author.

Cloyes, K. G. (2002). Agonizing care: Care ethics, agonistic feminism and a political theory of care. *Nursing Inquiry, 9*(3), 301–14.

Condon, E. H. (1992). Nursing and the caring metaphor: Gender and political influences on an ethic of care. *Nursing Outlook, 40*(1), 14–19.

Cooper, M. (1991). Principle-oriented ethics and the ethic of care: A creative tension. *Advances in Nursing Science, 4*, 22–31.

Crowley, M. A. (1989, April). Feminist pedagogy: Nurturing the ethical ideal. *Advances in Nursing Science, 11*(3), 53–61.

Dawson, K., & Singer, P. (1988). Australian developments in reproductive technology. *Hastings Center Report, 18*(2), 4.

Eskimo Old Age. (n.d.). *Revelations: The initial journey.* Retrieved from http://www.theinitialjourney.com/features/eskimos_01.html

Gilligan, C. (1988). *In a different voice* (pp. 5–23). Cambridge, MA: Harvard University Press.

Gilligan, C. (1995). Hearing the difference: Theorizing connection. *Hypatia, 10*(2), 120–27.

Grassian, V. (1981). *Moral reasoning: Ethical theory and some contemporary moral problems* (p. 3). Englewood Cliffs, NJ: Prentice-Hall.

Ives-Baine, L. (2007). A lasting and meaningful difference: Bereavement care. The Hospital for Sick Children, *Nursing Matters, 8*(3), 1. Retrieved July 21, 2008, from http://www.safekidscanada.ca/CentreforNursing/NursingMatters/2007/special07.pdf

Izumi S., Konishi E., Yahiro M., & Kodama, M. (2006, April/June). Japanese patients' descriptions of "the good nurse": Personal involvement and professionalism. *Advances in Nursing Science, 29*(2), E14–E26.

Kant, I. (2007). *Groundwork of the metaphysics of morals.* (P. Guyer, Ed.). New York: Continuum International Publishing Group. (Original work published in 1785.)

Landauer, J., & Rowlands, J. (2001). *Importance of philosophy.* Retrieved July 2008 from http://www.importanceofphilosophy.com/Ethics_Rationality.html

Lind, A., Wilburn, S., & Pate, E. (1986, Spring). Power from within: Feminism and the ethical decision-making process in nursing. *Nursing Administration Quarterly, 10*(3), 50–57.

Malmsten, K. (2000). Basic care, bodily knowledge and feminist ethics. *Medicine & Law, 19*(3), 613–22.

Mill, J. S. (1948). *On liberty and considerations on representative government.* Oxford: B. Blackwell.

Millette, B. E. (1994). Using Gilligan's framework to analyze nurses' stories of moral choices. *Western Journal of Nursing Research, 16*(6), 660–74.

Noddings, N. (1992). In defense of caring. *Journal of Clinical Ethics, 3*(1), 15–18.

Olsen, D. (1992). Controversies in nursing ethics: A historical review. *Journal of Advanced Nursing, 17*, 1020–1027.

Parker, R. S. (1990). Nurses' stories: The search for a relational ethic of care. *Advances in Nursing Science, 13*(1), 31–40.

Pellegrino, E. D. (1995). Toward a virtue-based normative ethics for the health professions. *Kennedy Institute of Ethics Journal, 5*(3), 253–77.

Peter, E., & Gallop, R. (1994). The ethic of care: A comparison of nursing and medical students. *Image: Journal of Nursing Scholarship, 26*(1), 47–52.

Peter, E., & Morgan, K. P. (2001). Explorations of a trust approach for nursing ethics. [Review]. *Nursing Inquiry, 8*(1), 3–10.

Reich, W. T. (Ed.). (1995). *Encyclopedia of bioethics* (p. 810). New York: Simon & Schuster/ Macmillan.

Rushton, C. H. (2008). Defining and addressing moral distress: Tools for critical care nursing leaders. *AACN Advanced Critical Care, 17*(2), 161–168.

Sherwin, S. (1992). *No longer patient* (p. 55). Philadelphia: Temple University Press.

Valentine, P. E. (1994). A female profession: A feminist management perspective. In J. M. Hibberd & M. E. Kyle (Eds.), *Nursing management in Canada* (pp. 372–390). Toronto, ON: W. B. Saunders.

Watson, J. (1985). *Nursing: Human science and human care.* Boulder, CO: Appleton-Century-Crofts.

Watson, J. (1992). Response to "caring, virtue theory, and a foundation for nursing ethics." *Scholarly Inquiry for Nursing Practice, 6*(2), 169–171.

Watson, M. J. (1988). New dimensions of human caring theory. *Nursing Science Quarterly, 1*(4), 175–181.

Wolf, S. M. (Ed.). (1996). *Feminism and bioethics: Beyond reproduction* (p. 8.). New York: Oxford University Press.

# Chapter 3

# Ethics Resources for Nurses

## Learning Objectives

The purpose of this chapter is to enable you to understand:

- The resources available to nurses to guide ethical practice
- The Canadian Nurses Association's *Code of Ethics for Registered Nurses* as a guide to ethical nursing care, to decision making, and to clarifying the ethical obligations and responsibilities of the nurse
- The interplay between professional standards and the ethical and legal principles that guide nursing practice
- The purpose of clinical ethics committees, the resources they offer to nurses, and how and when to consult with them
- The role of the clinical ethicist as a member of the health care team
- How ethical models or frameworks guide ethical reflection and decision making

## Introduction

STANDARDS OF ETHICAL PRACTICE for professionals are articulated in professional codes of ethics. As discussed earlier, professional groups accept the duty to serve the public interest and the common good. Members of professional bodies have this obligation because their roles, missions, and ethical foundations focus not only on the individuals they serve but also on society as a whole (Jennings, Callahan, & Wolf, 1987). Professional codes of ethics provide their members with guidelines and standards for working ethically. The possession of a code of ethics is often regarded as a key characteristic of a professional body. It is a public declaration of the profession's societal mission and a formal expression of the values and responsibilities of that profession (Wall, 1995).

Ethical principles generally found in codes of ethics include (Wall, 1995):

- Respecting a person's individuality (autonomy)
- Endeavouring to do good (beneficence)
- Not doing harm (nonmaleficence)
- Telling the truth (fidelity)
- Being fair (justice)

## The History of Codes of Ethics

Codes of ethics have a long history and are not unique to modern health care and professional bodies. The following are illustrations of earlier codes. Of interest are the foundational principles that ground each of them. Though these principles may have been interpreted differently over time, they continue to be relevant today.

### The Code of Hammurabi (1780 B.C.)

The Babylonian empire, guided by their king, Hammurabi, in power from 1795 to 1750 B.C., established the first recorded collection of laws or codes in history. The code established by this culture reveals an interpretation of key principles that is very different from how they are viewed in Canadian society today. It is an early and interesting example of how existing cultural values influence the law and ethical thinking. Some of the principles discussed in Chapter 2 are linked with the examples chosen from this code.

### Justice

In the code, there is evidence of a stern sense of justice, emphasis on the principle of "an eye for an eye," and a demand for severe punishment for crimes such as bribery, theft, dishonest weights and measures of grains and other produce, and damage to another's property. There appears to have been a sharp division of classes, in that harsher punishment was given when the offence was against a noble or priest than when against a common person—an artisan, merchant, farmer, or slave.

continued on following page >>

### Autonomy/Paternalism/Beneficence

Though the code demanded fair treatment of women by permitting them to own property and engage in business, it strictly regulated their behaviour. A woman was expected to be dependent on her husband, who had authority over the children but at the same time had the legal duty to support his wife and family.

As it was an advanced business society, the code also established regulations for protecting property and business contracts, limiting interest on loans, and setting wages for workers.

Source: Babylonians. (n.d.). Retrieved October 17, 2008, from http://home.cfl.rr.com/crossland/AncientCivilizations/Middle_East_Civilizations/Babylonians/babylonians.html; Horne, C.F., & Johns, C.H.W. (1911). Ancient history sourcebook: Code of Hammurabi, c. 1780 BC. In The Encyclopaedia Britannica (11th ed.). New York: Brittanica Books.

### The Hippocratic Oath (400 B.C.)

This oath, traditionally taken by physicians, is believed to have been written in the fourth century B.C. by Hippocrates, who is considered the father of medicine. Again, the key components, values, and laws of the original oath are consistent with the principles included in many contemporary codes.

#### Beneficence and Nonmaleficence

I will use those dietary regimens which will benefit my patients according to my greatest ability and judgement, and I will do no harm or injustice to them.

#### Sanctity of Life

I will not give a lethal drug to anyone if I am asked, nor will I advise such a plan; and similarly I will not give a woman a pessary to cause an abortion. In purity and according to divine law will I carry out my life and my art.

#### Competence

I will not use the knife, even upon those suffering from stones, but I will leave this to those who are trained in this craft.

#### Professional Integrity

Into whatever homes I go, I will enter them for the benefit of the sick, avoiding any voluntary act of impropriety or corruption, including the seduction of women or men, whether they are free men or slaves.

#### Privacy and Confidentiality

Whatever I see or hear in the lives of my patients, whether in connection with my professional practice or not, which ought not to be spoken of outside, I will keep secret, as considering all such things to be private.

Source: The Hippocratic oath. Retrieved October 17, 2008, from http://www.nlm.nih.gov/hmd/greek/greek_oath.html

## The Nuremberg Code (1947)

The *Nuremberg Code* was established in 1947 after the trials of Nazis accused of human experimentation at the end of the Second World War. It became clear during the deliberations that there were no laws to guide research on human subjects. Hence, the code was developed to address important issues such as informed consent, the competence of the investigator, and the balance of harm and benefit to the research subject. The following excerpts from the code clarify the relationship of its elements to key ethical principles:

### Principle of Informed Consent (Autonomy)

The duty and responsibility for ascertaining the quality of the consent rests upon each individual who initiates, directs, or engages in the experiment. The human subject must:

- Give voluntary consent
- Have the legal capacity to give consent
- Be able to exercise free power of choice, without the intervention of any element of force, fraud, deceit, duress, overreaching, or other ulterior form of constraint or coercion
- Have sufficient knowledge and comprehension of the elements of the subject matter involved to understand and make an enlightened decision
- Understand the nature, duration, and purpose of the experiment; the method and means by which it is to be conducted; all inconveniences and hazards reasonably to be expected; and the effects upon his health or person which may possibly come from his participation in the experiment
- Be at liberty to bring the experiment to an end if he has reached the physical or mental state where continuation of the experiment seems to him to be impossible

### Contribute to the Greater Good (Beneficence)

The experiment should:

- Yield fruitful results for the good of society, unprocurable by other methods or means of study, and not random and unnecessary in nature
- Be designed and based on the results of animal experimentation and a knowledge of the natural history of the disease or other problem under study that the anticipated results will justify the performance of the experiment

### Do No Harm (Nonmaleficence)

The experiment should:

- Be conducted as to avoid all unnecessary physical and mental suffering and injury
- Not be conducted where there is an a priori reason to believe that death or disabling injury will occur, except, perhaps, in those experiments where the experimental physicians also serve as subjects
- Ensure that proper preparations should be made and adequate facilities provided to protect the experimental subject against even remote possibilities of injury, disability, or death

continued on following page >>

### Risk Benefit (Beneficence versus Nonmaleficence)

The researcher should ensure that:

- The degree of risk to be taken should never exceed that determined by the humanitarian importance of the problem to be solved by the experiment
- The experiment be conducted by scientifically qualified persons
- The research be terminated at any stage if there is probable cause to believe that a continuation of the experiment is likely to result in injury, disability, or death to the experimental subject

Sources: The Nuremberg code. (n.d.) Retrieved August 7, 2008, from http://www.brown.edu/Courses/Bio_160/Projects2000/Ethics/THENUREMBURGCODE; The Nuremberg code [1947]. (1996). *British Medical Journal, 313*(7070), 1448. Retrieved from http://www.cirp.org/library/ethics/nuremberg; The Nuremberg code. (2005). Retrieved August 7, 2008, from http://www.hhs.gov/ohrp/references/nurcode.htm

The public trusts that professionals will use their knowledge and skills in the best interests of the individuals and communities they serve. To maintain this trust, it is essential that professionals maintain scrupulous standards of conduct and be held accountable to the public (Jennings, Callahan, & Wolf, 1987). To that end, professional codes of ethics articulate the professional's ethical standards and obligations to clients and to society (Jennings, Callahan, & Wolf, 1987). They define acceptable and unacceptable behaviour, rules of conduct, and responsibilities. Codes convey and clarify the principles that guide professionals' decisions and actions. When nurses enter the profession, they commit to a clearly articulated code of practice and conduct, which provides guidance in ethically appropriate practice.

These codes also establish a standard by which a nurse is assessed if disciplinary action is taken by a professional body or legal action is brought against the nurse in the courts.

Not only professional bodies but many health care organizations have their own codes of ethics. These include institutions such as hospitals, community agencies, professional associations, and regulatory bodies.

## The History of Nursing Codes of Ethics

A key characteristic of a profession is a code of ethics that makes clear the obligations and responsibilities of that profession to society. The evolution of codes of ethics in nursing has mirrored the growth of nursing as a profession (Viens, 1989). Early nursing codes focused on the character and behaviour of the nurse and had a strong foundation in Christian morality. For example, *Nursing Ethics for Hospital and Private Use* (Robb, 1900) placed emphasis on the conduct of nurses. The moral education of the nurse focused on obedience, compliance with rules, etiquette, and loyalty to the physician, not on judgement, reflection, or critical thinking (Kelly, 1981).

Florence Nightingale, recognized as the founder of nursing as a profession, promoted a moral education of nurses that was based on Aristotelian thinking (Sellman, 1997).

Nightingale's view of nursing and morality was also grounded in Christian morality. She saw nursing as a calling from God. Giving advice to nursing students in 1873, she made the following remarks:

> Nursing is most truly said to be a high calling, an honourable calling. But what does the honour lie in? In working hard during your training to learn and to do all things perfectly. The honour does not lie in putting on Nursing like your uniform. Honour lies in loving perfection, consistency and in working hard for it: in being ready to work patiently: ready to say not "how clever I am!" but "I am not yet worthy; and I will live to deserve to be a Trained Nurse." (Sellman, 1997)

Nightingale's ethics were also those of etiquette: "how proper young ladies behaved on the wards and in the halls of their residence. For years, pupil nurses were closely monitored by straight-laced house mothers who prowled the floors of the residence to be certain all was in order" (Levine, 1999, p. 214). It wasn't until the late 1960s that a shift in the ethical responsibilities of the nurse emerged (Levine, 1999). Nightingale had a strong belief in the importance of caring in nursing and has been viewed as a leader in influencing policy related to societal health and social inequity (Falk-Rafael, 2005). The 2008 revision of the Canadian Nurses Association's code of ethics, discussed in this chapter, addresses these issues.

This moral tradition, with a focus on character, behaviour, and loyalty to physicians, continued in the **Nightingale Pledge**. This pledge was written not by Nightingale but by a committee chaired by Lystra Gretter, an instructor of nursing at the old Harper Hospital in Detroit, Michigan, and was first used by its graduating class in the spring of 1893. It was, in fact, an adaptation of the Hippocratic oath taken by physicians:

> I solemnly pledge myself before God and in the presence of this assembly to pass my life in purity and to practice my profession faithfully. I will abstain from whatever is deleterious and mischievous, and will not take or knowingly administer any harmful drug. I will do all in my power to maintain and elevate the standard of my profession, and will hold in confidence all personal matters committed to my keeping and all family affairs coming to my knowledge in the practice of my calling. With loyalty will I endeavor to aid the physician, in his work, and devote myself to the welfare of those committed to my care. (Florence Nightingale: The "*Nightingale Pledge*")

Early nursing codes focused not only on the key principles that guide the ethical behaviour of the nurse in practice—the well-being of patients and clients, the prevention of harm, confidentiality—but on the virtues and character of the nurses themselves. Early in the development of the profession, there was a strong commitment to God and religion and an expectation that the nurse would live a pure and virtuous life. The nurse also deferred to the physician, who was considered the leader, contrary to today's environment, where the physician and nurse are collaborators within a broader health care team.

In Canada, the responsibility for developing nursing codes of ethics is assumed primarily by nursing associations and colleges. These are influenced by and aligned with the code of ethics developed by nursing's national body, the Canadian Nurses Association. The following section provides some background on this influential body.

## The Canadian Nurses Association

The Canadian Nurses Association (CNA) is a national nursing organization with links to 11 provincial and territorial nursing associations, which collectively represent more than 133,000 registered nurses (Canadian Nurses Association, 2008). The CNA assists and supports the provinces in the development of standards of nursing practice, education, and ethical conduct. It initiates and influences legislation, government programs, and national and international health policy. The CNA establishes and supports research priorities, facilitates information sharing, and represents the profession to health groups, government bodies, and the public.

## The CNA *Code of Ethics for Registered Nurses*

The *Code of Ethics for Registered Nurses* of the Canadian Nurses Association offers Canadian nurses a framework and guide for ethical practice. It affirms that each nurse must recognize his or her responsibility not only to individual patients or clients and their families but also to society, and must participate in activities that contribute to the community as a whole.

Since its first publication in 1980, the Code has been revised periodically (in 1985, 1991, 1997, 2003, and 2008) to respond to the constantly changing societal context, which can significantly influence the practice and work environment of nurses. Since the 2003 revision, Canadian nurses have experienced SARS; the Canadian military has become engaged in Afghanistan; worries about a looming pandemic have emerged; and concerns regarding healthy work environments, leadership, and violence in the workplace have grown. These conditions have influenced and informed the most recent (2008) revision, which continues to focus on "nurses in all contexts and domains of nursing practice and at all levels of decision-making" (CNA, 2008, p. 4).

There are two parts to the code of ethics. In Part I, "Nursing Values and Ethical Responsibilities," the focus is on the values and ethical responsibilities of nurses, and in Part II, "Ethical Endeavours," it is on the approaches nurses may take to address social inequality. As well as outlining the ethical responsibilities of nurses and their accountability to "individuals, families, groups, populations, communities and colleagues," it addresses the "broad societal issues" that influence health and well-being and encourages nurses to "maintain awareness of aspects of social justice that affect health and well-being and to advocate for change" (CNA, 2008, p. 2). This is significant since the social context of Canada is one of great diversity.

The Code provides a framework that nurses can integrate with the theory and content in this book to guide ethical reflection and decision making.

The entire Code is available at http://www.cna-aiic.ca/CNA/practice/ethics/code/default_e.aspx. The following sections will highlight the key values and responsibilities included in the Code. Case scenarios that can be discussed using the Code as a guiding framework can be found at http://evolve.elsevier.com/Canada/Keatings/ethical.

## Part I: Nursing Values and Ethical Responsibilities

Part I of the *Code of Ethics for Registered Nurses* is organized around seven primary values:

- Providing safe, compassionate, competent, and ethical care
- Promoting health and well-being
- Promoting and respecting informed decision making
- Preserving dignity
- Maintaining privacy and confidentiality
- Promoting justice
- Being accountable

The boxes in the following section summarize the values expressed in the Code and provide brief analyses of the responsibilities of nurses. The case scenarios found at http://evolve.elsevier.com/Canada/Keatings/ethical are intended to foster discussion on each primary value.

THE SEVEN PRIMARY VALUES

### Box 3.1: Providing Safe, Compassionate, Competent, and Ethical Care

*Nurses provide safe, compassionate, competent and ethical care.*

**Ethical Responsibilities**

1. Nurses have a responsibility to conduct themselves according to the ethical responsibilities outlined in this document and in practice standards in what they do and how they interact with persons receiving care as well as with families, communities, groups, populations and other members of the health-care team.
2. Nurses engage in compassionate care through their speech and body language and through their efforts to understand and care about others' health-care needs.
3. Nurses build trustworthy relationships as the foundation of meaningful communication, recognizing that building these relationships involves a conscious effort. Such relationships are critical to understanding people's needs and concerns.
4. Nurses question and intervene to address unsafe, non-compassionate, unethical or incompetent practice or conditions that interfere with their ability to provide safe, compassionate, competent and ethical care to those to whom they are providing care, and they support those who do the same.

continued on following page >>

5. Nurses admit mistakes and take all necessary actions to prevent or minimize harm arising from an adverse event. They work with others to reduce the potential for future risks and preventable harms.

6. When resources are not available to provide ideal care, nurses collaborate with others to adjust priorities and minimize harm. Nurses keep persons receiving care, families and employers informed about potential and actual changes to delivery of care. They inform employers about potential threats to safety.

7. Nurses planning to take job action or practising in environments where job action occurs take steps to safeguard the health and safety of people during the course of the job action.

8. During a natural or human-made disaster, including a communicable disease outbreak, nurses have a duty to provide care using appropriate safety precautions.

9. Nurses support, use and engage in research and other activities that promote safe, competent, compassionate and ethical care, and they use guidelines for ethical research that are in keeping with nursing values.

10. Nurses work to prevent and minimize all forms of violence by anticipating and assessing the risk of violent situations and by collaborating with others to establish preventive measures. When violence cannot be anticipated or prevented, nurses take action to minimize risk to protect others and themselves.

Canadian Nurses Association. (2008). *Code of Ethics for Registered Nurses* (pp. 8–9). Ottawa, ON: Author. Reprinted with permission from the Canadian Nurses Association.

In expressing this value, the Code makes explicit that the major focus of nursing is the health and well-being of the patient or client. The Code acknowledges that nurses do not function in isolation but in collaboration with the interprofessional team and other key stakeholders.

Interprofessional practice, as a model, responds to the growing demand for greater flexibility from professional workers so they can more effectively respond to changing health care needs in Canada. This model challenges the exclusivity of knowledge and recognizes that by respecting the knowledge, skills, and perspectives of team members, nurses are able to respond to the growing complexity and diversity of the patient community and society (CNA, 2008).

Consider this value when reflecting on the responsibilities of the nurse in the following case scenarios, found at http://evolve.elsevier.com/Canada/Keatings/ethical:

- *Case Scenario: A worried daughter; a father at risk*
- *Case Scenario: Differences, challenges, and opportunities*
- *Case Scenario: The accountable nurse within a complex system*
- *Case Scenario: Differences, but shared values*
- *Case Scenario: Challenges to caring*

As part of your discussion, think about the following questions:

1. What are the key moral issues raised by the scenario?
2. Does the *Code of Ethics for Registered Nurses* assist you in identifying these issues?
3. Does the *Code of Ethics for Registered Nurses* clarify the responsibilities of the nurse?
4. Do any of the theories presented in Chapter 2 assist in clarifying your thinking?

## Box 3.2: Promoting Health and Well-Being

*Nurses work with people to enable them to attain their highest possible level of health and well-being.*

### Ethical Responsibilities

1. Nurses provide care directed first and foremost toward the health and well-being of the person, family or community in their care.
2. When a community health intervention interferes with the individual rights of persons receiving care, nurses use and advocate for the use of the least restrictive measures possible for those in their care.
3. Nurses collaborate with other health-care providers and other interested parties to maximize health benefits to persons receiving care and those with health-care needs, recognizing and respecting the knowledge, skills and perspectives of all.

Canadian Nurses Association. (2008). *Code of Ethics for Registered Nurses* (p. 10). Ottawa, ON: Author. Reprinted with permission from the Canadian Nurses Association.

Consider this value when reflecting on the responsibilities of the nurse in the following case scenario, found at http://evolve.elsevier.com/Canada/Keatings/ethical:

- *Case Scenario: What outcome? What interventions?*

As part of your discussion, think about the following questions:

1. What are the key moral issues raised by the scenario?
2. Does the *Code of Ethics for Registered Nurses* assist you in identifying these issues?
3. Does the *Code of Ethics for Registered Nurses* clarify the responsibilities of the nurse?
4. Do any of the theories presented in Chapter 2 assist in clarifying your thinking?

## Box 3.3: Promoting and Respecting Informed Decision Making

*Nurses recognize, respect and promote a person's right to be informed and make decisions.*

### Ethical Responsibilities

1. Nurses, to the extent possible, provide persons in their care with the information they need to make informed decisions related to their health and well-being. They also work to ensure that health information is given to individuals, families, groups, populations and communities in their care in an open, accurate and transparent manner.

2. Nurses respect the wishes of capable persons to decline to receive information about their health condition.

3. Nurses recognize that capable persons may place a different weight on individualism and may choose to defer to family or community values in decision-making.

4. Nurses ensure that nursing care is provided with the person's informed consent. Nurses recognize and support a capable person's right to refuse or withdraw consent for care or treatment at any time.

5. Nurses are sensitive to the inherent power differentials between care providers and those receiving care. They do not misuse that power to influence decision-making.

6. Nurses advocate for persons in their care if they believe that the health of those persons is being compromised by factors beyond their control, including the decision-making of others.

7. When family members disagree with the decisions made by a person with health-care needs, nurses assist families in gaining an understanding of the person's decisions.

8. Nurses respect the informed decision-making of capable persons, including choice of lifestyles or treatment not conducive to good health.

9. When illness or other factors reduce a person's capacity for making choices, nurses assist or support that person's participation in making choices appropriate to their capability.

10. If a person receiving care is clearly incapable of consent, the nurse respects the law on capacity assessment and substitute decision-making in his or her jurisdiction (Canadian Nurses Protective Society [CNPS], 2004).

11. Nurses, along with other health-care professionals and with substitute decision-makers, consider and respect the best interests of the person receiving care and any previously known wishes or advance directives that apply in the situation (CNPS, 2004).

Canadian Nurses Association. (2008). *Code of Ethics for Registered Nurses* (pp. 11–12). Ottawa, ON: Author. Reprinted with permission from the Canadian Nurses Association.

In expressing this value, the Code makes explicit that nursing is dedicated to ensuring respect for persons and promoting and respecting informed decision making.

Whether written, verbal, or simply implied, a valid consent is one that must be (a) based on the relevant information required to make that choice, (b) free from coercion, and (c) made by someone capable of this level of decision. For example, a patient or client may be able to make decisions about activities of daily living yet may not be competent to decide whether surgery is in his or her best interest. The challenge for the nurse and the medical team is to assess competence and to ensure that choices are made in a noncoercive environment. Even if it is not the nurse's responsibility to obtain informed consent, it is his or her responsibility to take action if this standard is not met. Since decisions about health care are not always easy, nurses should also ensure, as much as is possible, that their patients or clients have the time and opportunity to reflect on and consider their options, and to make the choice they think is best for them.

The Code acknowledges recent legislation in the area of substitute decision making and the nurse's duty to ensure that the competent or incompetent client's wishes are respected (CNA, 2008). If a substitute decision maker has been designated, this person is best positioned to appreciate the values and beliefs of the patient who is no longer able to act on his or her own behalf. An important consideration in ensuring that the client's wishes are respected is the role of beneficence.

Consider this value when reflecting on the responsibilities of the nurse in the following case scenarios, found at http://evolve.elsevier.com/Canada/Keatings/ethical:

- *Case Scenario: Discovering the client's story*
- *Case Scenario: Heart-wrenching choices*
- *Case Scenario: My choice, my risks*

As part of your discussion, think about the following questions:

1. What are the key moral issues raised by the scenario?
2. Does the *Code of Ethics for Registered Nurses* assist you in identifying these issues?
3. Does the *Code of Ethics for Registered Nurses* clarify the responsibilities of the nurse?
4. Do any of the theories presented in Chapter 2 assist in clarifying your thinking?

## Box 3.4: Preserving Dignity

*Nurses recognize and respect the intrinsic worth of each person.*

### Ethical Responsibilities

1. Nurses, in their professional capacity, relate to all persons with respect.
2. Nurses support the person, family, group, population or community receiving care in maintaining their dignity and integrity.
3. In health-care decision-making, in treatment and in care, nurses work with persons receiving care, including families, groups, populations and communities, to take into account their unique values, customs and spiritual beliefs, as well as their social and economic circumstances.
4. Nurses intervene, and report when necessary, when others fail to respect the dignity of a person receiving care, recognizing that to be silent and passive is to condone the behaviour.
5. Nurses respect the physical privacy of persons by providing care in a discreet manner and by minimizing intrusions.
6. When providing care, nurses utilize practice standards, best practice guidelines and policies concerning restraint usage.
7. Nurses maintain appropriate professional boundaries and ensure their relationships are always for the benefit of the persons they serve. They recognize the potential vulnerability of persons and do not exploit their trust and dependency in a way that might compromise the therapeutic relationship. They do not abuse their relationship for personal or financial gain, and do not enter into personal relationships (romantic, sexual or other) with persons in their care.
8. In all practice settings, nurses work to relieve pain and suffering, including appropriate and effective symptom and pain management, to allow persons to live with dignity.
9. When a person receiving care is terminally ill or dying, nurses foster comfort, alleviate suffering, advocate for adequate relief of discomfort and pain and support a dignified and peaceful death. This includes support for the family during and following the death, and care of the person's body after death.
10. Nurses treat each other, colleagues, students and other health-care workers in a respectful manner, recognizing the power differentials among those in formal leadership positions, staff and students. They work with others to resolve differences in a constructive way.

Canadian Nurses Association. (2008). *Code of Ethics for Registered Nurses* (pp. 13–14). Ottawa, ON: Author. Reprinted with permission from the Canadian Nurses Association.

In expressing this value, the Code makes explicit that nursing is guided by consideration for the dignity of patients or clients. All persons deserve to be treated with respect and compassion. Disrespectful communication, disregard for client privacy, or failure to involve patients in discussions that relate to them violates the nurse's ethical responsibility (CNA, 2008). This value emphasizes that people need care during very difficult and meaningful periods in their lives, from birth to death.

This value is especially significant to the role of the nurse caring for dying patients and their families in ensuring that the process of dying is dignified and that the emotional, psychological, and physical needs of the patient, family, and significant others are met. It clarifies that nurses are obligated to provide optimal patient comfort and pain management, to deal compassionately in situations in which treatment is withdrawn, and to provide the patient and family with the opportunity for home care if and when possible. Based on this value, it would be the ethical obligation of the nurse to ensure, for example, that everything possible be done so that a patient does not die alone, unless he or she expresses this wish. The same priority should be given to these situations as that provided to emergencies. Assignments can be reorganized; help can be requested so that someone is with the patient.

Consider this value when reflecting on the responsibilities of the nurse in the following case scenarios, found at http://evolve.elsevier.com/Canada/Keatings/ethical:

- *Case Scenario: Dying—with dignity?*
- *Case Scenario: Do you know who I am?*

As part of your discussion, think about the following questions:

1. What are the key moral issues raised by the scenario?
2. Does the *Code of Ethics for Registered Nurses* assist you in identifying these issues?
3. Does the *Code of Ethics for Registered Nurses* clarify the responsibilities of the nurse?
4. Do any of the theories presented in Chapter 2 assist in clarifying your thinking?

### Box 3.5: Maintaining Privacy and Confidentiality

*Nurses recognize the importance of privacy and confidentiality and safeguard personal, family and community information obtained in the context of a professional relationship.*

#### Ethical Responsibilities
1. Nurses respect the right of people to have control over the collection, use, access and disclosure of their personal information.
2. When nurses are conversing with persons receiving care, they take reasonable measures to prevent confidential information in the conversation from being overheard.
3. Nurses collect, use and disclose health information on a need-to-know basis with the highest degree of anonymity possible in the circumstances and in accordance with privacy laws.
4. When nurses are required to disclose information for a particular purpose, they disclose only the amount of information necessary for that purpose and inform only those necessary. They attempt to do so in ways that minimize any potential harm to the individual, family or community.

continued on following page >>

5. When nurses engage in any form of communication, including verbal or electronic, involving a discussion of clinical cases, they ensure that their discussion of persons receiving care is respectful and does not identify those persons unless appropriate.

6. Nurses advocate for persons in their care to receive access to their own health-care records through a timely and affordable process when such access is requested.

7. Nurses respect policies that protect and preserve people's privacy, including security safeguards in information technology.

8. Nurses do not abuse their access to information by accessing health-care records, including their own, a family member's or any other person's, for purposes inconsistent with their professional obligations.

9. Nurses do not use photo or other technology to intrude into the privacy of a person receiving care.

10. Nurses intervene if others inappropriately access or disclose personal or health information of persons receiving care.

Canadian Nurses Association. (2008). *Code of Ethics for Registered Nurses* (pp. 15–16). Ottawa, ON: Author. Reprinted with permission from the Canadian Nurses Association.

In expressing this value, the Code makes explicit that fundamental to the nurse–client relationship is the professional obligation of respect for patient confidentiality and privacy. The promise of confidentiality ensures that the patient can fully disclose information essential to achieving the goals of care, and that this information will not be revealed.

A limitation to this rule arises if harm to the client or to others might result if confidentiality were maintained, or in a situation in which statute law or legislation requires disclosure (e.g., reporting child abuse or providing information to workers' compensation boards) (CNA, 2008).

Consider this value when reflecting on the responsibilities of the nurse in the following case scenarios, found at http://evolve.elsevier.com/Canada/Keatings/ethical:

- *Case Scenario: Confidentiality—a sacred trust?*
- *Case Scenario: Privacy and the best interests of my friend*

As part of your discussion, think about the following questions:

1. What are the key moral issues raised by the scenario?
2. Does the *Code of Ethics for Registered Nurses* assist you in identifying these issues?
3. Does the *Code of Ethics for Registered Nurses* clarify the responsibilities of the nurse?
4. Do any of the theories presented in Chapter 2 assist in clarifying your thinking?

## Box 3.6: Promoting Justice

*Nurses uphold principles of justice by safeguarding human rights, equity and fairness and by promoting the public good.*

### Ethical Responsibilities

1. When providing care, nurses do not discriminate on the basis of a person's race, ethnicity, culture, political and spiritual beliefs, social or marital status, gender, sexual orientation, age, health status, place of origin, lifestyle, mental or physical ability or socio-economic status or any other attribute.

2. Nurses refrain from judging, labelling, demeaning, stigmatizing and humiliating behaviours toward persons receiving care, other health-care professionals and each other.

3. Nurses do not engage in any form of lying, punishment or torture or any form of unusual treatment or action that is inhumane or degrading. They refuse to be complicit in such behaviours. They intervene, and they report such behaviours.

4. Nurses make fair decisions about the allocation of resources under their control based on the needs of persons, groups or communities to whom they are providing care. They advocate for fair treatment and for fair distribution of resources for those in their care.

5. Nurses support a climate of trust that sponsors openness, encourages questioning the status quo, and supports those who speak out to address concerns in good faith (e.g., whistle-blowing).

Canadian Nurses Association. (2008). *Code of Ethics for Registered Nurses* (p. 17). Ottawa, ON: Author. Reprinted with permission from the Canadian Nurses Association.

In expressing this value, the Code makes explicit the importance of justice and equity in the right to health care. If the principles of the *Canada Health Act* are to be upheld, then issues related to fair distribution and equal access to health care must be constantly addressed by nurses and other health care professionals. To gain access to the system and good health care, consumers must be knowledgeable and informed about good health practices and the health care resources available to them. Ensuring fair distribution becomes a challenge for nurses as health care resources are diminished through financial constraints and downsizing. The structures and systems put into place in response to these changes need to ensure that fairness is maintained.

Consider this value when reflecting on the responsibilities of the nurse in the following case scenarios, found at http://evolve.elsevier.com/Canada/Keatings/ethical:

- *Case Scenario: Great needs, limited resources*
- *Case Scenario: How do I communicate?*

As part of your discussion, think about the following questions:

1. What are the key moral issues raised by the scenario?
2. Does the *Code of Ethics for Registered Nurses* assist you in identifying these issues?
3. Does the *Code of Ethics for Registered Nurses* clarify the responsibilities of the nurse?
4. Do any of the theories presented in Chapter 2 assist in clarifying your thinking?

## Box 3.7: Being Accountable

*Nurses are accountable for their actions and answerable for their practice.*

### Ethical Responsibilities

1. Nurses, as members of a self-regulating profession, practise according to the values and responsibilities in the *Code of Ethics for Registered Nurses* and in keeping with the professional standards, laws and regulations supporting ethical practice.
2. Nurses are honest and practise with integrity in all of their professional interactions.
3. Nurses practise within the limits of their competence. When aspects of care are beyond their level of competence, they seek additional information or knowledge, seek help from their supervisor or a competent practitioner and/or request a different work assignment. In the meantime, nurses remain with the person receiving care until another nurse is available.
4. Nurses maintain their fitness to practise. If they are aware that they do not have the necessary physical, mental or emotional capacity to practise safely and competently, they withdraw from the provision of care after consulting with their employer or, if they are self-employed, arranging that someone else attend to their clients' health-care needs. Nurses then take the necessary steps to regain their fitness to practise.
5. Nurses are attentive to signs that a colleague is unable, for whatever reason, to perform his or her duties. In such a case, nurses will take the necessary steps to protect the safety of persons receiving care.
6. Nurses clearly and accurately represent themselves with respect to their name, title and role.
7. If nursing care is requested that is in conflict with the nurse's moral beliefs and values but in keeping with professional practice, the nurse provides safe, compassionate, competent and ethical care until alternative care arrangements are in place to meet the person's needs or desires. If nurses can anticipate a conflict with their conscience, they have an obligation to notify their employers or, if the nurse is self-employed, persons receiving care in advance so that alternative arrangements can be made.
8. Nurses identify and address conflicts of interest. They disclose actual or potential conflicts of interest that arise in their professional roles and relationships and resolve them in the interest of persons receiving care.
9. Nurses share their knowledge and provide feedback, mentorship and guidance for the professional development of nursing students, novice nurses and other health-care team members.

Canadian Nurses Association. (2008). *Code of Ethics for Registered Nurses* (pp. 18–19). Ottawa, ON: Author. Reprinted with permission from the Canadian Nurses Association.

In expressing this value, the Code makes explicit the responsibility of nursing to protect patients and clients from harm. For example, when the facts of a situation indicate incompetence on the part of another nurse or health professional, a nurse must take the most appropriate action, given the circumstances, to ensure the safety of patients. When a nurse is aware of incompetence and neglects to take action, then he or she shares responsibility for the consequences of that incompetence.

In nonemergencies requiring specialized skills that the nurse does not have, or situations in which the provision of care conflicts with the nurse's moral beliefs, the nurse is required to refer that patient to another nurse. In emergencies, or situations in which there is a lack of alternative resources, any nurse may be called on to provide care (CNA, 2008).

When delegating responsibility to others, the nurse must be assured that this delegation is appropriate and that those delegated to (e.g., students, the family, other health care assistants) are competent to fulfill the delegated functions (CNA, 2008).

Finally, the nurse must represent the profession when serving on committees dealing with health care issues. Nurses should also participate in activities that fulfill the profession's obligation to society (e.g., community groups or public organizations that shape health care policy) (CNA, 2008).

Consider this value when reflecting on the responsibilities of the nurse in the following case scenarios, found at http://evolve.elsevier.com/Canada/Keatings/ethical:

- *Case Scenario: The nurse's obligation*
- *Case Scenario: Supportive transitions*
- *Case Scenario: What makes a nurse?*

As part of your discussion, think about the following questions:

1. What are the key moral issues raised by the scenario?
2. Does the *Code of Ethics for Registered Nurses* assist you in identifying these issues?
3. Does the *Code of Ethics for Registered Nurses* clarify the responsibilities of the nurse?
4. Do any of the theories presented in Chapter 2 assist in clarifying your thinking?

## Part II: Ethical Endeavours

### Box 3.8: Part II: Ethical Endeavours from the CNA *Code of Ethics for Registered Nurses* (2008)

There are broad aspects of social justice that are associated with health and well-being and that ethical nursing practice addresses. These aspects relate to the need for change in systems and societal structures in order to create greater *equity* for all. Nurses should endeavour as much as possible, individually and collectively, to advocate for and work toward eliminating social inequities by:

continued on following page >>

i. Utilizing the principles of **primary health care** for the benefit of the public and persons receiving care.

ii. Recognizing and working to address organizational, social, economic and political factors that influence health and well-being within the context of nurses' role in the delivery of care.

iii. In collaboration with other health-care team members and professional organizations, advocating for changes to unethical health and social policies, legislation and regulations.

iv. Advocating for a full continuum of accessible health-care services to be provided at the right time and in the right place. This continuum includes **health promotion**, disease prevention and diagnostic, restorative, rehabilitative and palliative care services in hospitals, nursing homes, home care and the community.

v. Recognizing the significance of **social determinants of health** and advocating for policies and programs that address these determinants.

vi. Supporting environmental preservation and restoration and advocating for initiatives that reduce environmentally harmful practices in order to promote health and well-being.

vii. Working with individuals, families, groups, populations and communities to expand the range of health-care choices available, recognizing that some people have limited choices because of social, economic, geographic or other factors that lead to inequities.

viii. Understanding that some groups in society are systemically disadvantaged, which leads to diminished health and well-being. Nurses work to improve the quality of lives of people who are part of disadvantaged and/or **vulnerable groups** and communities, and they take action to overcome barriers to health care.

ix. Advocating for health-care systems that ensure accessibility, universality and comprehensiveness of necessary health-care services.

x. Maintaining awareness of major health concerns such as poverty, inadequate shelter, food insecurity and violence. Nurses work individually and with others for social justice and to advocate for laws, policies and procedures designed to bring about equity.

xi. Maintaining awareness of broader **global health** concerns such as violations of human rights, war, world hunger, gender inequities and environmental pollution. Nurses work individually and with others to bring about social change.

xii. Advocating for the discussion of ethical issues among health-care team members, persons in their care, families and students. Nurses encourage ethical reflection, and they work to develop their own and others' heightened awareness of ethics in practice.

xiii. Working collaboratively to develop a moral community. As part of the moral community, all nurses acknowledge their responsibility to contribute to positive, healthy work environments.

Canadian Nurses Association. (2008). *Code of Ethics for Registered Nurses* (pp. 20–21). Ottawa, ON: Author. Reprinted with permission from the Canadian Nurses Association.

This section of the Code makes it explicit that nurses and the profession of nursing play an important role in advocating for social justice as it influences the health of the population. Moreover, the Code challenges the profession to be sensitive to the international challenges that influence the health and well-being of the world population, and to play a strong role in addressing issues of poverty, homelessness, vulnerability, and globalization. Essentially, nurses are citizens of the world who must collectively work with others to address and resolve the growing international health challenges.

The addition of Part II to the Code demonstrates the growing diversity and complexity of the nursing profession. Today, nurses work with the homeless in Canadian communities; they work, too, within the military, caring not only for the men and women in uniform but also for citizens of other countries devastated by war. Nurses play a role in developing policy for national, territorial, provincial, and municipal governments and contribute to programs related to health care, human resources, poverty, transitioning new immigrants into Canadian society, and so on.

This section of the Code has further significance as Canadians become more diverse and have different health care needs. Consider the recent census data from one of Canada's largest cities, Toronto. According to Statistics Canada (2005), Toronto is the destination of 45.7% of all new immigrants to Canada. This represents an increase from 43.7% 5 years ago and places Toronto among those world cities that are home to very high numbers of residents born outside the country. English remains the dominant language (i.e., the first language learned) in Toronto for 54.1% of the population. Canada's other official language, French, is the first language of 1.2% of Toronto's population, meaning that 44.7% of Toronto's residents may have another language as their first language.

Immigrants who come to Canada have high hopes for themselves and their families. However, despite this optimism, research indicates that many are at risk of experiencing deteriorating health as part of the transition to living in Canada. Evidence from the National Population Health Survey (Statistics Canada, 2005) shows that recent immigrants from non-European countries are twice as likely as Canadian-born citizens to report a decline in their health over an 8-year period. This finding is echoed in the conclusion of the Ontario Health Quality Council's first yearly report. This arm's-length government advisory group for Queen's Park concluded that "some groups, in particular the poor, immigrants, rural residents and aboriginals face greater difficulties in getting care" (Ontario Health Quality Council, 2006, p. 5).

Indicators suggest that there are significant health disparities among the population regarding functional health, early childhood tooth decay, emotional and behavioural problems, obesity, respiratory conditions, readiness to learn at school entry, abuse, injury, and so on. These disparities are related to factors that include having English as a Second Language (ESL), living below the poverty line, and living in a single-parent household (McKeown, 2007). Poverty has been shown to be a significant risk factor for newcomers to Canada, and, not surprisingly, children from immigrant families who are visible minorities are among those hit disproportionately hard by it. Poverty is increasingly defined along ethno-racial lines, and there are indications that systemic barriers confront visible minorities (Access Alliance Multicultural Community Health Centre, 2005). A recent review of patients at the Hospital for Sick Children shows that children from high-poverty neighbourhoods (i.e., 120 of approximately 500 neighbourhoods in Toronto) constitute:

- 56% of total admissions
- 62% of total length of stay (measured in days)
- 7.6 versus 6.0 average length of stay (measured in days)
- 2.0 versus 1.5 Resource Intensity Weighting (i.e., medical complexity rating) (McNeill, 2008a, 2008b)

These statistics are alarming and point to the toxic effect of poverty on children's health.

Consider the extent to which ethical endeavours influence the responsibilities of the nurse and nursing in the following case scenarios, found at http://evolve.elsevier.com/Canada/Keatings/ethical:

- *Case Scenario: Should I go home?*
- *Case scenario: A global responsibility?*

As part of your discussion, think about the following questions:

1. What are the key moral issues raised by the scenario?
2. Does the *Code of Ethics for Registered Nurses* assist you in identifying these issues?
3. Does the *Code of Ethics for Registered Nurses* clarify the responsibilities of the nurse?
4. Do any of the theories presented in Chapter 2 assist in clarifying your thinking?

## Who Is Vulnerable?

The Code draws attention to those who are vulnerable in our society, including children, older adults, visible minorities, and the homeless.

Reducing health disparities among these vulnerable people is critical, both for those whose opportunities in life might otherwise be compromised and for Canadian society, which has a responsibility to nurture a social environment in which all citizens can sustain health and realize their potential by achieving academic success, economic independence, and constructive interactions with others. It is a matter of fairness and social justice that every Canadian has the opportunity for health and a good quality of life.

The code of ethics of the CNA not only provides clarification of the ethical standards and responsibilities of nurses but is a key resource to guide decision making. In the 2008 document, the CNA has also provided examples of decision-making documents that are available to nurses. Decision-making frameworks provide a process or approach to help nurses narrow the focus of relevant questions and issues and to guide them in ethical decision making.

## Ethical Decision-Making Models As a Resource for Nurses

The 2008 CNA *Code of Ethics for Registered Nurses* "points to the need for nurses to engage in ethical reflection and discussion." Ethical frameworks or models assist nurses and the interprofessional team in addressing ethical problems and concerns. They provide a guide to facilitate communication and discussion of the issues and can serve as useful tools to "guide nurses in their thinking about a particular issue or question" (CNA, 2008, p. 28).

> Ethical reflection (which begins with a review of one's own ethics) and judgment are required to determine how a particular value or responsibility applies in a particular nursing context. There is room within the profession for disagreement among nurses about the relative weight of different ethical values and principles. More than one proposed intervention may be ethical and reflective of good ethical practice. Discussion and questioning are extremely helpful in the resolution of ethical problems and issues. (CNA, 2008, p. 28)

In the 2008 publication of the Code, the CNA has provided examples of guidelines that assist in ethical reflection and decision making. These can be found on the CNA Web site.

The following framework is offered as a tool that attempts to integrate the key concepts, theories, and principles introduced in this book. As well, it ensures the proper collection of the data relevant to the process of ethical decision making and considers all aspects of the situation. This framework may be used to guide discussion and reflection on the many case scenarios provided.

## An Ethical Decision-Making Process

### 1. DETERMINE WHO IS INVOLVED
Who should be participating in the discussion of this issue? The patient? The health care team? The family? Others? Who should make the decision?

### 2. DESCRIBE THE ISSUE
Determine whether the situation constitutes an ethical issue or an ethical violation, or whether some significant gap in the care process, such as a breakdown in communication, has led to the problem. Who brought the concern forward? Are there conflicts within the team? Within the family? Between the team and the patient or family?

### 3. ASSESS THE SITUATION
What is the patient's diagnosis? Prognosis? Age? What is the patient's cultural background and religion? Are there family members or significant others involved? What is their relationship? Who is involved in the patient's care? Who within the team has the most significant relationship with the patient and the family? Is the patient competent? Has a proxy decision maker been appointed? Is there a living will? Are there other complexities, other factors external to the team and family (e.g., child welfare groups) that may influence this situation?

### 4. CLARIFY VALUES
What are your beliefs about the situation? What are the values of the patient, the family and other members of the team? Will the patient's cultural and religious background influence what is happening and who should be involved in dealing with this problem?

## 5. EXPLORE THE STORY AND NOTE REACTIONS

Share the story from each perspective. How is everyone responding to the situation? What are their behaviours? Are there any emotive reactions? How is this influencing care?

## 6. IDENTIFY ETHICAL PRINCIPLES

Which principles apply to this situation? Are any of these principles in conflict? Does one principle (or more) have priority over the others? Are other ethical perspectives more relevant?

## 7. CLARIFY LEGAL RULES

Are there any legal rules that govern this situation (e.g., release of confidential information)?

## 8. EXPLORE OPTIONS AND ALTERNATIVES

How many options are available? Evaluate each in relation to ethical theories and principles. What are the potential consequences of each alternative? Are there rules that apply to these alternatives? Are they in conflict? How do they apply to the CNA's *Code of Ethics for Registered Nurses*?

## 9. DECIDE THE COURSE OF ACTION

Is one course of action more consistent with ethical theories, principles, and rules? Is there one consistent with your own values and beliefs? How do you feel about making this choice? Can you accept the consequences of your decision?

## 10. DEVELOP AN ACTION PLAN

Once the choice has been made, how will it be carried out? How will the choice and the reasons behind it be communicated to others? Who will be involved? What are the responsibilities of the patient, the family, the nurse, and the health care team?

## 11. EVALUATE THE PLAN

Review the situation regularly. Modify the plan or strategy as required. In retrospect, is there anything you would have done differently? How might you improve this process next time? Is there anything in this process that should be incorporated into a guideline that could help others deal with a similar situation in the future?

## Ethics Committees

Another resource available to nurses in some settings is a clinical ethics committee. Ideally, most ethical issues and challenges are resolved, and most decisions are made, in collaboration with the patient, the family, and the health care providers most involved in that patient's care. However, the decision maker(s) may need support from those with knowledge about ethics and the skills to facilitate discussion and decision making. The issues health care teams and families face are often extremely complex and not easily resolved, or they may have larger implications for the agency, the community, or society. Ethics committees exist to provide education, guidelines, advice, and support in dealing with these issues. Where they exist, ethics committees usually have representation from nurses and other members of the inter-professional team who have some knowledge of and experience with clinical ethics. Such groups may also include patients or family members who have experienced challenging ethical issues. There is value in the committee representing various views of or "lenses" on the issues.

## Clinical Ethics Committees

A clinical ethics committee is defined as "any committee that is recognized as being primarily involved in ethical issues regarding patient care" (Storch, Griener, Marshall, & Olineck, 1990). Unlike research ethics committees, which have the function of reviewing the ethical aspects of research proposals, clinical ethics committees deal primarily with the ethical perspectives of patient care. Ethics committees can take a passive role and wait for issues to be brought to them or take an active role in influencing practice across an organization (Piette, Ellis, St. Denis, & Sarauer, 2002). The latter is done, for example, by building ethics into organizational processes and making the ethics committee visible through the establishment of educational programs, presenting at rounds, and so on. The roles of clinical ethics committees vary and may include one or more of the following functions.

### CONSULTATION

Rarely are ethics committees in Canada involved in decisions regarding patient care. Rather, they offer advice about how a situation may be approached or assist those seeking help in working through the decision process. Essentially, it is the patient, the family, and the caregivers who must make decisions and act on them, but they can obtain support and assistance from ethics committees. Patients, families, physicians, nurses, other caregivers, and administrators can make referrals to ethics committees.

### EDUCATION

Many clinical ethics committees play a role in the education of staff. In fact, this is their most important function, given the increased need for staff to be knowledgeable about these issues. Education is provided through interest sessions or in-services, workshops, case presentations, and internal publications.

### POLICY

Ethics committees may have the responsibility of establishing policies or guidelines to assist staff in dealing with complex issues or to help clarify the ethical values and duties within an organization or agency. These may include policies on confidentiality and guidelines about resuscitation, withdrawal of treatment, use of reproductive technologies, and consent. New approaches regarding non–heart-beating organ donors and new language related to "allowing a natural" versus DNR are discussed in Chapter 8. These issues would usually be discussed by an ethics committee, which would be a key stakeholder in the approval and implementation of such approaches. Guidelines developed by ethics committees can also serve as educational tools for staff if the ethical rules and principles involved in developing the guidelines are made explicit.

RESEARCH

Ethics committees may also conduct research on ethical issues. For example, a committee may survey provider attitudes on withdrawal of treatment or organ donation in order to develop guidelines in these areas, or they may be interested in determining the extent of ethical problems that caregivers face and the decision processes they use.

## Composition of Ethics Committees

Most ethics committees have representation from nurses, physicians, chaplains, lawyers, administrators, social workers, and other care providers. Some also include ethicists, board members, and community representatives. Ethics committees tend to report either to the board of directors of a hospital or to the professional advisory committee.

There is growing interest in the need for expanding the traditional ethics committee focus to encompass discussions regarding organizational ethics. Further, as the focus on quality improvement in most settings grows, there is interest in integrating ethics into existing leadership and quality processes (Piette, Ellis, St. Denis, & Sarauer, 2002), such as an organization's approach to disclosure of adverse events, organizational practices regarding human resources, and allocation of resources. Clinical ethics committees have continued to advance and grow in these areas over the past number of years (Singer, Pellegrino, & Siegler, 2001).

## Implications for Nurses

Nurses, more than any other health care professional, have prolonged exposure to the patient. Consequently, they are more likely than any other member of the health care team to understand the patient's situation and perspective. This knowledge is critical when making ethical decisions. Further, nurses are involved in the outcomes of these decisions, in that they are the ones acting on the proposed plan of care.

Nurses are aware of the extent of ethical problems and violations because they face them daily. Therefore, they must participate or be represented in ethics committees. Involvement in these processes is essential so that the voice of nurses directly facing these challenges is heard. Nurses need to be aware that (in some settings) when they have unresolved ethical concerns, they have access to ethics committees. Furthermore, as professionals who are held accountable for their practice, nurses have the right (and often the responsibility) to go directly to ethics committees for advice and consultation. These committees can also support nurses in determining the most appropriate process to follow and in providing the information or knowledge required. Representatives from ethics committees may also be invited to participate in discussions with other care providers, patients, and families in direct care environments. Some ethics committees have a framework for consultation by which members with specific skills or education join front-line health care teams to facilitate ethical discussion and decision making. This consulting process should also be available to patients and their families.

## Clinical Ethicists

Within the past few decades, the role of clinical ethicist has been introduced to some health care environments. This role provides not only a worthwhile resource for nurses but an interesting career opportunity for them.

First introduced in the 1980s, the role of clinical ethicist was intended to be an expert resource for the health care team, patients and patients' families to support and facilitate ethical decision making. Those in this role are expected to have knowledge of ethical theory, clinical experience, and the skills to manage conflict and aid in decision making (Chidwick et al., 2004). Professionals in a variety of disciplines—for example, nursing, medicine, social work, law, or philosophy—may pursue a career as a clinical ethicist. The curriculum in ethics studies usually complements the professional background of the students but focuses on ethical theories, frameworks, and consultation methods.

ROLE

The role of clinical ethicists in different settings may vary and have diverse areas of focus. However, there are common elements that will always be present (Singer, Pellegrino, & Siegler, 2001):

*Consultations*

Clinical ethicists may be consulted by a health care team or an individual team member. They are also available to patients, families, and students. They may be approached for advice or assistance in understanding the components of various types of ethical problems. Clinical ethicists help to identify, analyze, and resolve issues through facilitated discussion with an individual or a team. In most circumstances, they do not make decisions but guide discussions, pose meaningful questions, and help the team understand the principles involved. They aid in value clarification and allow each perspective or voice to be heard.

*Education*

Many clinical ethicists are involved in education, which may be organized around a structured curriculum or administered through case discussions and rounds. In some settings, clinical ethicists participate in clinical rounds and help the team to identify ethical issues and to discuss them both as part of the care plan and as a learning opportunity.

*Participation on Ethics Committees*

Where an ethics committee exists in an organization, clinical ethicists participate. They do not usually chair the committee but are active contributing members of the team.

*Research*

The role of the clinical ethicist might involve participation on research ethics boards. Also, there is growing exploration into the field of research ethics that might include evaluation of various decision-making guidelines, evaluation of policy implementation, and so on.

*Organization*

Ethicists may also be involved in organizational issues such as resource allocation, managing conflict, and supporting staff who are experiencing moral distress. They may be vital in supporting an organization undergoing a key strategic challenge that has an ethical component to it—for example, disclosing to multiple patients the potential for harm from exposure to an infectious agent (Gibson, 2008).

## Other Resources Available to Nurses

The scope of this book does not allow its authors to cite all ethics resources available to nurses. However, guidelines, tools, and resources are available through most provincial colleges and associations. Regulatory colleges also have practice consultants available as confidential resources for nurses facing ethical and professional challenges. Many faith groups and cultural organizations also provide information to assist in clarifying their various values and beliefs. These resources can usually be accessed through their respective Web sites.

## Summary

This chapter offered readers the opportunity to become familiar with the many resources available to nurses dealing with everyday ethical challenges and other complex issues. The CNA *Code of Ethics for Registered Nurses*, which makes clear the significant values and responsibilities of professional nurses, was summarized. The Code provides guidance to the nurse as a moral agent and provides a model to support ethical nursing practice. A number of case scenarios that reflect nursing challenges were presented to encourage ethical discussion and reflection. Through the discussion of these scenarios, students should be able to identify and understand key moral issues. To guide these discussions, ethical decision-making frameworks were provided or referenced.

Additional resources available to nurses, such as access to clinical ethics committees and clinical ethicists, were described. Since they are not available in all settings, nurses are also invited to explore other resources available through professional associations, colleges, and cultural and faith organizations. It is hoped that enhanced awareness of these resources will help guide the ethical practice of the nurse.

# Critical Thinking

## Discussion Points

1. Have you had experiences with ethical challenges in the past? Would the *Code of Ethics for Registered Nurses* have helped you in addressing these challenges?
2. As you review the Code, are any of the theories presented in Chapter 2 evident to you?
3. Take the opportunity to work with other students to simulate an ethics committee. Does discussion among various team members help to identify the most appropriate action to be taken? Does using an ethical decision-making framework assist you? Do individual team members offer different or unique perspectives?
4. What ethical resources are available through your own provincial or territorial college or association?

## References

### Texts and Articles

Access Alliance Multicultural Community Health Centre. (2005). *Racialised groups and health status: A literature review exploring poverty, housing, race-based discrimination and access to health care as determinants of health for racialised groups.* Retrieved August 7, 2008, from http://ceris.metropolis.net/events/seminars/2005/August/LiteratureReviewRGHS.pdf

*Babylonians.* (n.d.). Retrieved October 17, 2008, from http://home.cfl.rr.com/crossland/AncientCivilizations/Middle_East_Civilizations/Babylonians/babylonians.html

Canadian Nurses Association. (2008). *Code of ethics for registered nurses.* Ottawa, ON: Author.

Canadian Nurses Protective Society. (2004). Consent of the incapable adult. *InfoLaw, 13*(3), 1–2.

Chidwick, P., Faith, K., Godkin, D., et al. (2004). Clinical education of ethicists: The role of a clinical ethics fellowship. *BMC Med Ethics, 5,* 6.

Falk-Rafael, A. (2005, July–September). Speaking truth to power: Nursing's legacy and moral imperative. *Advances in Nursing Science, 28*(3), 212–23.

*Florence Nightingale: The "Nightingale pledge."* Retrieved August 7, 2008, from http://www.countryjoe.com/nightingale/pledge.htm

Gibson, J. L. (2008). Clinical ethicists' perspectives on organizational ethics in healthcare organizations. *Journal of Medical Ethics, 34,* 320–323.

*The Hippocratic oath.* Retrieved October 17, 2008, from http://www.nlm.nih.gov/hmd/greek/greek_oath.html

Horne, C. F., & Johns, C. H. W. (1911). Ancient history sourcebook: Code of Hammurabi, c. 1780 BCE. In *The Encyclopaedia Britannica* (11th ed.). New York: Brittanica Books.

Jennings, B., Callahan, D., & Wolf, S. (1987, February). The professions: Public interest and common good. *Hastings Centre Report* (special supplement), 3–10.

Kelly, L. Y. (1981). *Dimensions of professional nursing* (4th ed.). New York: Macmillan.

Levine, M. E. (1999). On the humanities in nursing. *Canadian Journal of Nursing Research, 30*(4), 213–217.

McKeown, D. (2007). *The health of Toronto's young children.* Toronto Public Health Report. Retrieved August 7, 2008, from http://www.toronto.ca/health/hsi/hsi_young_children.htm

McNeill, T. (2008a). *Children, poverty and health care utilization: Research and implications.* Halifax, NS: Canadian Public Health Association.

McNeill, T. (2008b). *Children, poverty and health.* Report presented at Session 92 of the Social Work National Conference held May 22–25, 2008, in Toronto, ON.

*The Nuremberg code.* Retrieved August 7, 2008, from http://www.brown.edu/Courses/Bio_160/Projects2000/Ethics/THENUREMBURGCODE

*The Nuremberg code.* Retrieved August 7, 2008, from http://www.hhs.gov/ohrp/references/nurcode.htm

*The Nuremberg code [1947].* (1996). *British Medical Journal, 313*(7070), 1448. Retrieved from http://www.cirp.org/library/ethics/nuremberg/

Ontario Health Quality Council. (2006). *2006 First Yearly Report.* Toronto, ON: Queen's Printer for Ontario.

Piette, M., Ellis, J. L., St. Denis, P., & Sarauer, J. (2002 October). Integrating ethics and quality improvement: Practical implementation in the transitional/extended care setting. *Journal of Nursing Care Quality, 17*(1), 35–42.

Robb, I. H. (1900). *Nursing ethics for hospital and private use.* Cleveland, OH: E. C. Koeckert.

Sellman, D. (1997). The virtues in the moral education of nurses: Florence Nightingale revisited. *Nursing Ethics, 4*(1), 3–11. Retrieved August 7, 2008, from http://www.spartacus.schoolnet.co.uk/REnightingale.htm

Singer, P., Pellegrino, E. P., & Siegler, M. (2001). Clinical ethics revisited. *BMC Medical Ethics 2,* 1.

Statistics Canada. (2005). *National population health survey* [Pdf file]. Available from http://www.statcan.ca/english/concepts/nphs/index.htm

Storch, J. L., Griener, G. G., Marshall, A., & Olineck, B. A. (1990, Winter). Ethics committees in Canadian hospitals: Report of the 1989 survey. *Healthcare Management Forum, 3*(4), 3–8.

Viens, D. C. (1989). A history of nursing's Code of Ethics. *Nursing Outlook, 37*(1), 45–48.

Wall, A. (1995, May). Best behaviour. *Health Service Journal: Ethics and probity—Health Management Guide,* 1–3.

# Chapter 4

## The Canadian Legal System

**Learning Objectives**

The purpose of this chapter is to enable you to understand:

- The differences between the two primary legal systems in Canada—French civil law and English common law—and appreciate their sources
- The legislative process
- The difference between tort law and criminal law
- The Constitution and the *Charter of Rights and Freedoms*

## Introduction

THE LEGAL SYSTEM IS seen by most laypeople as an arcane, complicated institution with its own language and rituals, shrouded in mystery. The law is also misunderstood. It is seen by many as being infallible, but we must realize that it is not. As a creation of the human mind, the law is never perfect because human circumstances are never black and white or as cut and dried as one would like or popular culture often leads us to believe. Very often an absolute solution to a problem is elusive, and usually, legal rules and principles yield an imperfect compromise solution. Nevertheless, a good understanding of the law's basic machinery is valuable for nurses. The legal and social interrelationships between individuals and institutions are becoming more complex in Canadian society. Thus, nurses with a working knowledge of the legal system are better able to deal with the myriad rules and regulations that govern their profession, their relationships with physicians and other health practitioners, and the health care system.

## Foundations of Canada's Legal System

The Canadian legal system, excluding that of Quebec, is derived from English common law. Historically, the term **common law** describes a system based on rules, principles, and doctrine developed by English judges over time that was meant to be applicable to all the people in England. These legal rules and principles are contained in a large collection of judgements, or "case law," derived through centuries of judicial rulings. The judges who made these rules and principles over the centuries never actually claimed to be making law—since that was the exclusive purview of, first, the king and, later, the king and Parliament—but, rather, claimed that they were divining it from the ancient body of unwritten principles that existed throughout England. These rules were often based on common sense or common practices that had evolved over the centuries and were deemed to have always existed and been accepted or understood by society.

Canada is a confederation of former British colonies and territories, first settled largely by French colonists in the 16th, 17th, and early 18th centuries and later by English, Scottish, Welsh, and Irish colonists in the 18th and 19th centuries. These settlers brought with them not only their language, religions, and culture but also the legal structures, rules, and principles of their "mother countries." The province of Quebec was initially settled by French settlers and, for a large part of its history, was ruled by the kings of France under French **civil law**.

### French Civil Law

What is today Quebec was governed exclusively under French civil law until the French colonies in the St. Lawrence River Valley were ceded by France to Great Britain in 1763 under the Treaty of Paris, which concluded the Seven Years' War. French civil law was based upon the Roman civil law system, which is still prevalent in western Europe and many other countries around the world. This is one of the legacies of the ancient Roman

Empire, which controlled much of Europe until its collapse in the sixth century A.D. In Roman civil law systems, legal rules and principles that establish the rights and responsibilities of individuals, including the various principles governing land ownership, contracts, civil wrongs (called delicts), marriage laws, the laws of inheritance, and so forth, are formally written—or, as lawyers say, **codified**—in a single document known as a **civil code**. Lawyers and judges view this code as the chief source of all rules and principles necessary to resolve disputes or legal issues.

## English Common Law

Unlike civil law systems, the majority of the common law is not formally written down or codified.

In the common law system, many of the essential rules and principles that govern day-to-day life, such as the laws of negligence (e.g., professional misconduct, malpractice; discussed further in Chapter 7) and of contract, are contained in an extensive body of precedent, usually referred to as **case law**, developed through centuries of judicial rule-making in countless previously decided court cases. Written by a judge, a **precedent** is a set of reasons for a decision in a particular case. Precedents usually contain the facts of the case, the legal issues that had to be decided, the legal principles that were applied, and a reasoned discussion of how these principles applied to the case at hand. Legal principles and rules are distilled and developed from these precedents, and then applied to relevant cases by judges. These legal principles and rules are often derived from common sense and ethical principles. For example, the law holds that touching a person without the consent of that person is an assault. The need for consent is based on the principle of autonomy (discussed in Chapter 2), in which a person's independence and sense of personhood encompasses the right to control his or her body and to determine his or her own destiny. The law of assault is also derived from the principle of nonmaleficence—that one should do no harm.

## Sources of Common Law

The two primary sources of law in the common law legal system are case law and statute law. **Statute law** is a formal written set of rules passed by a **parliament** or other legislative body to regulate a particular area, such as Ontario's *Regulated Health Professions Act* (1991), which regulates all of the health professions in Ontario.

A secondary source of law is found in textbooks and journals written by legal scholars and experts. These experts may address specific topics, such as contracts or property law, and their scope may be narrow or broad. Though invaluable to common law scholarship and legal education, this scholarly writing, or doctrine, is not as authoritative or persuasive to common law courts as it is to their civil law counterparts, and it is subordinate to statute and case law. As discussed further below, in the civil law system, doctrine, highly respected by the courts in their judicial decision making, is usually considered authoritative.

**Custom** constitutes another, less prominent source of law in common law systems. As its name suggests, custom means that in the absence of specific and applicable legal principles in case law, statutes, or doctrine, the courts will be guided by the longstanding practices of a particular industry, trade, or other endeavour.

Table 4.1 lists the four major sources of common law.

## Case Law (Precedent)

Case law is a collection or body of judges' decisions rendered over centuries of judicial consideration and refinement. Case law is found in many nations—including Canada, the United States, Australia, and New Zealand—that have embraced English common law. In each case, a judge applies a legal principle to resolve a legal issue arising in a situation that is similar to that of a past case based on the presence of similar or identical facts. These principles are usually derived from ethical principles.

### Table 4.1: Sources of Common Law (in Decreasing Order of Authority)

| Source and Degree of Authority | Definition and Characteristics |
| --- | --- |
| **Statute law and regulations**<br>Most authoritative, overrides case law in court. | Formal written laws and regulations passed by legislature or cabinet that set forth rules and principles governing a particular subject. |
| **Case law**<br>Very authoritative; depends on level of court that rendered the decision and its relationship to the court considering the precedent. | Individual court decisions constitute a body of precedent in which rules, definitions of legal concepts, and legal principles fashioned by judges over centuries are found. Applied in similar-fact situations. |
| **Doctrine**<br>Seldom seen as authoritative by common law judges; depends on the respect accorded to, and the stature of, the author of the work by the legal community and, in particular, by judges. | Articles, texts, treatises, and other materials by legal scholars and academics elucidating a particular area of law. Authors comment on statute and case law, and elaborate upon and interpret the legal principles found in these sources. |
| **Custom**<br>Least authoritative; must be a complete absence of guidance from other sources before courts will resort to custom. Rarely invoked. | Principles and rules of a particular trade. The courts will elevate accepted practice in a particular trade to a rule of law when statutes and the common law are silent on a particular issue. |

For example, one particular legal principle holds that a party (person) suing another for negligence must prove three things: that he or she has suffered **damages** (i.e., either physical or mental injury to the person suing or damage or loss to that person's property); that the other party owed him or her a duty of care (e.g., a nurse toward a patient or a teacher toward a pupil); and that the damages were caused by the other's breach or failure to perform that duty. This rule evolved from early cases in which someone was harmed as a result of another person's carelessness. The courts sought to protect people generally from carelessness while not imposing unreasonable restrictions. Therefore, they developed the requirement to show the existence of these three elements to prove negligence in law. The principles of negligence are discussed in more detail in Chapter 7.

The use of precedent and case law is best illustrated in the example of a lawsuit. Each party to the suit, called a **litigant** (usually represented by a lawyer), cites case law to the court containing facts similar to the case at hand. Each litigant relies on cases containing a principle or rule of law that, if applied in this case, will yield a result favourable to him or her. In our example in the previous paragraph, if the person bringing the suit cannot present enough **evidence** that he or she suffered any damages, the case would, following precedent, be dismissed. If damages are proved, case law might be used to establish their amount. For example, the law might place a higher value of damages on a brain-damaged child than on an adult who lost a limb due to a negligent medical procedure.

The court must select from among these precedents those that are most relevant and most authoritative or binding. It then applies the principles stated in the precedents to the facts of the case before it. The court may elaborate upon the principles derived from previous cases, thus further developing the law. In this sense, common law is fashioned by judges, who have to observe established legal rules in developing it. The decision itself then becomes a further precedent, which serves to bolster or destroy a future litigant's case. For example, in the recent Ontario Superior Court decision of *Latin v. Hospital for Sick Children* (2007), the court considered a case involving an infant who suffered severe brain damage following a series of seizures while she was in the hospital's emergency department. In this lawsuit, the mother of the child alleged that the charge nurse on duty on the day she brought her daughter—who was suffering from a high fever and "jerking" episodes—into the hospital had negligently classified her as an "urgent" case rather than as an "emergent" one. The plaintiff believed that the child's brain damage had been caused by oxygen deprivation and that if she had been classified as an "emergent" case, a physician would have recognized signs of early shock and would have taken appropriate measures to prevent a status of epilepticus.

In considering the standard of care, the court applied the legal principles in a previous decision of the Supreme Court of Canada: *Wilson v. Swanson* (1956). In that case, the Supreme Court held that while the law does not require a standard of perfection, it does require the exercise of such care and skill that would be reasonably expected of a prudent and careful hospital and a prudent and careful nurse in the same circumstances. In the 2007 case, the court ultimately ruled that the hospital and the actions of the nurses involved (who were also defendants in the action) were not responsible for the infant's brain damage.

In English common law, unlike in Roman civil law systems, when any applicable existing precedent of a **superior court** exists, an **inferior court** is bound to decide cases using the same legal principles and rules pronounced in a case with similar circumstances. This is called the doctrine of **stare decisis**. *Stare decisis* is a Latin phrase that means "to abide by the decision" (Stuart, 1982, p. 7). Since an inferior court (usually a trial court) is judicially subordinate to an appellate (appeal) court in the hierarchical court structure, it is bound to follow the decisions and precedents of that higher court. (Jurisprudence, or written judges' decisions—similar to common law decisions in the common law provinces—is often used in similar ways by lawyers in Quebec; however, the bulk of legal argument that takes place in court usually relies heavily on the many articles and sections of the *Civil Code of Quebec* itself. The concept of stare decisis does not apply to Quebec civil law.)

The application of precedent in English common law is designed to achieve two primary objectives. First, the law strives to be as consistent as possible. Review of relevant case law is necessary to determine which judicial pronouncements have the force of law and which have been overruled by subsequent higher court decisions. Consistency is achieved by applying the same legal principles in similar circumstances in a similar manner over time. Consequently, a degree of certainty is a characteristic of the common law system.

Second, the common law strives to be as predictable as possible. If lower courts were not bound to follow the decisions and precedents of higher ones, then the outcome of a given case would be unpredictable. A court would be free to decide the case on the basis of any principle of its own choosing, regardless of existing legal principles and rules previously found and applied in case law in similar-fact situations. This would defeat the requirement of consistency, as we would never know which principles would be applied in a given situation.

In the common law tradition, predictability and consistency of the law are seen as conducive to a well-ordered society in which people know their rights and obligations toward one another. For example, A can enter into a **contract** with B because A knows that the law will enforce the contract in favour of A if B attempts to break it. This certainty follows from a primary legal principle established in case law that people who freely enter into contracts should and will be bound to perform their obligations, unless the contract is contrary to existing law or public policy or was obtained through misrepresentation or fraud. Within such a legal framework, a society flourishes both politically and economically, as people can predict the likely legal consequences of their activities, which lends greater stability to their social and economic endeavours.

This body of precedent spans roughly nine centuries and has become quite large and comprehensive. Over time, case law has developed and adapted, albeit slowly, to changing social, moral, and economic conditions and situations.

## Statutes and Regulations

Case law can be a rather slow means of altering and fashioning the law to meet changing social and economic conditions. Yet, the impact of court decisions on society is significant and far-reaching.

Courts by nature tend to be conservative institutions. Traditionally, they have defined their role as interpreting and applying an existing body of laws and regulations rather than creating law from abstract principles. The court, as the impartial arbiter of societal conflicts, is usually loath to infringe upon Parliament's power to make the nation's laws. In more recent years, however, courts have occasionally taken a more activist role in interpreting and applying the law—for example, in cases concerning the rights of same-sex couples and the parental roles in blended families.

Perhaps the best example of this is found in laws dealing with **abortion** and **assisted suicide**. Until recently, the courts upheld laws that prohibit abortions except in special cases. The *Criminal Code of Canada* (1985) made it an offence for anyone to perform such a procedure unless it was intended to preserve the life of the mother and was deemed necessary by a hospital committee. In a legal challenge of the provision within the *Criminal Code*, the Supreme Court of Canada in *R. v. Morgentaler* (1988) ruled the law unconstitutional, a violation of a woman's right to life and personal security. Abortion is therefore regulated by provincial health legislation and no longer prohibited through federal criminal law.

With respect to the controversial issue of assisted suicide, the *Criminal Code of Canada* (1985) makes it an offence for anyone to assist or counsel a person to take his or her own life. The decision of the Supreme Court of Canada in the case of Sue Rodriguez (described more fully in Chapter 8) illustrates the court's reluctance to strike down statutory provisions respecting assisted suicide (*Rodriguez v. British Columbia*, 1993). But in *R. v. Latimer* (1997), the trial court, at the end of a new trial ordered by the Supreme Court of Canada, concluded that, while the accused was guilty of the second-degree murder of his daughter, who suffered from a severe form of muscular dystrophy, sentencing him to the maximum prison term prescribed by law would violate his Charter right to be free from cruel and unusual punishment. Instead, he was sentenced to time served, with eligibility for parole after 2 years. On appeal to the Saskatchewan Court of Appeal, however, a 10-year sentence was substituted. Latimer's subsequent appeal to the Supreme Court of Canada in 2001 was dismissed. The Supreme Court of Canada ruled that Latimer could not invoke the defence of necessity (as he had tried to do in his second trial and as he subsequently argued on appeal in the Saskatchewan Court of Appeal) because (a) he did not lack a legal alternative, (b) there was no imminent peril, and (c) the harm he had inflicted was out of all proportion to the harm he sought to avoid.

## The Legislative Process

The slower pace of preindustrial life may have been well suited to the gradual and incremental introduction of common law courts; however, a modern and swiftly changing society demands more rapid response, which our legal institutions are ill suited to provide.

Canada's government comprises three branches: the judicial branch, or the courts that apply the law impartially to resolve disputes between individuals or an individual and the state; the executive branch, or the Queen and her ministers, who enforce the law; and the legislative branch, which consists of Parliament and the provincial legislatures. Figure 4.1 illustrates the three branches of government in Canada.

In Canada, the power to make law (or pass legislation) rests with Parliament or, in the case of a province or territory, the **legislative assembly**. Parliament and the provincial and territorial legislatures make statute laws, which are also called acts or statutes. These take priority over common law and may confirm, clarify, alter, limit, or rescind common law as determined by the courts. Further, Parliament and the legislatures can adopt urgently needed laws more quickly and comprehensively than can the courts if sufficient political will exists and is brought to bear. When this does not happen, however, activist judges sometimes will take on the task of developing precedents to deal with new situations. The legislatures may also create laws in areas in which the courts have not yet pronounced, thereby pre-empting judicial "lawmaking" that might steer the law in a direction other than that desired by elected lawmakers. Or they may formalize into legislation rules developed by the courts through common law. For example, the common law principle that one must consent to being touched has been formally codified in the health consent statutes now in force in many provinces and territories.

### Figure 4.1: The Three Branches of Government *

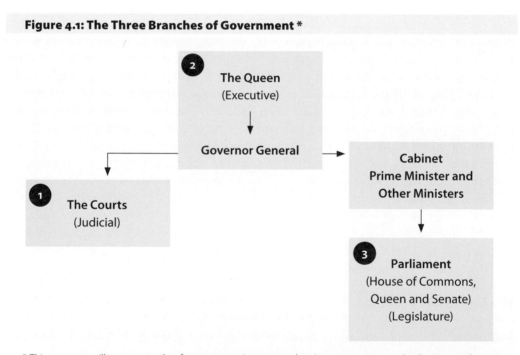

* This structure will vary somewhat from one province to another. In some provinces, the Superior trial court and Court of Appeal are combined to form one supreme court for the province. In Ontario, the Superior trial court has a second branch called the Divisional Court which itself hears appeals from that province's administrative tribunals. In Quebec, on the other hand, municipal courts also exist to hear certain by-law offences and local matters.

Cabinet ministers, including the prime minister, who is the head of the government, are usually elected members of the political party that holds the majority of seats in the House of Commons. Ministers can also be chosen from the Senate, but this is a rare occurrence. By unwritten **constitutional convention** (a practice that is not part of the **Constitution** yet is followed by tradition derived from British parliamentary practice), such members are entitled to form a government since with their majority in Parliament, they are said to command the confidence of the House. For example, in December 2005, the minority Liberal government of Paul Martin was defeated in a motion of nonconfidence in the House of Commons because his government did not have a majority of parliamentary votes. As a consequence, he was required by constitutional convention to recommend to the governor general (the Queen's representative in Canada) that Parliament be dissolved (i.e., dismissed) and that a general election be called to elect a new government.

Government ministers and the prime minister (who will be the leader of the party holding the most seats in the House of Commons) are formally appointed and chosen to form a government by the governor general. Provincial and territorial governments are formed in the same way; however, the provincial lieutenant governor or territorial commissioner, the Queen's representative in that province or territory, makes the formal appointment.

Before it can become law, a statute must pass the scrutiny of Parliament or, in the case of a provincial law, the legislative assembly. The draft version of a proposed law, called a **bill**, is usually prepared by a legislative committee made up of members of Parliament in order to address a specific area of concern to the government, special interest groups, constituents of a particular geographic region, or the general public. It can deal with any subject within the **jurisdiction** of the assembly in which it is to be proposed—criminal law, taxation and government spending, agricultural policy, health care, education, foreign policy, defence, or a host of other areas of concern to various sectors of society. The subject matter of the proposed legislation will depend on whether it comes within an area of federal or provincial or territorial jurisdiction according to the Constitution.

The procedure followed in Parliament (Dawson, 1970, pp. 356–357) and in the provincial and territorial legislatures when passing a bill into law is essentially the same, with a few variations across provincial and territorial boundaries.

The bill is first introduced in the legislature and given a formal reading. If approved in principle, the bill is then taken to a committee of the legislature for detailed study. Public hearings may be held, at which witnesses—private individuals, special interest groups, and others—may provide information or suggest changes, deletions, or additions. On second reading, a bill is again taken to a vote, through which the legislature may approve it in principle. After further debate and refinement, the bill is then put to a third reading, at which time the legislature considers the committee's report. Usually, each of the bill's provisions is debated until it is put to a third and final vote. If passed, the bill is then submitted to the lieutenant governor for royal assent in the case of provincial legislation. A bill of the House of Commons would be laid before the Senate, where it would proceed in the same fashion. If passed by the Senate, the bill is then submitted to the governor general for royal assent.

Figure 4.2 illustrates the process by which a bill becomes law in Canada.

A bill becomes law—an act of Parliament or of the provincial legislature—on proclamation or on a specific date after it receives royal assent. In many cases, an act has the force of law upon proclamation and publication in an official government publication called a gazette.

At this point, all citizens are deemed to know the law and to be governed by it. As unreasonable as this may seem, the purpose of this rule is to ensure the efficient and impartial enforcement of the law. Otherwise, ignorance would be used as a defence, the law would be unenforceable, and chaos would ensue. Thus, the rule that "ignorance of the law is no excuse" is fundamental to any society's ability to govern itself and maintain order.

**Figure 4.2: Legislative Process Involved in a Bill's Becoming Law**

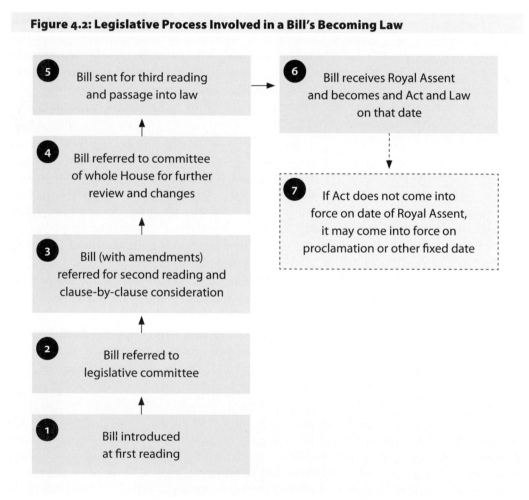

Parliamentary and provincial statutes usually contain a short title—for example, the *Regulated Health Professions Act* (1991). They may have a preamble that briefly states why the act was passed and its purpose. The act will also contain one or more numbered and detailed sections or clauses setting forth definitions, conditions, and prohibitions that are to be regulated by the act. As comprehensive as such provisions may seem, they cannot provide for every situation that the government wants to regulate. Additional legislative details may be set forth in written regulations.

**Regulations**, also known as *subordinate legislation*, have the same force of law as statutes but are inferior to the act from which they flow. The statute takes priority. In the event that a regulation goes beyond the authority granted in the statute, a court may strike down such a regulation and refuse to enforce it. The government of the day, therefore, must always ensure that any regulations passed are consistent with the act that gives it the authority to make such regulations.

Since the legislative branch of government has the ultimate power to make law (subject, of course, to any restrictions contained in the Constitution), it follows that statute law will take precedence over the common (i.e., judge-made) law. If there is a conflict or contradiction between a principle of common law and a provision found in a statute of Parliament or of a provincial or territorial legislature, then a court is bound to apply the statute. The court presumes that it was the intent of the legislature to alter the common law by enacting the statutory provision. For example, before the passage of the **negligence** statutes by the legislatures of common law provinces, the common law held that a person suing another for negligence could not recover any damages whatsoever regardless of fault if the person claiming the damages (the **plaintiff**) had in any way, however slight, contributed to the accident or occurrence that caused his or her injury or damage. Thus, even if the **defendant** (the person being sued) was 99% to blame for the plaintiff's injuries, the claim would fail since the plaintiff was 1% at fault. This was found to be manifestly unjust, yet the courts continued to uphold the common law rule. It took the passage of negligence statutes in the provinces early in this century to change it. Section three of Ontario's *Negligence Act* (1990), for example, provides that:

> In any action for damages that is founded upon the fault or negligence of the defendant if fault or negligence is found on the part of the plaintiff that contributed to the damages, the court shall apportion the damages in proportion to the degree of fault or negligence found against the parties respectively.

So, a plaintiff who is, for example, 20% responsible for his or her injuries is still entitled to recover 80% of the damages from the defendant (provided the defendant has been found liable to that extent). If there is more than one defendant, the court will apportion **liability** among the various defendants (and the plaintiff, if liable in any way) to the extent to which each is to blame for the occurrence.

## The Quebec *Civil Code*

Despite some similarities with common law, Quebec civil law is sufficiently different that it deserves a separate discussion. It has many features and characteristics that are unique to civil law countries. While Quebec's legal system is principally derived from the French one, for historical, social, and geographical reasons, it has also been influenced (to some degree) by English common law.

In the Quebec system, the primary source of law is the *Civil Code*: a lengthy, detailed, and comprehensive statute that sets out a variety of legal rules and principles dealing with matters that include contracts, civil wrongs or "delicts" (e.g., trespassing, slander, assault), negligence, family relations, children's rights, marriage, property rights, wills and the laws of inheritance, corporate law, and insurance law. Quebec's legal system, like that of the common law provinces, has a body of precedent called **jurisprudence**. In the Quebec legal system, however, jurisprudence is subordinate to the *Civil Code*. Jurisprudence is merely evidence of how previous courts have treated a particular provision of the Code; it is not binding on a subsequent court since the doctrine of stare decisis does not apply in the Quebec civil law system.

Quebec also has a body of statute law, but the *Civil Code* takes precedence unless the relevant statute expressly states otherwise. Ultimately, the principles set out in the Code, derived and developed from doctrinal writings of legal scholars, common sense, and ethical principles, are the primary source of law to resolve civil disputes.

**Doctrine**, or the scholarly writings of law experts, is another guide that has the force of law for the civil court. It takes precedence over even the jurisprudence of a higher court in helping a judge to interpret a provision of the *Civil Code* and to apply it in a particular situation. Doctrine may take the form of law review articles, textbooks, or, frequently, multivolume treatises on various areas of civil law. The more respected the author, the more respected, relevant, and authoritative that author's works will be in the eyes of the court.

While a Quebec civil court is not strictly bound by the decisions of a higher court, this does not mean that it can ignore jurisprudence. A court in Quebec is still required to treat such decisions with utmost respect and must have a sound reason, in the Code itself, in accepted doctrine, or in earlier decisions, for departing from a precedent. This is a requirement more so in Quebec than in other civil law jurisdictions because of the influence of English common law on Quebec's judicial traditions. An added consequence of the nonbinding nature of civil law jurisprudence is that the courts have somewhat greater leeway in applying the Code's various provisions to new situations. Because of this, civil law has often been said to have greater flexibility and adaptability than common law.

Table 4.2 lists the three major sources of civil law.

An interesting illustration of the court's deliberative process is found in the controversial decision of the Quebec Superior Court in the case of *Nancy B. v. Hôtel-Dieu de Québec* (1992). This case involved a young woman of 25 stricken with Guillain-Barré syndrome, a

### Table 4.2: Sources of Civil Law (in Decreasing Order of Authority)

| Source and Degree of Authority | Definition and Characteristics |
| --- | --- |
| **_Civil Code of Quebec_, Statues, and Regulations**<br>Binding on all courts, the Code is often used as an aid in interpreting statutes and takes precedence, unless the statute says otherwise. | The Code embodies rules, definitions, and legal principles regulating many areas of provincial law. Other statutes and regulations supplement the Code and usually regulate a specific area (e.g., highways). |
| **Doctrine**<br>Usually given wide deference and seen as persuasive and authoritative in civil law courts. | Articles, books, treatises, and other written materials by legal scholars; used by courts as an aid to interpreting ambiguous provisions of the Code or statutes. |
| **Jurisprudence**<br>Persuasive but not binding; accorded less authority in some cases than doctrine; seen as evidence of how courts have interpreted and applied law in past cases. | Resembles common law case law (see Table 4.1) but is not strictly binding on civil law courts. Doctrine of _stare decisis_ does not apply in Quebec. |

rare and sometimes incurable neurological disease, which, in its final stages, leaves a person completely paralyzed and dependent on a respirator. Patients can survive for years; however, they are incapable of physical activity. Nancy B.'s life was limited to lying in bed and watching television. Her mental faculties were keen, yet she felt trapped in a useless body, an existence that she found unbearable. She expressed a wish to die a natural death and requested that her intravenous feedings be discontinued and her respirator turned off. The physician and hospital involved in her care had difficulty complying with her request and took the matter to a higher authority.

Nancy retained a lawyer and brought an application to the Quebec Superior Court for an **injunction** (a court order) directing the hospital and physician to cease all treatment, nourishment, and use of the respirator so that she might die. The court considered a provision of the _Civil Code_ then in effect (Article 19.1, _Civil Code of Lower Canada_, no longer in force), which stipulated that no one could be made to undergo medical treatment of any kind without giving consent. It held that this provision applied to this case, and thus Nancy had the right to refuse further treatment. The court also considered certain doctrine that held that, absent of a threat to the rights of others or a threat to public order, the right was effectively absolute. To supplement the Code, the court relied on further doctrine stating that the act of placing a person on a respirator constituted medical treatment and thus fell within the meaning of the provision of the Code.

In dealing with the argument that to remove Nancy from the respirator would be a violation of the *Criminal Code of Canada* (insofar as the physician and hospital would be assisting her in committing suicide or could arguably be committing murder), the court stated that the discontinuation of treatment would merely allow a natural death to occur. It noted, referring as well to U.S. case law, that a natural death is a consequence of neither murder nor suicide. Thus, the removal of the respirator could not be classified as assisted suicide or murder.

The court further reasoned that these particular provisions of the *Criminal Code* could not reasonably be interpreted in such a way as to make removal of the respirator an offence. To interpret it so would hamper the medical profession in that any course of treatment, no matter how ineffective, could never be discontinued once undertaken. This, the court held, could not have been the intent of Parliament in enacting these provisions. It thus ruled that Nancy had the right to withhold consent to her treatment, and accordingly granted her the injunction. Once the time for an appeal of the decision had lapsed, the respirator was disconnected, and Nancy died shortly after.

This example, in which doctrine was used to uphold a patient's right to autonomy, demonstrates the civil court's use of doctrine and case law from another jurisdiction in interpreting a crucial provision of the *Civil Code*, and illustrates how the courts of Quebec tend to value doctrine to a far greater extent than do their common law counterparts. Examples of how a common law court might have resolved the issue are found in the Supreme Court of Canada decisions in the cases of Sue Rodriguez and Robert Latimer mentioned above and discussed in greater detail in Chapter 8.

In 1992, the *Civil Code* was entirely revised. This new Code came into force on January 1, 1994. The new Code has added provisions dealing with areas of law unforeseen in the nineteenth century, when the former Code was enacted. It includes explicit provisions for the patient's right to consent to medical treatment, enshrines the right to refuse treatment, expands children's rights to have a say in their treatment, and introduces a host of other new provisions dealing with mentally incompetent or terminally ill persons, organ donation, substitute decision making, and so on.

## Natural Justice and Procedural Fairness

During the Enlightenment of the mid-eighteenth century, thinkers and philosophers advanced the concept of a "higher law"—a set of overarching principles that govern human society and interaction. This higher law, usually called "natural law," is viewed as being either divinely ordained or derived from nature, depending upon one's philosophical or spiritual perspective. Since human beings, unlike other animals, have the capacity to reason and think, they can use this ability to discern the natural and universal rules according to which they govern themselves, their societies, and their relationships with others. Humans, therefore, use reason to discern what is "good," "just," and "morally right" behaviour.

One of the main principles of this natural law is that all human beings must be treated fairly and consistently. Thus, for example, the rules of natural justice require that prior to being subjected to any moral or legal punishment for alleged wrongdoing, a person must be given an opportunity to defend himself or herself and to have his or her "side of the story" considered or heard by the persons or body charged with reviewing or adjudicating upon that person's conduct. As we shall see in Chapter 5, this natural justice gives rise to certain procedural rights and fairness in both disciplinary and legal proceedings. These rights include the right to be informed of the allegations of misconduct, to be informed of the time and place at which that conduct will be reviewed, to be given an adequate opportunity to prepare and present evidence and arguments in defence of one's actions, and to have one's case heard before an impartial and objective decision-making body.

Consider the following scenario.

### Paul's Story

Paul is a registered nurse working in the pediatric unit of a hospital in a small prairie town. One morning, before commencing his shift, he is called into his supervisor's office and told that serious allegations of sexual misconduct have been brought against him in connection with a 6-year-old diabetic girl receiving dialysis treatment in the unit. These allegations, he is informed, were made by a colleague, who learned of his actions from the girl's mother. He is further told that the matter has been reported to the local police, that his employment at the hospital is being terminated immediately, and that the provincial nursing college, which governs nurses in that province, has been informed of his conduct.

In such a case, to which requirements of procedural fairness would Paul be entitled?

- He should be given details of the allegations made against him and the evidence in support of those allegations.
- He should be advised of the date, time, and place of any disciplinary hearing and the procedures that will be followed.
- He should be given the opportunity to consult with a lawyer, not only in connection with the disciplinary proceedings but also for advice on any criminal proceedings that may ensue and to protect his legal rights.
- He should also consult an employment lawyer with respect to any possible claim for wrongful dismissal that he may have against his employer.
- His case should be heard by an unbiased and impartial disciplinary decision-making body. This should not include anyone personally connected with the case or to whom he reports.

## Due Process and Rule of Law

Flowing from the concept of natural justice discussed above are the principles of due process and rule of law. These are common to both common law and civil law in Canada. As in other democratic countries with highly developed legal systems, these principles permeate the legal system and give it legitimacy. In Paul's case above, this means he has the right to know the procedures that will be followed in any disciplinary proceedings before his professional college and to know that those procedures will be followed in letter and spirit. In terms of any legal proceedings, Paul is entitled to due process and to have his legal rights under the *Charter of Rights and Freedoms* respected and enforced. These rights are discussed in more detail below.

**Due process** is a feature of justice that encompasses the notion that all people are equal before the law and are entitled to the same rights and benefits arising from the law. In the past, the applicability of rules and laws was often determined by a person's social status, ancestry, religion, race, or wealth. A basic tenet of the Canadian legal system is that any person, no matter how rich, poor, powerful, famous, or unknown, and regardless of that person's race, sex, sexual orientation, physical or mental disability, or religion or creed, is entitled to be treated by the law in exactly the same manner as any other person. For example, if the son of a government minister were arrested for drunk driving, he should and would receive no special or preferential treatment by the criminal justice system simply because his father is a member of the government.

The **rule of law** means that those who are charged with administering and enforcing laws will behave in accordance with them, that they will not overstep or act beyond their legal authority, and that their decisions will be respected and complied with by members of society and persons in positions of authority. This gives a court order or judgement its finality and authority, or the decision of a government official (e.g., a judge, tribunal officer, or minister of the Crown) its force. If it were otherwise, while a society might have the best written law, chaos and disorder would ensue. Rule of law ensures that contracts are enforceable, for example, and encourages a stable, democratic society and a prosperous economy.

## Civil Law As Distinct from Criminal Law

The term *civil law* has several distinct meanings to lawyers and judges. In one sense, it describes a legal system based on Roman law, such as Quebec's, in which legal principles and rules are codified and form the primary source of law.

In another sense, *civil law* refers to a body of rules and legal principles that govern relations, respective rights, and obligations among individuals, corporations, or other institutions. It is separate and distinct from **criminal law**, which is chiefly concerned with relations between the individual and the state and the breach of criminal statutes. Civil law includes law related to contracts, property, family, marriage and divorce, tort and negligence, health, wills and inheritance, the creation and administration of business and nonprofit corporations or partnerships, insurance, copyright, trademarks and patents, employment, and labour.

To give a simple example of a civil law relationship in a nursing setting, suppose that a nurse is called upon one night to administer an antibiotic to a patient suffering acute appendicitis. In error, the nurse administers the wrong antibiotic. Furthermore, it is noted in the chart that this patient is allergic to that particular antibiotic. The patient consequently suffers an anaphylactic reaction resulting in brain damage. He emerges from a coma two weeks later, at which time it is determined that he has suffered partial paralysis of his left side. The brain damage is later shown to be permanent and irreversible. In such a case, the patient and his family would have the right to sue the nurse, and even the hospital, for professional negligence.

This case is essentially a private dispute between two sets of individuals seeking redress in the courts. The state (or more specifically, society) is not directly interested in the outcome of the case. Since the court's decision may later be applied in similar cases, however, society is indeed indirectly interested in the outcome, which may form the impetus for amending or creating legislation to regulate the particular nursing practice that gave rise to the negligence.

Another distinction between civil law and criminal law is that of substantive and procedural laws. **Substantive laws** create rights and obligations between individuals—for example, laws governing the creation of a contract, the rights of a spouse within a marriage, an employee's rights versus an employer's, or the creation and governance of a corporation. **Procedural laws**, on the other hand, regulate how those rights are preserved and enforced in the courts. Procedural laws include the rules of court governing how a lawsuit is started, when it may be started, what documents must be filed, and to which court the suit pertains.

## What Is a Lawsuit?

Thus far, we have dealt with the rights and duties of individuals and with the mechanics and workings of tort law. A **tort** is a civil (as opposed to criminal) wrong committed by one person against another, such as, for example, an assault, defamation (e.g., spreading false gossip about a person so as to damage his or her reputation in the community), or conversion (i.e., the civil law equivalent of theft). The person who is wronged can bring a lawsuit against the offending party for damages to restore the injured party to the position he or she would have been in had the tort not occurred. This area of law has perhaps the greatest significance for nurses. Tort law affects the nursing process directly insofar as nurses are professionals whose conduct must meet a standard of care. (Collective agreements and other employment matters that affect the daily working lives of nurses are discussed in detail in Chapter 11.)

Individual rights are adjudicated and enforced by means of the court **action**. In Canada, a **lawsuit** is not usually the first step in an attempt to resolve a contractual, tort, or other legal dispute. Informal attempts to resolve the problem may include discussions between the parties, mediation or arbitration, or other complaint mechanisms. Lawyers should be engaged in the early stages to resolve the dispute without resorting to the courts. If this fails, a court action must be started by the aggrieved party.

## The Action (Lawsuit) and Pleadings

The process for starting a lawsuit, similar in all provinces, is controlled by a code usually referred to as the **rules of civil procedure**, or the rules of court, which are detailed regulations setting out how a court action is conducted; which documents must be filed in which court and by whom; and detailed provisions governing examinations of parties, summonses to witnesses (subpoenas), the manner of serving notice, the conduct of the actual trial, appeals, and other such matters.

A lawsuit is initiated by filing a **statement of claim**, or writ of summons, in the appropriate court. This document, which is usually filed by a lawyer acting on behalf of the plaintiff, is also referred to as an **originating process** since it starts the action. It sets out the plaintiff's version of the facts, which support the claim made against the defendant(s). (See, for example, rule 25.06(1) of the *Ontario Rules of Civil Procedure* [ORCP]).

The statement of claim is issued by the court in which it is filed, and a court file is opened at the court office for that action. This file will contain all court documents relevant to this action. Once the claim is issued, the lawsuit officially commences. A copy of the statement of claim must then be served on (given to personally) the defendant(s) within a specified period of time. This time limit varies from province to province. In Ontario, for example, the statement of claim must be served within 6 months of its issue (see rule 14.08(1), ORCP). In British Columbia, a writ of summons must be served within 12 months (see rule 9(1), *British Columbia Supreme Court Rules*).

The defendant then has the right to file a **statement of defence** to the plaintiff's claim within a specified time. Failure to file a statement of defence will prevent the defendant from participating in the action. Further, a defendant who fails to file a defence to the action may be deemed, by the rules of court of the particular province, to have admitted the truth of the allegations contained in the statement of claim (e.g., rule 19.02(1)(a), ORCP). The statement of defence, like the statement of claim, sets forth the facts upon which the defendant relies in his or her defence to the claim. This statement of defence must, in turn, be served on the plaintiff and filed in the court office where the action was commenced within a specified time. Failure to file in time may mean the defendant will lose all opportunity to defend the action. The statements of claim and defence are collectively known as **pleadings**.

## The Examination for Discovery

Assuming the defendant has filed a defence, the next step requires the parties to exchange all relevant documents upon which they intend to rely to help prove their respective cases. The intent of the rules of civil procedure is that each party to a lawsuit fully *disclose* to the others all relevant evidence, both oral (i.e., from witnesses) and documentary, in that party's possession or control. This policy is designed to eliminate the element of surprise in litigation. Policymakers believe that avoiding surprise is less costly in the long run and promotes settlement of cases without the need for expensive trials. If both parties to a lawsuit are fully aware of the strength of the other's case, each can assess his or her chance of success more realistically.

Thus, a party who realizes that an opponent has the evidence necessary to prove his or her case is more likely to be willing to settle the matter out of court than risk paying a higher sum of damages at the conclusion of the trial. A key provision of the law of **costs** is a further incentive: the unsuccessful party not only must pay his or her own legal fees but will usually be ordered to pay those of the victorious opponent. (See, for example, Ontario's *Courts of Justice Act*, 1990, s. 131(1).)

**Disclosure** is achieved through two mechanisms: documentary discovery and the oral examination for discovery (rule 30.02(1), ORCP). In **documentary discovery**, each party shows that he or she has disclosed all relevant documents by swearing an **affidavit**, which lists all such documents. Failure to disclose the existence of a document relating to the action means that the party cannot rely upon it at trial. In the example of a medical negligence action, a defendant hospital being sued by a patient would have to disclose all medical records, charts, and other clinical notes it might have in its possession pertaining to the patient's care.

In an **examination for discovery**, each party, in the presence of his or her lawyer, is asked a series of questions relevant to any matter raised in the pleadings by the opposing party's lawyer. The questions and answers are recorded either by means of audio tape or by a stenographer at an official examiner's office. The party being examined answers under oath as if giving testimony in open court; however, no judge is present at this stage—an examination for discovery is not a trial. The answers given at the examination enable each party to know the other's position and the kind of testimony that the other is likely to give at trial. They can also be used to test the credibility of a party whose answer at discovery differs from that given at trial. If the parties are unable to settle the action at this stage, the matter proceeds to trial. Each party summons all necessary witnesses and documents to prove his or her case. Meanwhile, a trial date is set.

Before the trial, however, one last effort will be made to encourage the parties to settle: the **pretrial conference**. The parties' lawyers, in the presence of a judge, advance (put forth) their clients' respective positions on liability, the amount of the damages, and the prospects of settling the case. With limited evidence, the judge then indicates how the matter might be decided at trial. To prevent bias, the pretrial judge is not the one who will try the case. If a settlement is still not achieved, the parties prepare for trial.

## The Trial

A civil action may be tried by judge alone or by a court consisting of judge and **jury**, according to the wishes of any one of the parties. However, certain types of actions, because of their nature or complexity, may only be tried by a judge alone. A civil trial jury is composed of fewer **jurors** than the 12 required in a criminal trial; however, the number of jurors varies from province to province. For example, Ontario requires no more than six persons, while Newfoundland and Labrador requires nine. Civil jury trials were abolished in Quebec several years ago.

During the trial, the **burden of proof** is upon the plaintiff. It is not up to the defendant to prove that he or she is not liable. The plaintiff must present enough evidence to show that the injury or harm was caused, on a balance of probabilities, by the defendant. If at the end of the trial the plaintiff has failed to prove his or her case, or the evidence is at best inconclusive, the defendant will be found not liable, and the action will be dismissed.

If the plaintiff wins, the court grants a judgement, a court order stating that the defendant is to pay to the plaintiff a certain sum of money as damages. Damages—monetary compensation for the harm incurred by a plaintiff as a result of the defendant's negligence, willful tort, or breach of contract—are one remedy the court may award. The court may also issue an injunction, an order directing the defendant to do or to refrain from doing something that is causing damage to the plaintiff. Damages compensate for losses due to pain and suffering, medical expenses incurred, loss of earnings, and loss of future income.

## Enforcing Judgement

Many defendants do not pay a judgement once it has been awarded. A plaintiff often has to expend further sums to recover on the judgement by means of a **judgement debtor examination**, during which a defendant debtor (called a **judgement debtor** because he or she owes money according to a court order) is asked questions about his or her financial resources, property, and ability to pay the judgement. The plaintiff can have any of the defendant's assets (e.g., the defendant's home, land, bank accounts, securities, automobiles, jewellery) seized and sold by the **sheriff** (a court official) at an auction in order to realize the necessary funds to satisfy the judgement. The defendant's wages can also be subjected to **garnishment**, meaning that the defendant's employer (or any other debtor of the defendant) will be required to pay a portion of the defendant's weekly or monthly wages (or the debt itself, in the case of a debt owed to the defendant) to the sheriff for the benefit of the plaintiff and any other creditors of the defendant. Through these mechanisms, the law permits a successful plaintiff to bring considerable pressure to bear on a delinquent judgement debtor.

## Criminal Law

Thus far, we have been discussing court actions involving one or more individuals asserting private claims. These are classed as civil law. Other cases—those that involve a breach of fundamental values and rules that threatens the peace, stability, order, and well-being of all citizens—concern society collectively. This is the focus and province of criminal law.

Most criminal law is contained in the *Criminal Code of Canada* (1985), which was originally enacted by Parliament in 1892. It is a lengthy statute containing a comprehensive and detailed list of criminal offences and a code of criminal procedure governing arrests, laying of charges, release on bail, preliminary hearings, trials, and sentencing. It also contains provisions for appeals from verdicts and sentences, and for release pending appeal.

## Classes of Criminal Offences

There are three classes of criminal offences in the *Criminal Code of Canada* (1985):

- Indictable offences
- Summary conviction offences
- Dual procedure (or hybrid) offences

**Indictable offences** are generally the most serious type of offence. These include murder (both first- and second-degree) (see *Criminal Code*, s. 235(1)). Murder is in the first degree if the accused has deliberately planned the act. Murder that is not planned and deliberate but is, for example, committed in the heat of the moment, qualifies as second-degree murder. Regardless of planning and deliberation, however, the murder of a police officer, prison guard, or prison employee, or murder committed as a result of a kidnapping, sexual assault, aircraft hijacking, or hostage-taking is first-degree murder (see *Criminal Code*, s. 231). Other indictable offences include manslaughter (*Criminal Code*, s. 236), attempted murder (*Criminal Code*, s. 239), **criminal negligence** causing death (*Criminal Code*, s. 239), robbery (*Criminal Code*, s. 344), theft of property having a value of over $1000 (*Criminal Code*, s. 344(a)), treason (*Criminal Code*, s. 47), and conspiracy to commit an indictable offence (*Criminal Code*, s. 465(1)(c)).

Given their serious nature, the procedure for trying indictable offences is more complex than that for summary conviction offences. Depending on the type of offence, the accused will be tried by a provincial court judge alone (e.g., for offences such as theft of or possession of stolen property of a value under $1000, counselling such an offence, keeping a gaming or betting house, betting, bookmaking, placing bets, organizing lotteries and games of chance without a government licence, keeping a common bawdy house, cheating at play, fraud in relation to fares, and driving while disqualified (see *Criminal Code*, s. 553)), or may elect a mode of trial as allowed under the Code for certain indictable offences—that is, those not listed in *Criminal Code* sections 553 and 469. Section 469 offences include treason; intimidating Parliament or a legislature; inciting to mutiny; seditious offences; piracy; piratical acts; murder; being an accessory after the fact to high treason, treason, or murder; bribery of a judicial office holder; attempting to commit any of these offences; or conspiring to commit any of these offences (see *Criminal Code*, s. 554). If the indictable offence is one that allows the accused to elect, the choices are:

- Trial by a provincial court judge without a jury and without a **preliminary inquiry**
- A preliminary inquiry and trial by a judge (other than a provincial court judge) without a jury
- A preliminary inquiry and trial by a court composed of a judge and jury

If the accused fails to make an election, the third option is automatically assigned (*Criminal Code*, s. 536(2)). For those indictable offences listed in section 469 of the Code (treason, etc.), the accused automatically has a preliminary inquiry and is tried by a court composed of a judge and jury. The accused is given no choice, although he or she may, if the Crown prosecutor agrees, be tried by a judge without a jury (*Criminal Code*, s. 473(1)). The jury is composed of 12 Canadian citizens over 18 years of age.

The purpose of the preliminary inquiry is to determine whether the Crown has sufficient evidence such that a reasonable jury, reasonably instructed in the law, could (not would) convict the accused of the offence (*United States of America v. Sheppard*, 1977). It is not a trial. If the provincial court judge, after conducting the hearing, concludes that the evidence is deficient, the accused will be discharged. This means that there is insufficient evidence to satisfy the standard (test) described above and that the accused will not be made to stand trial.

Generally, an accused person cannot be charged with and tried for the same criminal offence more than once. If after a preliminary inquiry, however, the Crown obtains additional evidence that suggests that a separate and different offence was committed, the accused can be charged again with the offence or with a new offence. If the Crown's new evidence is insufficient, the charge may be dismissed as an abuse of the court's process. Or the charge may be dismissed because laying it violates the accused's rights under the *Canadian Charter of Rights and Freedoms* (discussed on pages 111–113).

**Summary conviction offences** are those of a minor or relatively less serious nature. They include such offences as causing a disturbance (*Criminal Code*, s. 175(1)(a)), discharging a firearm in a public place (*Criminal Code*, s. 175(1)(d)), loitering (*Criminal Code*, s. 175(1)(c)), trespassing at night (*Criminal Code*, s. 177), and vagrancy (*Criminal Code*, s. 179). Such offences are tried before a provincial court judge.

The third class of offence under the Code is that of **dual procedure**, or **hybrid offences**. These are sometimes referred to as "offences triable either way" (Marrocco, 1989–90, pp. 1–3). They are hybrid in that the Crown may choose to try the accused summarily or indictably. An example is found in section 266, which reads: "Every one who commits an assault is guilty of (a) an indictable offence and liable to imprisonment for a term not exceeding five years; or (b) an offence punishable on summary conviction." Until the Crown attorney prosecuting the case makes the choice, the offence will be deemed to be indictable. (See *Interpretation Act*, s. 34(1)(a).) If the Crown elects to proceed summarily, the accused will be tried by a provincial court judge alone. Should the Crown choose to proceed by indictment, the accused will be called upon to elect the mode of trial in accordance with the procedure outlined above.

## The Presumption of Innocence

In Canada, as in most Western democracies, an accused person is considered innocent until proven guilty. Not only is this principle enshrined in the *Criminal Code* (s. 6(1)(a)) but, more significantly, it is also a fundamental right guaranteed in the *Canadian Charter of Rights and Freedoms* (1982). Section 11(d) of the Charter reads:

11. Any person charged with an offence has the right: . . . (d) to be presumed innocent until proven guilty according to law in a fair and public hearing by an independent and impartial tribunal.

The *Canadian Charter of Rights and Freedoms* has been an integral part of the Canadian Constitution since 1982. It sets forth the basic legal, mobility, language, equality, and democratic rights of citizens, rights that the state cannot abridge (limit), violate, or infringe upon without breaching the Constitution. (The Constitution and the *Charter of Rights and Freedoms* are discussed more fully later in this chapter.)

Two consequences flow from the **presumption of innocence**. First, the Crown must prove all the essential elements of a case. It is up to the Crown to prove the offence and not for the accused person to disprove the charge against him or her. This is known as the *burden of proof*. The degree of proof that the Crown must meet in order to secure a conviction is proof beyond a **reasonable doubt**. Second, while the accused may refuse to lead (present) any evidence, more frequently the focus of the defence is to establish a reasonable doubt in the mind of either the judge or the jury, depending upon the mode of trial.

## Elements of a Criminal Offence

Most criminal offences have two main elements: a *physical element* and a *mental element*. The physical element is known in law by the Latin term **actus reus**. Thus, for example, in the offence of assault, the actual physical conduct of striking the victim constitutes the *actus reus*. The mental component, known by the Latin term **mens rea**, is the element of *intent*. In most cases, a person must intend to commit the act with which he or she is charged. Thus, in an assault, the *mens rea* is the perpetrator's intention to strike the victim. The perpetrator's willful direction of his or her body to commit the actual physical act is the *actus reus*.

The link between these two elements, insofar as proving the offence is concerned, is that a conscious rational person, thinking rationally, always intends the consequences of his or her physical conduct. This means that a sane person, acting voluntarily and rationally, who is seen physically striking another, is presumed to have intended that action. In other words, such conduct is the product of a conscious mind acting voluntarily. The two elements of the offence must therefore both be present (see *Fowler v. Padget*, 1798; but see *R v. Bernard*, 1961).

For example, suppose a woman suffers a head injury in an automobile accident. She is released from the hospital a few weeks later, seemingly recovered from her injuries. One night she gets out of bed, proceeds to the kitchen, and obtains a carving knife, which she uses to stab her sleeping husband repeatedly. The husband dies. The woman discovers the murder the next day and, to her horror, concludes from the physical evidence at the scene that she committed the deed. However, she has absolutely no recollection of it. She and her husband loved each other. She had no motive nor any wish to see her husband dead and cannot fathom how she could have done such a thing. It may be that her head injury caused her to act involuntarily: that is, her actions were not the product of her *conscious* mind but merely the automatic movement of her body resulting from the injury to her brain. In such a case, the accused could not be found guilty of murder, as she clearly was not aware of the circumstances, she was not conscious, and she was not acting voluntarily. This defence is known in law as the defence of automatism (Stuart, 1982, pp. 77–91). Strange as it may sound, it has been accepted in Canadian courts as a legitimate defence since the Supreme Court of Canada's decision in *R. v. Rabey* (1980). In *R. v. Rabey*, the accused was convicted at trial of assaulting a woman with whom he was infatuated and who had rebuffed him. He had no recollection of having done so. The Supreme Court of Canada recognized (in a split decision) that a person might suffer a psychological blow that could cause him or her to act unconsciously. This decision seems less strange, however, when one considers the basic principle that persons should be held responsible only for intentional acts that are the product of a rational mind acting voluntarily.

One must not conclude that an accused in an unconscious state is necessarily insane. In our example of the case of the woman with the head injury, if the accused had been conscious, she would not have voluntarily committed the act, would have been fully capable of discerning right from wrong, and would have been aware of the consequences of her actions. A truly insane person is afflicted with a disease of the mind and is not legally capable of appreciating the nature and quality of his or her actions and their consequences. Such a person, therefore, is incapable of formulating the necessary intent or *mens rea*. Since one of the elements necessary to prove guilt is absent, such a person would be acquitted (found not guilty). Specifically, this situation would attract a verdict of not guilty by reason of insanity, as provided in sections 16(1) and (2) of the *Criminal Code*:

16. (1)  No person shall be convicted of an offence in respect of an act or omission on his part while that person was insane.

   (2)  For the purposes of this section, a person is insane when the person is in a state of natural imbecility or has disease of the mind to an extent that renders the person incapable of appreciating the nature and quality of an act or omission or of knowing that an act or omission is wrong.

Breach of a criminal law through **malfeasance** (doing something that is one's duty to do, but doing it poorly), such as criminal negligence causing death (*Criminal Code*, s. 220), or **nonfeasance** (failure to act altogether when a duty to do so exists), such as criminal negligence causing death (*Criminal Code*, s. 220) or a parent failing to provide the necessities of life for his or her child (*Criminal Code*, s. 215), is also punishable.

For example, suppose an accused were driving his car at excessive speed on a residential street and struck and killed a child. The accused's behaviour was clearly out of step with the standard of reasonable behaviour. His negligent departure from that standard is the mental element required to prove the offence. In other words, he was aware that he was driving at excessive speed, and he knew or ought to have known that injury could result from his carelessness. The law would punish such reckless behaviour in the interest of protecting the public from gross carelessness.

## The Constitution

### History of the Constitution

Unlike the United States and several other countries with colonial histories, Canada became an independent and sovereign nation by evolution, not revolution.

Canada's Constitution was originally passed by the British Parliament in 1867 as the *British North America Act* (1867). At that time, and until well into the twentieth century, Canada was a self-governing colony of the United Kingdom. Britain, however, possessed ultimate legislative power over Canada, so it alone could provide supreme legislation to which all colonial parliaments in British North America, and later the Parliament of Canada, were subject.

With the enactment of the *Canada Act, 1982,* by the Parliament of the United Kingdom, Canada was given the power to amend its Constitution.

### Supremacy of the Constitution

It is a fundamental requirement of any democracy that its government and institutions be subject to a higher law. The constitution of a country is essentially a set of supreme laws that define and regulate the various branches of government, their powers, and restrictions on those powers. Canada's Constitution includes a *Charter of Rights and Freedoms*, which sets forth the basic legal and democratic rights of Canadians. These are rights the government cannot infringe upon unless it has a justifiable reason. Any governmental action or law that breaches the Constitution or a person's constitutional rights is itself illegal and invalid. A government is neither above the law, nor is it immune from the law's reach. It must always act legally. This is an adjunct to the principle of the rule of law and of due process, discussed above.

### The *Charter of Rights and Freedoms*

FUNDAMENTAL RIGHTS

Canada's ***Charter of Rights and Freedoms*** is an entrenched (integral) part of its Constitution. It codifies as constitutional law many of the **fundamental rights** and freedoms enjoyed by everyone in Canadian society, including freedom of religion and conscience (*Charter*, s. 2(a)), freedom of thought and expression (*Charter*, s. 2(b)), freedom of the press (*Charter*, s. 2(b)), freedom of peaceful assembly (*Charter*, s. 2(c)), and freedom of association (*Charter*, s. 2(d)).

DEMOCRATIC RIGHTS

The Charter also protects **democratic rights**, such as the right of citizens (i.e., noncitizens are not entitled to these particular rights) to vote (*Charter*, s. 3), the provision that no Parliament or provincial legislature may continue for more than 5 years from the date of the last election (*Charter*, s. 4(1)), and the requirement that Parliament or a provincial or territorial legislature sit at least once every 12 months (*Charter*, s. 5). These particular rights are meant to ensure that governments remain responsible and accountable to the electors and do not become tyrannical.

MOBILITY RIGHTS

As well, Canadian citizens have the right to enter, remain in, and leave Canada, as well as to move and to take up residence in any province to pursue a livelihood (subject to laws providing for reasonable residency requirements in that province) (*Charter*, s. 6). These are called **mobility rights**.

LEGAL RIGHTS

Perhaps the most important rights enshrined in the Charter are **legal rights**. These rights are guaranteed to all persons in Canada regardless of citizenship. These include the right to life, liberty, and security of the person (*Charter*, s. 7), the right to be secure against unreasonable search and seizure (*Charter*, s. 8), and the right not to be arbitrarily detained or imprisoned (*Charter*, s. 9). Thus, for example, the police in Canada do not have the right to arrest a person because they do not agree with that person's political views or fear that such person may engage in behaviour that is not illegal but which the police, other government officials, or politicians might find objectionable or offensive. Likewise, the authorities do not have the right (as they do in many totalitarian countries) to apprehend a person and hold him or her in prison for an indefinite period of time without a trial or specific criminal charges being laid.

Any person in Canada who has been arrested or **detained** (held in police custody) has the right to be informed of the reasons for the arrest (*Charter*, s. 10(a)), to speak with a lawyer without delay and to be informed of that right (*Charter*, s. 10(b)), to have the validity or lawfulness of the detention determined by a court, and to be released if the detention is unlawful (*Charter*, s. 10(c)).

Rights accorded to all accused persons in a criminal trial or other proceeding include the right to be informed without delay of the specific offence (*Charter*, s. 11(a)), to be tried within a reasonable time (*Charter*, s. 11(b)), not to be forced to give testimony against himself or herself (*Charter*, s. 11(c)), to be presumed innocent until and unless proven guilty (*Charter*, s. 11(d)), to reasonable bail (*Charter*, s. 11(e)), and to be tried by a jury if the punishment for the offence is imprisonment for five years or more (*Charter*, s. 11(f)).

If tried and acquitted of an offence, a resident of Canada has the right not to be tried for it again. If found guilty and punished, he or she has the right not to be punished a second time for the same offence (*Charter*, s. 11(h)), not to be subjected to cruel and unusual punishment (*Charter*, s. 12), not to have evidence given as a witness in a proceeding subsequently used against him or her in another proceeding (*Charter*, s. 13), and to an interpreter if he or she does not understand or speak the language in which the proceedings are being conducted, or is deaf (*Charter*, s. 14).

EQUALITY RIGHTS

Finally, all persons in Canada are equal before the law regardless of race, sex, national or ethnic origin, colour, religion, age, and mental or physical disability (*Charter*, s. 15(1)). The Supreme Court of Canada has also held that discrimination on the basis of a person's sexual orientation is prohibited under this section of the Charter of Rights. This provision is subject to the enactment of laws implementing affirmative action programs for the benefit of disadvantaged groups in society (*Charter*, s. 15(2)).

It is important to note that the absence of any right from those specifically enshrined as **equality rights** in the Charter does not mean that such unwritten right does not exist and is not otherwise enforceable.

THE NOTWITHSTANDING CLAUSE

While any statute law enacted in Canada is subject to the Charter, it is possible for Parliament or a provincial or territorial legislature to override the Charter by invoking the *notwithstanding clause* of the Constitution. This clause provides that a law, even one contravening the Charter, may apply for up to five years. The five-year limit is designed to ensure that rights are not permanently infringed (violated) by a law. After five years, the notwithstanding clause expires insofar as it applies to that particular law, unless it is invoked again.

LANGUAGE RIGHTS

The Charter also contains minority language education rights and states that French and English are the official languages of Canada (*Charter*, s. 16(1)).

SUPREMACY OF THE CHARTER

Since the Charter is part of the Canadian Constitution (*Charter*, s. 52(2)), and the Constitution is the supreme law of Canada (*Charter*, s. 52(1)), any law that is inconsistent with that supreme law has no force or effect. This means that any such law is as if it had never been passed, and any action taken pursuant to it may be declared illegal by the court that rules upon its constitutionality. However, all laws are presumed to be constitutionally valid until the law is determined to be invalid by a court.

## Division of Legislative Powers

The federal government plays an active role in health care through its funding activities, transfer payments to the provinces, and federal/provincial arrangements. A major federal law in this area is the *Canada Health Act* (1985). Health care, however, is largely an area of provincial responsibility under the Canadian Constitution (*Constitution Act, 1867*, s. 92(7)). (Specific provincial legislation regulating the nursing profession is discussed in Chapter 5.) The provinces, through their ministries of health, administer and regulate health care systems within their boundaries. This includes such matters as the establishment, administration, and funding of hospitals and clinics; regulations governing public hospitals and private health care institutions such as nursing homes, long-term care facilities, and the like; and public health insurance. The provinces also regulate health care professionals and professional self-governing bodies through their powers to make laws governing property, civil rights, and hospitals.

## The Court System

The Constitution also provides for the establishment of a court system to adjudicate upon criminal and civil matters and to interpret the laws (*Constitution Act, 1867*, ss. 92(14) and 96–101). Our court system is organized primarily at the provincial level, where the bulk of litigation occurs. The Constitution gives the provinces the power to establish and maintain provincial civil and criminal courts and to set the rules of civil procedure in these courts. (Recall that criminal procedure is set out in the federally enacted *Criminal Code of Canada*.) The specific court structure varies somewhat from province to province; however, there are fundamental similarities, discussed below.

### Provincial and Superior Courts

Each province has two basic levels of court: a trial level and an appellate (appeals) level. The organizational structure and number of trial courts vary among provinces, but their jurisdiction (i.e., the types of matters they can hear and the orders and judgements they can make) is much the same. Trial courts are further split into two types: a provincial court and a superior court.

### Administrative Tribunals

The provinces have established boards and commissions, which, although not courts in the strict sense, nevertheless **adjudicate** upon the respective rights and obligations of the parties who come before them. Examples of such boards or commissions, known as **administrative tribunals**, include the various provincial human rights commissions, labour boards, energy boards, provincial securities commissions, municipal boards, assessment review boards, and **health disciplines boards** (which regulate and govern nurses and other health professionals).

For example, the health disciplines boards established by the various provinces (discussed in greater detail in Chapter 5) establish and enforce minimum standards of competence for health professionals. They may have the power to grant permission to practise a given profession or use a professional title (such as RN) within the province, and to discipline members who breach the standards or ethical rules of that profession. Thus, they operate like a court in that they have a duty to decide on such matters fairly and impartially and to give the parties before them a full opportunity to be heard and to present their case.

Figure 4.3 illustrates the structure of the provincial court system.

**Figure 4.3: Typical Provincial Court System\***

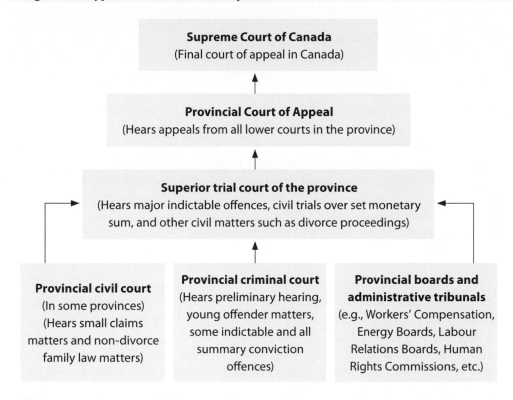

* This structure will vary somewhat from one province to another. In some provinces, the superior trial court and Court of Appeal are combined to form one Supreme Court for the province. In Ontario, the superior trial court has a second branch called the Divisional Court, which itself hears appeals from the province's administrative tribunals. In Quebec, on the other hand, municipal courts exist, as well, to hear certain bylaw offences and local matters.

## Roles of Trial Courts and Appellate Courts

A **trial court** hears matters as a court of **original jurisdiction** or a **court of first instance**. This means that it is the first court to hear a case. Once a trial court makes a decision or renders a verdict, that decision or verdict may be appealed to an **appellate court**, which reviews the proceedings of the lower trial court to ensure that no procedural, evidentiary, or other rules of law were breached or misapplied, that the trial court acted within its powers or jurisdiction, and that the accused's constitutional rights were not violated (especially in the case of a criminal trial).

An appeal is not a new trial. There are no witnesses, and new evidence is seldom heard. It is simply a review of the trial proceedings to ensure that no errors of law were made and that **findings of fact** are based on properly admitted evidence. Appeals courts review the decisions of trial courts if a party to the case appeals the decision because he or she believes the decision is unsound in law or unsupported by the evidence at trial.

### The Supreme Court of Canada

Under the Constitution, the Parliament of Canada may establish courts for the administration of the laws of Canada—that is, laws made specifically by Parliament or matters over which the federal government has constitutional authority (except matters governed by the *Criminal Code*), not provincial laws. Under this provision, the federal government has established the Federal Court of Canada (*Federal Court Act*, 1985, c. F-7), which is divided into a trial and an appellate division.

The Supreme Court of Canada, established in 1875, is Canada's highest court and the final interpreter of the meaning and scope of the Constitution and Charter. The Court hears appeals from all provincial and territorial appellate courts and from the Federal Court of Canada (*Supreme Court Act*, 1985, c. S-26). Its decisions are final until and unless the law is changed by Parliament or the Constitution is amended to reverse the Court's interpretation of one of its provisions. Furthermore, all decisions of the Supreme Court are binding on all lower courts. This is in accordance with the principle of stare decisis, discussed earlier.

The Supreme Court is made up of nine judges, who serve until age 75 and are appointed by the governor general on the advice of the prime minister. They, like all other federally appointed judges, may be removed from office only by resolution of Parliament. In this way, their independence is assured. They need not fear removal if they do not rule upon matters as the government of the day might wish. However, they may be removed if they have broken the law. No federally appointed judge has ever been removed in this fashion since Confederation, though a few judges have resigned following controversy impugning their integrity or impartiality.

Figure 4.4 illustrates the structure of the federal court system.

### Summary

In this chapter we have gained a basic understanding of the workings of the Canadian legal system. We have discussed the sources of the law in Canada's two main legal systems: the English common law and French civil law. A good knowledge of these is an invaluable asset to any nurse today.

The chapter has also briefly reviewed the structure of the provincial and federal court systems and described how laws are passed. Finally, the workings of the Canadian Constitution, *Charter of Rights and Freedoms*, and criminal law have rounded off our overview of the legal system.

The key points introduced in this chapter include:

• The two primary legal systems in Canada—French civil law and English common law—and their sources

**Figure 4.4: Federal Court Structure***

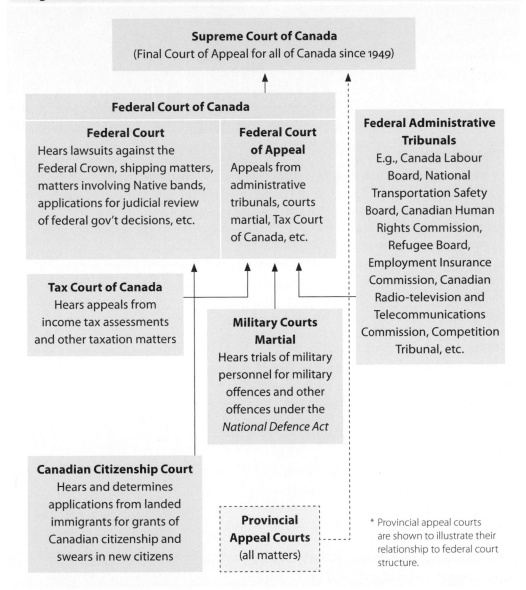

* Provincial appeal courts are shown to illustrate their relationship to federal court structure.

- The legislative process
- The distinction between tort law and criminal law
- An overview of Canada's federal court structure, Canada's Constitution, and the *Charter of Rights and Freedoms*
- The basic structure and functions of the Canadian court system

# Critical Thinking

## Discussion Points

1. Compare and contrast the key elements of English common law and French civil law.
2. Describe the concept of due process and the rule of law in Canada. Discuss the benefits and advantages of due process and the rule of law in modern society.
3. What is a lawsuit, and how does an action typically progress through the court system?
4. What is Canada's Constitution, and what is its function?
5. What is the purpose of the *Canadian Charter of Rights and Freedoms*? Apply your discussion to a nursing setting.

## References

### Statutes

*British North America Act, 1867*, 30 & 31 Vict., c. 3, now known as the *Constitution Act, 1867* (U.K.).

*Canada Act, 1982* (1982), c. 11 (U.K.).

*Canada Health Act*, R.S.C. 1985, c. C-6 (Canada).

*Charter of Rights and Freedoms*, Part I of the *Constitution Act, 1982*, being Schedule B to the *Canada Act 1982* (U.K.), 1982, c. 11.

*Civil Code of Lower Canada*, 1866 (Quebec).

*Civil Code of Quebec*, C.C.Q. 1994, (Quebec).

*Constitution Act, 1867*, 30 & 31 Vict., c. 3 (U.K.).

*Courts of Justice Act*, R.S.O. 1990, c. C. 43 (Ontario).

*Criminal Code of Canada*, R.S.C. 1985, c. C-46 (Canada).

*Federal Court Act*, R.S.C. 1985, c. F-7 (Canada).

*Interpretation Act*, R.S.C. 1985, c. I-21 (Canada).

*Negligence Act*, R.S.O. 1990, c. N.1 (Ontario).

*Ontario Rules of Civil Procedure*, R.R.O. 1990, Regulation 194, as amended (Ontario).

*Regulated Health Professions Act*, S.O. 1991, c. 18, as amended (Ontario).

*Supreme Court Act*, R.S.C. 1985, c. S-26, as amended (Canada).

## Case Law

*Fowler v. Padget* (1798), 7 TR 509; 4 RR 511; 101 ER 1103 (KB).

*Latin v. Hospital for Sick Children et al.* (2007) CanLII 34 (ON S.C.).

*Nancy B. v. Hôtel-Dieu de Québec et al.* [1992] RJQ 361; (1992), 86 DLR (4th) 385; (1992), 69 CCC (3d) 450 (SC).

*R v. Bernard* (1961), 130 CCC 165; 47 MPR 10 (NBCA).

*R. v. Latimer* (1997), 121 CCC (3d) 226 (Sask. QB), aff'd (1998), 131 C.C.C. (3d) 191, 172 Sask. R. 161, 185 W.A.C. 161, 22 C.R. (5th) 380, [1999] 6 W.W.R. 118, [1998] S.J. No. 731 (QL),; aff'd. [2001] 1 S.C.R. 3; (2001), 193 D.L.R. (4th) 577; [2001] 6 W.W.R. 409; (2001), 150 C.C.C. (3d) 129; (2001), 39 C.R. (5th) 1; (2001), 80 C.R.R. (2d) 189; (2001), 203 Sask. R. 1.

*R. v. Morgentaler* [1988] 1 SCR 30; (1988) 63 or (2d) 281 (note); 82 NR 1; 26 OAC 1; 62 CR (3d) 1; 44 DLR (4th) 385; 31 CRR 1 (sub. nom *Morgentaler v. R.*), 37 CCC (3d) 449, rev'g. in part (1985), 52 or (2d) 353; 22 DLR (4th) 641; 22 CCC (3d) 353; 48 CR (3d) 1; 17 CRR 223 (ca), rev'g. (1984), 47 or (2d) 353; 12 DLR (4th) 502; 14 CCC (3d) 258; 41 CR (3d) 193; 11 CRR 116 (HCJ).

*R. v. Rabey* [1980] 2 SCR 513; (1981) 54 CCC (2d) 1; 15 CR (3d) 225; 114 DLR (3d) 193; 32 NR 451.

*Rodriguez v. British Columbia* (AG), [1993] BCWLD 347; (1992), 18 WCB (2d) 279 (SC), aff'd. (1993), 76 BCLR (2d) 145; 22 BCAC 266; 38 WAC 266; 14 CRR (2d) 34; 79 CCC (3d) 1; [1993] 3 WWR 553, aff'd. [1993] 3 SCR 519; *R. v. Latimer* (1997), 121 CCC (3d) 226 (Sask. QB), aff'd. (1998), 131 C.C.C. (3d) 191, 172 Sask. R. 161, 185 W.A.C. 161, 22 C.R. (5th) 380, [1999] 6 W.W.R. 118, [1998] S.J. No. 731 (QL), aff'd. [2001] 1 S.C.R. 3; (2001), 193 D.L.R. (4th) 577; [2001] 6 W.W.R. 409; (2001), 150 C.C.C. (3d) 129; (2001), 39 C.R. (5th) 1; (2001), 80 C.R.R. (2d) 189; (2001), 203 Sask. R. 1.

*United States of America v. Sheppard* [1977] 2 SCR 1067; (1976), 30 CCC (2d) 424; 34 CRNS 207; 9 NR 215; 70 DLR (3d) 136.

*Wilson v. Swanson* (1956) CanLII 1 (S.C.C.), [1956] S.C.R. 804.

## Texts and Articles

Dawson, R. (1970). *The government of Canada* (5th ed., N. Ward., Ed.) Toronto, ON: University of Toronto Press.

Marrocco, F. (1989–90). The classification of offences and trial jurisdiction. Law Society of Upper Canada Bar Admission Course lecture notes (pp. 1–3).

Stuart, D. (1982). *Canadian criminal law.* Toronto, ON: Carswell.

Chapter 5

# Regulation of the Nursing Profession

## Learning Objectives

The purpose of this chapter is to enable you to understand:

- The laws, procedures, and structures regulating the nursing profession across Canada
- The role, function, and responsibility of nursing governing bodies
- Some of the rules and standards regulating the nursing profession
- The processes and procedures used by governing bodies for complaints, discipline, and quality assurance
- The role of regulatory bodies in defining standards of professional practice

## Introduction

ALONG WITH OTHER CANADIAN health professionals, nurses are held to an ever-escalating standard of accountability. Over the past few decades, new structures and mechanisms have been implemented to make professional regulatory bodies more responsive to their duty to ensure competent and safe nursing standards for practice, education, research, and leadership. Nurses must be aware of the basic organization of the self-regulatory bodies in the nursing profession. While the structure of these regulatory bodies may vary across the country, their main objectives are to be accountable, responsible, flexible, and adaptable to rapid changes in the evolution of nursing, while remaining focused on the safety and well-being of the public.

Nurses throughout the country are held accountable for making decisions that result in safe, effective, and ethical practice. This must be accomplished within the context of a complex system in which they face many challenging issues. Regulatory bodies offer support to nurses by clarifying the scope and standards of practice, and by providing advice and education to nurses on a regular basis. Their roles are outlined in this chapter.

Self-regulation is a privilege, *not a right*, granted by the provincial or territorial government to a profession (e.g., nursing, medicine, dentistry, law, accounting), allowing it to govern its own members, set standards of entry into the professions, establish educational requirements for students of the profession, set standards of practice, receive and investigate complaints, and administer a disciplinary process for its members. This privilege reflects the trust the public has put in these professions. In many other countries, these professions are regulated by civil servants in a government department; nonmembers of the profession are essentially responsible for regulation and oversight of those professions. Many believe this results in a loss of professional autonomy. Thus, historically, there has been a long-standing preference in Canada for self-regulation, and, in turn, a requirement that these bodies govern their professions in the public interest. Otherwise, they run the risk of losing the public's trust and, hence, their privilege of self-regulation.

The provincial and territorial regulatory bodies must be distinguished from nurses' unions, such as United Nurses of Alberta, the Nova Scotia Nurses' Union, or the Ontario Nurses' Association. The latter exist as collective bargaining agents and act solely in the interests of members as employees of various health facilities. (Labour issues, as they relate to nurses, are discussed more fully in Chapter 11.)

As Canadians become increasingly aware of their legal rights, they question the ability of health professionals to regulate themselves in the public interest. Thus, the primary purpose of the governing bodies of nursing and other health disciplines is to serve as watchdog and to promote the welfare of the public. This is done through the setting and enforcing of practice standards and codes of ethics that protect the public from incompetent, unqualified, or unethical health care professionals and provide the benchmarks against which professional practice may be measured.

This chapter will summarize the structures and systems of the regulatory bodies governing the nursing profession in Canada, including organizational structures, methods of regulation, licensing systems, establishment of educational standards, evaluation of the qualifications and skills of nurses, and management of complaints and disciplinary procedures.

## The History of Nursing Regulation in Canada

The profession of nursing across Canada has been regulated since approximately World War I. In some provinces—for example, British Columbia (1918), Manitoba (1913), and Prince Edward Island (1922)—the profession has always been self-regulated, while in others, government regulation gradually gave way to self-regulation. In Ontario, for example, nursing has been a self-regulated profession only since 1963. In Quebec, until the 1960s, regulation of the nursing profession was primarily within the purview of the Catholic Church since most nurses were members of religious orders. The secularization of the profession came in the early 1970s with the establishment of Quebec's Ordre des infirmières et infirmiers.

## Definitions of Nursing Practice

Within their respective statutes, most provinces and territories have enacted legal definitions of the term *nursing*. The purpose of such definitions is to describe the nature and scope of nursing practice by delimiting those acts and procedures that constitute nursing practice. This provides a framework to determine whether certain actions comprise the practice of nursing and allows a distinction to be drawn between nursing and other professional practices. The definition also aids the courts in interpreting other sections of the respective provincial and territorial statutes. These definitions are set out in Table 5.1.

## Legal and Organizational Structure of Nursing Bodies

The laws regulating nursing in the provinces and territories of Canada are broadly similar in their purpose and objectives. They seek to ensure an orderly and well-regulated process for entry into the nursing profession, to ensure maintenance of nursing skills and standards of practice among all practising nurses, and to ensure a fair and thorough complaints procedure and disciplinary process to protect the public from professional misconduct and poor-quality nursing care. They do this through the creation of regulatory bodies, discussed below.

### Categories of Nurses

In Canada, there are generally two classes of registered nurse: *registered nurses* (RNs) and extended-class RNs called *nurse practitioners* (RN, NPs), discussed in more detail below. Another category of nurse is the practical nurse, in Ontario called *registered practical nurses*, (RPN), and *licensed practical nurses* (LPN) in all other provinces. Although the terminology differs, the nature of practice undertaken by practical nurses is essentially the same across Canada. The main difference between RNs and practical nurses is that RNs have more

**Table 5.1: Definitions of Nursing Across Canada**

| Province | Nursing Definition |
|----------|--------------------|
| Alberta | No set legal definition. The *Registered Nurses Profession Regulation*, Alta. Reg. 232/2005, made under the *Health Professions Act*, R.S.A. 2000, c. H-7 provides that "registered members on any register (i.e., Registered Nurses, Certified Graduate Nurses, Nurse Practitioners, and nurses registered in the Temporary or Courtesy registers) may, within the practice of registered nursing and in accordance with the standards of practice governing the performance of restricted activities approved by the Council, perform specified and restricted activities including such procedures as cutting a body tissue, administer anything by an invasive procedure on body tissue or to perform surgical or other invasive procedures on body tissue below the dermis or the mucous membrane; insert or remove instruments, devices, fingers or hands, reduce a dislocation of a joint except for a partial dislocation of the joints of the fingers and toes; dispense, compound, provide for selling or sell certain drugs within the meaning of the *Pharmaceutical Profession Act*; among other acts."<br><br>There are also regulations governing registered psychiatric and mental deficiency nurses. |
| British Columbia | The *Nurses (Registered) and Nurse Practitioners Regulation*, B.C. Reg. 233/2005, made under the *Health Professions Act*, R.S.B.C. 1996, c. 183 provides that "'nursing' means the health profession in which a person provides or performs the following services: (a) health care for the promotion, maintenance and restoration of health, and (b) prevention, treatment and palliation of illness and injury, primarily by<br>(i)   assessment of health status, planning and implementation of interventions, and<br>(ii)  coordination of health services."<br>There are also definitions for registered psychiatric nurses. |
| Manitoba | The *Registered Nurses Act*, C.C.S.M., c. R40, s. 2(1) provides that "the practice of nursing is the application of nursing knowledge, skill and judgment to promote, maintain and restore health, prevent illness and alleviate suffering, and includes, but is not limited to,<br>(a) assessing health status;<br>(b) planning, providing and evaluating treatment and nursing interventions;<br>(c) counselling and teaching to enhance health and well-being; and<br>(d) education, administration and research related to providing health services. |

continued on following page >>

## Table 5.1: Definitions of Nursing Across Canada *continued*

| Province | Nursing Definition |
| --- | --- |
| Manitoba *(continued)* | Nursing practice includes<br><br>(2) In accordance with any requirements set out in the regulations, a registered nurse may do any of the following in the course of engaging in the practice of nursing:<br><br>(a) order and receive reports of screening and diagnostic tests designated in the regulations;<br><br>(b) prescribe drugs designated in the regulations;<br><br>(c) perform minor surgical and invasive procedures designated in the regulations." |
| New Brunswick | Section 2(1) of the New Brunswick *Nurses Act*, 1984, provides that nursing means "the practice of nursing and includes the nursing assessment and treatment of human responses to actual or potential health problems and the nursing supervision thereof." |
| Newfoundland and Labrador | No legal definition, but the Association of Registered Nurses of Newfoundland & Labrador has adopted the Canadian Nurses Association's definition: "Registered Nurses are self-regulated health care professionals who work autonomously and in collaboration with others. RNs enable individuals, families, groups, communities and populations to achieve their optimal health. RNs coordinate health care, deliver direct services and support clients in their self-care decisions and actions in situations of health, illness, injury and disability in all stages of life. RNs contribute to the health care system through their work in direct practice, education, administration, research and policy in a wide array of settings" (CNA, 2007, p. 6). |
| Northwest Territories | Section 2(1) of the Northwest Territories' *Nursing Profession Act*, S.N.W.T. 2003, c. 15 provides that "(1) A registered nurse is entitled to apply nursing knowledge, skills and judgment<br><br>(a) to promote, maintain and restore health;<br><br>(b) to prevent and alleviate illness, injury and disability;<br><br>(c) to assist in prenatal care, childbirth and postnatal care;<br><br>(d) to care for the terminally ill and the dying;<br><br>(e) in the coordination of health care services;<br><br>(f) in administration, supervision, education, consultation, teaching, policy development and research with respect to any of the matters referred to in paragraphs (a) to (e); and<br><br>(g) to dispense, compound and package drugs where the bylaws so permit." |

continued on following page >>

**Table 5.1: Definitions of Nursing Across Canada** *continued*

| Province | Nursing Definition |
|---|---|
| Nova Scotia | Section 1 of the *Registered Nurses Act*, S.N.S. 2001, c. 10 defines the scope of nursing practice as "the performance of professional services requiring substantial specialized knowledge of nursing theory and the biological, physical, behavioural, psychological and sociological sciences as the basis for<br>(i) assessment, planning, intervention and evaluation in<br>   (A) the promotion and maintenance of health,<br>   (B) the facilitation of the management of illness, injury or infirmity,<br>   (C) the restoration of optimum function, or<br>   (D) palliative care, or<br>(ii) research, education, management or administration incidental to the objectives referred to in subclause (i), and includes the practice of a nurse practitioner." |
| Nunavut | No set definition. Scope is outlined in practice standards documents of the Registered Nurses Association of the Northwest Territories and Nunavut. |
| Ontario | Section 3 of the *Nursing Act*, 1991, S.O. 1991, c. 32 defines the practice of nursing as "the promotion of health and the assessment of, the provision of care for and the treatment of health conditions by supportive, preventive, therapeutic, palliative and rehabilitative means in order to attain or maintain optimal function." |
| Prince Edward Island | The *Registered Nurses Act*, R.S.P.E.I., 1988, c. 8.1, s.1(s) defines the practice of a registered nurse in the same manner as Nova Scotia's statute (see above). |
| Quebec | Section 36 of the *Nurses Act*, R.S.Q., c. I-8 provides that "the practice of nursing consists of assessing a person's state of health, determining and carrying out of the nursing care and treatment plan, providing nursing and medical care and treatment in order to maintain or restore health and prevent illness, and providing palliative care." |
| Saskatchewan | Section 2(k) of the *Registered Nurses Act*, 1988, S.S. 1988–89, c. R-12.2 provides that "the practice of 'registered nursing' means the performance or co-ordination of health care services including but not limited to:<br>(i) observing and assessing the health status of clients and planning, implementing and evaluating nursing care; and<br>(ii) the counselling, teaching, supervision, administration and research that is required to implement or complement health care services; for the |

continued on following page >>

**Table 5.1: Definitions of Nursing Across Canada** *continued*

| Province | Nursing Definition |
|---|---|
| Saskatchewan *(continued)* | purpose of promoting, maintaining or restoring health, preventing illness and alleviating suffering where the performance or co-ordination of those services requires skills or training as defined in that Act." |
| Yukon | Section 1 of the *Registered Nurses Profession Act*, R.S.Y. 2002, c. 194 provides that nursing means "the application of professional nursing knowledge or services for compensation for the purpose of<br>(a) promoting, maintaining, and restoring health,<br>(b) preventing illness, injury, or disability,<br>(c) caring for persons who are sick, injured, disabled, or dying,<br>(d) assisting in pre-natal care, childbirth, and post-natal care,<br>(e) health teaching and health counselling,<br>(f) coordinating health care, or<br>(g) engaging in administration, teaching, or research to implement a matter referred to in paragraphs (a) to (f)." |

in-depth education with a strong focus on critical thinking, evidence-informed practice, and so on. RNs are usually prepared at the university, or baccalaureate, level, while practical nurses follow a more basic educational program, usually at a community college. The scope of practice of RNs and practical nurses differs in that practical nurses care for less complex and more predictable client populations. Within the practice of registered nurses, there is the opportunity to specialize, for example, in pediatrics, critical care, psychiatry, and so on. In some jurisdictions, some nurses enter their practice with a specialized designation—for example, registered psychiatric nurses in Alberta.

## Single-Tiered Systems

There are two different regulatory systems governing nursing in Canada. One is a single-tier system, such as that found in all three territories and most provinces, including British Columbia, Alberta, Saskatchewan, Manitoba, New Brunswick, Nova Scotia, Prince Edward Island, and Newfoundland and Labrador. In a single-tier system, a provincially created regulatory body, such as the College & Association of Registered Nurses of Alberta, the Nurses Association of New Brunswick, or the College of Registered Nurses of Manitoba, has a complete legislative mandate to regulate entry of candidates into the nursing profession and to perform other functions as described below (see "Objectives of Nursing Regulatory Bodies").

## Two-Tiered Systems

In two-tiered systems, in place in Ontario and Quebec, the first tier consists of a nursing regulatory body such as those found in the other provinces. A higher-level body, the Health Professions Appeal and Review Board (HPARB) in Ontario and the Office des professions in Quebec, makes up the second tier. The functions and duties of Ontario's HPARB are confined to hearing appeals from complaints, registration, and accreditation committees of the lower-tier health professions colleges (i.e., those of nurses, physicians and surgeons, chiropractors, psychiatrists, dentists, etc.). In contrast, Quebec's Office des professions regulates all professions, both health- and nonhealth-related. In Quebec's system, however, the Office is not directly involved in appeals from disciplinary or registration matters. Its primary mandate is to ensure that the province's 45 self-regulated professions carry out their legal responsibilities in accordance with their governing legislation, that they self-regulate in the public interest, and that they adopt proper regulatory and professional standards for their respective professions. Disciplinary matters in Quebec are appealed to the Professional Tribunal, a government-appointed administrative tribunal that closely resembles Ontario's HPARB. Thus, there are notable structural and functional differences between the two-tiered Ontario and Quebec systems. Quebec appears to have the most unified system of professional regulation in Canada.

## Regulatory Bodies

In most provinces, separate classes of nurses are regulated by different regulatory bodies. For example, in Alberta, registered nurses are governed by the College & Association of Registered Nurses of Alberta, whereas licensed practical nurses are governed by the College of Licensed Practical Nurses of Alberta, and registered psychiatric and mental deficiency nurses are regulated by the College of Registered Psychiatric Nurses of Alberta. Governance is the same in British Columbia, Saskatchewan, and Manitoba. In Quebec (which has a two-tiered system), New Brunswick, Nova Scotia, Prince Edward Island, and Newfoundland and Labrador, psychiatric nurses do not answer to a separate body, although practical nurses have a different regulator than do RNs and NPs. In Yukon, registered nurses are governed by the Yukon Registered Nurses Association, and licensed practical nurses are governed by the Yukon government directly, with the aid of an advisory body of licensed practical nurses. The same holds true in the Northwest Territories. Nunavut, whose registered nurses are governed by the Registered Nurses Association of Northwest Territories and Nunavut, does not appear to provide for licensed practical nurses.

As stated above, in both the single- and two-tiered systems, there is a principal college or professional association charged with regulating nurses. (See Alberta: *Health Professions Act*, 2000, c. H-7; British Columbia: *Health Professions Act*, 1996, c. 183; Manitoba: *Registered Nurses Act*, c. R40; New Brunswick: *Nurses Act*, 1984, c. 71; Newfoundland: *Registered Nurses Act*, 1990, c. R-9; Northwest Territories and Nunavut: *Nursing Profession Act*, 2003, c.15; Nova Scotia: *Registered Nurses Act*, 2001, c. 10; Ontario: *Nursing Act*, 1991, c. 32; Prince Edward Island: *Registered Nurses Act*, 2004, c. 15; Quebec: *Nurses Act*, c. I-8; Saskatchewan: *Registered Nurses Act*, 1988, c. R-12.2; Yukon: *Registered Nurses Profession Act*, 2002, c. 194.) Each such college or association is governed by a board composed of members of the profession and registered with the college or association. It may or may not, depending on the province, also include laypersons appointed by the government. The board of a nursing college is usually granted powers and responsibilities to govern the nursing profession in the interest of the public and to protect the public from incompetent, unethical, or unprofessional conduct by its members. It must ensure its members are properly educated and meet the standards required to practise nursing in the province.

In some provinces (i.e., Nova Scotia, Ontario, Manitoba, and British Columbia), the regulatory bodies are formally and legally called "colleges." In some other provinces and territories (i.e., Yukon, Northwest Territories, Nunavut, Saskatchewan, New Brunswick, Prince Edward Island, and Newfoundland and Labrador), they are legally referred to as "associations." Alberta's regulatory body has both terms in its name: the College & Association of Registered Nurses of Alberta. It should also be noted that in most provinces, the regulatory arm (i.e., the bureaucratic structure of the college or association responsible for regulating entry to practice, licensing, continuing competence, and complaints and discipline) and the professional arm (i.e., the structure of the college or association responsible for advocacy for members of the nursing profession) are combined. In Ontario, these "arms" are completely separate: The regulatory aspect is entrusted solely to the Ontario College of Nurses. The professional advocacy aspect, including the provision of professional malpractice insurance, the lobbying of governments in nurses' professional interests, and political action, is undertaken by a completely separate entity called the Registered Nurses' Association of Ontario.

There is also a national professional organization of nurses, known as the Canadian Nurses Association, whose mandate is to represent nurses nationally and to support a high-quality and publicly funded public health care system. The CNA has no direct regulatory role akin to that of the provincial and territorial regulatory bodies, but its functions include the promotion and advancement of nursing regulation provincially and territorially in the public interest.

In Ontario, because the professional nursing association is separate from the College, the duty to self-regulate in the public interest cannot conflict with advocacy and lobbying on behalf of nurses in terms of work conditions, contracts, benefits, and so forth. However, these arms are combined in most other provinces and territories, so mechanisms must be available to resolve such potential conflicts. The foremost duty of all the regulatory bodies is to govern in the public interest. Since self-regulation is, as stated earlier, a privilege, not a right, a regulatory body that were to favour its professional self-interest over the public interest would soon lose the privilege of self-regulation. This knowledge helps ensure such conflicts are kept in check.

## Objectives of Nursing Regulatory Bodies

As discussed earlier, the objectives of the various **regulatory bodies** are to regulate nursing roles, education, entry into the profession, scope of practice, standards of practice, complaints processes, and discipline of members not in compliance (See Northwest Territories: *Nursing Profession Act*, s. 3; Yukon: *Registered Nurses Profession Act*, s. 3; British Columbia: *Health Professions Act*, s. 16; Prince Edward Island: *Registered Nurses Act*, s. 6; Newfoundland: *Registered Nurses Act*, s. 5). It is the duty of the professional association, as a servant and protector of the public, to regulate the nursing profession and to discharge its responsibilities consistent with the public interest, while balancing the need for autonomy in the functioning of its professionals.

## Board or Council's Role

Each regulatory body is headed by a board of directors or council, which governs the day-to-day affairs of the regulatory body and provides the mechanism to establish entry criteria and standards of practice. As the primary rule-making body, the council or board enacts rules and bylaws regarding nursing practice standards; standards for admission to nursing schools; the curricula and teaching standards of such schools (although the provinces also have a say in this); student membership; continuing education; reinstatement and renewal of membership; licensing, membership, and other fees; rules governing types of duties; and so forth. In many provinces (e.g., British Columbia *Act*, s. 44(1); Yukon *Act*, s. 52(1); Saskatchewan *Act*, s. 34(1); Manitoba *Act*, s. 38(1); New Brunswick *Act*, s. 34(1); Nova Scotia *Act*, s. 43; Prince Edward Island *Act*, s. 27(1)), the provincial regulatory body's board or council also hears **appeals** of decisions made by its disciplinary or professional conduct committee.

## Registration, Licensing, and Entry to Practice

All provincial and territorial laws require applicants for membership (registration and licensing, discussed below) in their respective regulatory body to have graduated from an approved school of nursing and to have passed the requisite nursing registration examination before they may be admitted as members of the regulatory body.

## Registration Versus Licensing

Although the terms *registration* and *licensing* mean two different things, provincial and territorial regulatory bodies often use them interchangeably. Regardless, the use of these credentials assures the public that these nurses meet the appropriate standards of the regulatory body and can safely practise.

**Registration** refers to a prospective registered nurse (or registered practical nurse or psychiatric nurse) enrolling as a member of a provincial or territorial nursing college or association. Through registration, the member is recognized as a person who is then authorized to practise nursing in the particular province or territory concerned. Registration allows the regulatory body to record the nurse's contact information, educational background, and qualifications. In this process, the qualifications for an applicant are carefully reviewed to ensure that all requirements related to education and hours of practice are met. Since listing the complete requirements for each governing body is beyond the scope of this book, the reader is urged to consult the Web site of his or her provincial or territorial governing body for its requirements.

### Provincial and Territorial Nursing Colleges and Associations

At time of writing, the respective Web sites of the provincial and territorial colleges and associations were as follows:

Yukon Registered Nurses Association: **http://www.yrna.ca**

Registered Nurses Association of Northwest Territories and Nunavut: **http://www.rnantnu.ca**

College of Registered Nurses of British Columbia: **http://www.crnbc.ca**

College & Association of Registered Nurses of Alberta: **http://www.nurses.ab.ca/Carna/ index.aspx**

Saskatchewan Registered Nurses' Association: **http://www.srna.org**

College of Registered Nurses of Manitoba: **http://www.crnm.mb.ca**

College of Nurses of Ontario: **http://www.cno.org**

Ordre des infirmières et infirmiers du Québec: **http://www.oiiq.org**

Nurses Association of New Brunswick: **http://www.nanb.nb.ca/index.cfm**

College of Registered Nurses of Nova Scotia: **http://www.crnns.ca**

Association of Registered Nurses of Prince Edward Island: **http://www.arnpei.ca**

Association of Registered Nurses of Newfoundland and Labrador: **http://www.arnnl.nf.ca**

*This information can also be found at http://evolve.elsevier.com/Canada/Keatings/ethical

Once a nurse has successfully passed the Canadian Registered Nurse Examination and met any other requirements imposed by the provincial or territorial regulatory body, he or she is granted a licence or issued a certificate of registration or permit, depending on the region, to practise nursing in that province or territory. This is called the **licensing** process.

In the case of applicants who have received their education in a province other than the one in which they are applying, the curriculum must be either equivalent to that association's educational standards or from a board-approved institution. The requirements for Canadian-trained and foreign-trained nurses are generally set out in each provincial or territorial act: See Alberta *Act*, section 28(2)(b); Saskatchewan *Act*, section 19(1)(i)(A)(II); Manitoba *Act* (for registration as a graduate nurse specifically), section 9(2)(a)(ii) and Man. Reg. 128/2001, subparagraph 4(1)(a)(ii) and subsection 4(2); Nova Scotia, N.S. Reg. 155/2001, Section 7; Prince Edward Island *Act*, sections 13 and 14, and E.C. 93/06, *Registration and Licensing of Nurses Regulations*, sections 3, and 6; and Newfoundland *Act*, section 8. In British Columbia, the College of Registered Nurses of British Columbia's bylaws set out the requirements for Canadian-trained and foreign-trained nurses. In some provinces, applicants who are already registered and licensed to practise nursing in another province, who demonstrate that they are competent, and who are not currently the subject of disciplinary or competency proceedings in any other jurisdiction will be entitled to registration in the province in which they are applying. Student nurses—that is, students who are undertaking formal nursing education and do not yet qualify for registration as nurses—are usually granted student membership in these regulatory bodies. Student nurses are required to have practised a specified number of hours before they can become full-fledged members. These hours vary by province and territory but are usually over 1100 hours' practice time within the previous four or five years.

## Access to the Nursing Profession

To address public concerns regarding fair access to regulated health professions, some provinces have put in place legal and supervisory mechanisms to ensure that all socioeconomic and cultural groups, particularly visible minorities, are given full opportunities to enter the health professions, including nursing. Ontario, for example, passed amendments to its *Health Professions Procedural Code* (HPPC) (1991) under the *Regulated Health Professions Act* that impose a duty on the College "to provide registration practices that are transparent, objective, impartial and fair" (*Regulated Health Professions Act* [RHPA], 1991, s. 22.2). To ensure such openness, a fairness commissioner appointed by the government is required to:

- Assess the registration practices of a college based on its obligations under the code and the regulations
- Specify audit standards, the scope of audits, times when fair registration practices reports and auditors' reports must be filed, the form of all required reports and certificates, and the information that they must contain
- Establish eligibility requirements that a person must meet to be qualified to conduct audits
- Establish a list of persons who in the opinion of the Fairness Commissioner have satisfied the eligibility requirements
- Consult with colleges on the cost, scope, and timing of audits
- Monitor third parties relied on by a college to assess the qualifications of individuals applying for registration by the college to help ensure that assessments are based on the obligations of the college under the code and the regulations
- Advise a college or others relied on by a college to assess qualifications and matters related to registration practices under the code and the regulations
- Provide advice and recommendations to the Minister of Health and Long-Term Care, including advice and recommendations that the college do or refrain from doing any action respecting a contravention by a college if the fairness commissioner finds that the college is not performing its obligations. The policy aim here is to ensure that any systemic barriers that may exist in the colleges' administrative structures for registration and licensing are removed (RHPA, s. 22.5; *Fair Access to Regulated Professions Act, 2006*, c. 31).

## Internationally Educated Nurses

In recent years, the issue of the registration and licensing of internationally educated nurses (IEN) has gained a great deal of attention. When shortages of health care professionals become acute across the country, pressure is put on Canada's regulatory bodies to admit to practice internationally educated professionals. Recognizing that not all international education programs will meet Canadian standards, regulatory bodies have begun to develop methods of evaluating credentials and experience. Unfortunately, however, the application process for these nurses can be daunting, discouragingly lengthy, and emotionally draining.

Most of the regulatory bodies' Web sites include information for new immigrants. Systems and procedures in use tend to be ad hoc and inconsistent across Canada. Quebec's Ordre des infirmières et infirmiers requires that all applicants for membership and licensing be proficient in the French language. There are similar English proficiency requirements in the other provinces and territories. British Columbia's College of Registered Nurses, for example, provides a fairly detailed information document for IENs, which gauges whether they are ready for registration in that province (see http://www.crnbc.ca). A detailed step-by-step chart outlines each requirement, including proficiency in English, registration in the country in which he or she studied nursing, and registration in every other country in which he or she has practised. It also requires applicants to disclose information about any disciplinary or competency issues faced, their postsecondary nursing education, any criminal records or pardons, and so forth. The requirements in the other provinces are essentially the same—that is, IENs must provide evidence of a nursing education at the postsecondary level (or at the secondary/community college level for RPNs or LPNs), provide evidence of safe nursing practice in their country of origin, be fluent in English (or French in Quebec), have a good character (i.e., lack of a criminal record or outstanding criminal charges in their home country), and so on. Each application is examined on its own merits and, depending on the applicant's qualifications or lack thereof, can take a considerable time to process.

## Unauthorized Practice and Use of Titles

As discussed, all provinces and territories restrict the practice of nursing, the use of the title "registered nurse" and the initials "RN" or "RegN," and the use of the title "nurse practitioner" and the initials "NP" to members of the regulatory body who hold a registration certificate or licence and who are members in good standing.

A member of a regulatory body who is under suspension or whose certificate of registration has been revoked or suspended may be deemed, for the duration of such suspension or **revocation**, not to be a member of the regulatory body. Such a person then ceases to be a registered nurse and is not entitled to practise nursing. If the nurse nevertheless continues to practise, he or she may be charged with unauthorized practice. Continuing practice while under suspension constitutes **professional misconduct** under most provincial laws (see, for example, Saskatchewan's *Act*, s. 26(2)(q)).

## Disciplinary and Competency Matters

It should be stressed from the outset that disciplinary proceedings against nursing professionals are a matter entirely separate and different from criminal proceedings. Criminal proceedings would normally be initiated against a nurse if it is alleged that he or she has committed an offence under the *Criminal Code*. Criminal charges would normally be laid by the police following a complaint filed either by a member of the public (for instance, a patient) or by a police investigator who has found sufficient grounds to allege that a criminal offence of some kind has been committed. A finding of guilt following a criminal trial would lead to a fine or perhaps a sentence in a correctional institution. (In some provinces, a nurse convicted of an indictable offence under the *Criminal Code*, or an offence under the *Controlled Drugs and Substances Act* or the *Food and Drugs Act*, may be liable to suspension from nursing practice, in some cases, without any hearing.)

Professional disciplinary proceedings, on the other hand, are entirely an internal matter governed by the nursing regulatory body and are designed to ensure nurses' professional conduct conforms to the *Code of Ethics for Registered Nurses* and the regulations of the professional body. Any findings of misconduct would normally be punished by a range of measures from a **reprimand** to outright cancellation of a nurse's licence to practice.

Disciplinary and competency matters are examined by an investigator. If criteria are met, the matter is referred to the professional conduct or disciplinary committee of the provincial or territorial association. Committee members are usually appointed by the board of directors or council of that association, and include laypersons. This preserves the public input aspect of self-regulation. The procedures for disciplinary hearings and the findings and penalties that can be assessed by the committee are fairly similar in all provinces and territories and are essentially as follows:

### Step 1: Complaint in Writing

In most cases, a complaint relating to alleged professional misconduct will be filed with the registrar or executive director of the provincial or territorial association to which the member belongs. The complaint must be in writing, must be signed and dated by the person making the complaint, and should name the health professional who is alleged to have acted in an unprofessional manner. (However, failure to name him or her will not necessarily invalidate the complaint.) Further, it must outline the facts and particulars of the alleged misconduct. A complaint that is not in writing and that is made anonymously is not considered.

**Complainants** (i.e., the persons who make a complaint) can be nursing colleagues, patients receiving care from a nursing professional or members of their immediate family, physicians or surgeons on the health care team, and even employers. Nursing regulatory bodies prefer that employers (usually a health care institution such as a hospital, nursing home, or health clinic) attempt to handle professional competence and conduct issues internally first. Thus, the colleague, manager, or supervisor of a nurse whose conduct is in question would first file a complaint with the employer pursuant to existing procedures in the health care organization concerned. Very often, this is sufficient to resolve any issues concerning a nurse's professional competence, ability to meet the standard of practice, and any minor concerns relating to conduct. If an employer's internal disciplinary or performance review procedures are not able to resolve the issue, the employer would be required to file a formal complaint with the provincial or territorial regulatory body. Ontario's *Regulated Health Professions Act* (1991, c.18) and Alberta's *Health Professions Act* (2000, c. H-7) require that members' employers file a detailed report outlining incidents or events giving rise to termination or the intention to terminate, whether they involved misconduct, incapacity, or a failure to observe the standards of practice, as well as the response of the member to these incidents and the ultimate action taken by the employer against the nurse. Similar requirements are in place in Saskatchewan and Manitoba.

As discussed above, ultimately, it is the ethical and, in many cases, the legal obligation of nurses to report improper professional conduct or incidents that involve a nursing colleague's failure to meet the standard of professional practice, whether that colleague has acted in an unprofessional manner; has a lack of skill, knowledge, or judgement that poses a threat to the safety of patients in the nurse's care; or is, by reason of addiction to alcohol or drugs, or mental or physical illness, unable to discharge his or her nursing duties competently or safely. In Alberta, New Brunswick, and many other provinces, failure to report such conduct or situation will constitute professional misconduct on the part of the nurse whose duty it was to disclose it. Ontario law specifically requires a member of the College of Nurses to report a nursing colleague who the member has reasonable grounds to believe has committed an act of sexual abuse of a patient. The report must be filed in writing with the registrar of the Ontario College of Nurses. Where nonsexual improper conduct is concerned, the nurse would first report the matter to his or her employer in order to invoke the internal practice review or disciplinary procedures prior to lodging a formal complaint with the regulatory body. British Columbia's *Health Professions Act* (1996, c. 183), as well as Alberta's statute, contain similar requirements but also require mandatory reporting of all conduct or situations in which a health professional's conduct, fitness to practise, competence to practice, or sexual misconduct poses a threat to the safety of the public. British Columbia's legislation additionally requires a medical practitioner in charge of a public hospital to report to the College a registrant (i.e., a member) who has been admitted to the practitioner's institution for psychiatric care or treatment.

The duty to disclose unprofessional conduct or incompetence is accompanied by a potentially conflicting duty to observe the nurse–patient or nurse–client relationship and to keep confidential any information disclosed by the patient in the course of treatment and the provision of nursing care. If, in the course of providing treatment to a patient, a nurse gained knowledge from that patient that another nurse was acting in an unskilled manner, that nurse may not be entirely free to disclose such information, if to do so would in any way compromise the confidentiality of the conversation. There are provisions in many provincial nursing and health professions statutes that authorize disclosure of a patient's identity in a complaint only with the patient's consent or that of a substitute decision maker (in the case of a patient who is mentally incapable of consenting).

It will usually be possible to disclose the information without divulging the identity of the patient or other details that would readily identify him or her. The patient who feels strongly about the professional's conduct may choose to waive privacy rights and authorize full disclosure.

## Step 2: Investigation

Usually, a complaint will be investigated in a preliminary way by a complaints committee, an investigator, or the registrar of the association in order to ascertain whether it is well founded or merely frivolous or malicious (i.e., brought deliberately to injure a person's reputation) (Nova Scotia *Act*, section 34 and N.S. Reg. 155/2001, s. 31; Manitoba *Act*, s. 21; Yukon *Act*, s. 24; New Brunswick *Act*, s. 29 and Part IV.1).

By statute, members whose conduct or competence is the subject of an investigation must be notified immediately upon receipt of a written complaint by their provincial or territorial association. They may also be entitled to make submissions to the committee or individual conducting a preliminary investigation (e.g., see Yukon *Act*, s. 24(4); Manitoba *Act*, ss. 29 (3) and 35(1)). At this stage, the complaint may be dismissed if it is unwarranted or unsupported by the results of the investigation. An investigator will have powers under the governing statute to inspect nursing records, conduct interviews, enter the nurse's place of practice, inspect equipment, conduct tests, and so forth.

Nurses must recognize that they are under a legal duty to cooperate with an investigator and to allow him or her to make examinations without interference. But patient confidentiality must be protected. It is also entirely appropriate, and recommended, that a nurse avail himself or herself of all legal and procedural rights during an investigation, including seeking a lawyer without delay. Legal counsel will be able to apply to an appropriate court for a ruling on whether such a search or seizure is lawful and made according to the procedural safeguards contained in the legislation. In many cases, nurses' professional organizations, or provincial or territorial nursing regulatory bodies in those provinces where the regulatory and advocacy "arms" are combined, will provide for the services of a lawyer to represent the nurse in such proceedings.

## Step 3: Interim Investigation

If well founded, the complaint may be referred to a disciplinary committee or a professional conduct committee (depending on the province or territory) for further investigation, and then to a hearing, if necessary. If the allegations show that the nurse being investigated poses a threat to the safety or security of patients, the committee usually has the power to order that the nurse's right to practise be suspended or restricted pending the conclusion of the disciplinary proceedings. This effectively halts the nurse's practice for the duration of the matter and may be a source of financial or other hardship to the nurse.

## Step 4: Disciplinary Committee

Before a hearing is scheduled to consider the matter, the disciplinary committee (in some provinces, the practice review committee) must first notify the nurse against whom the complaint was brought. The date and time of the hearing will usually be coordinated with the nurse's lawyer, if any. The notice usually specifies the nature of the conduct being reviewed, and the date, place, and time of the hearing by the committee.

The committee, after hearing the evidence, will make its decision. Among the possible findings it may make are:

- That the nurse is innocent of any wrongdoing
- That the nurse involved is incompetent, unskilled, or otherwise lacking in essential knowledge
- That he or she is guilty of professional misconduct
- That the nurse is habitually impaired by the use of alcohol or drugs such that he or she is unable to discharge nursing duties and obligations safely

Many of the provincial statutes specify acts that constitute professional misconduct. Such definitions are not meant to be exclusive but serve to identify many common situations.

Recall the case scenario of nurse Paul in Chapter 4. He was alleged to have engaged in sexually abusive behaviour toward a child in his care. His employment had been terminated and his conduct reported to the police and to his provincial regulatory body. Paul has the right to due process and natural justice. The procedures above, which would likely be followed, provide for notice to him and an opportunity to be heard and to defend himself. They are designed to respect and ensure that the requirements of natural justice are met. Failure to follow these procedures opens any disciplinary proceedings brought against Paul to attack on the grounds that he has been denied due process. Of course, any criminal charges brought against him by the police would also entitle him to procedural and legal rights in a court of law. But in the case of disciplinary proceedings to determine his continued status as a nurse, he would also be entitled to due process.

A 1993 British Columbia court decision involving a licensed practical nurse illustrates how provincial human rights laws may intervene to protect an applicant's right to membership despite that person's prior criminal record (*Mans v. Council of Licensed Practical Nurses*, 1990). Although the case involved legislation applying specifically to practical nurses, the principle is equally applicable to RNs. In this case, a woman had applied for a licence as an LPN after having worked unlicensed as such for a number of years. The Council of Licensed Practical Nurses of British Columbia refused her application on the grounds that she had a prior criminal record consisting of a conviction for shoplifting in the early 1970s, nearly 20 years earlier. The B.C. *Human Rights Act* then in force (now named the *Human Rights Code*, 1996, c. 21) prohibited discrimination in employment based on a person's past criminal record unless such a record was related to the person's intended occupation. The practical nurse took her complaint to the B.C. Human Rights Council, claiming that the

Licensed Practical Nurses' Council had illegally discriminated against her on this basis. The Human Rights Council found in the nurse's favour and ordered the LPN Council to grant the nurse a licence.

The LPN Council appealed, and the case ultimately found its way to the B.C. Court of Appeal, which upheld the Human Rights Council's decision and confirmed its view that the *Human Rights Act* superseded the statute granting the LPN Council authority to deny a licence to applicants who are not deemed fit to be licensed. The court further stated that the Human Rights Council was correct in asserting that the prior criminal record, in this case, was unrelated to the applicant's intended occupation as a licensed practical nurse and that the discrimination was therefore unlawful. The requirement of criminal record checks for nursing applicants is now governed by statute in British Columbia and several other provinces. This is discussed more fully below. The B.C. statute sets forth specific criminal offences that are deemed to be relevant to the practice of nursing and for which a nurse will be denied registration as a nurse. These offences include assault, sexual assault, fraud, and so forth—offences that suggest that a potential nursing candidate has a propensity to conduct that might pose a threat to the safety of the public.

It is arguable that such a ruling as that by the B.C. Court of Appeal could apply to other provinces, since most provincial human rights laws contain similar provisions with respect to discrimination on the basis of a criminal record. Of course, employers and professional bodies cannot deny employment or the awarding of a licence or registration on the basis of race, creed, ethnic origin, sex, religion, marital status, physical or mental disability, or sexual orientation either.

A recent disciplinary decision from New Brunswick illustrates the type of matters considered and disciplinary action that may be taken against a nurse. In this particular case, the Nurses Association of New Brunswick's discipline committee considered the case of a nurse who had treated at least two patients in his care in a rough manner, had used verbal and nonverbal inappropriate behaviour against other nursing staff and patients, and had demonstrated a serious lack of judgement in the care of patients and lack of respect for their dignity. The association ordered that his registration be revoked and that the nurse pay costs of $10,000 to the association prior to any application for readmission to the practice of nursing in New Brunswick. The committee further ruled that he could not reapply for admission for the next three years (see the Nurses Association of New Brunswick Web site for a summary of this case: http://www.nanb.nb.ca/index.cfm?include=protection2).

## Penalties

The penalties faced by the nurse who has been found guilty of professional misconduct, or who has been found incompetent, include:

- Censure or reprimand before the committee or in writing
- Conditions placed on the nurse's right to practise, including a requirement that he or she take additional courses or education and pass further examinations

- Suspension from practice for a specified period of time (e.g., for the completion of such additional training or education)
- Revocation of the nurse's right to practise and expulsion from the nursing association, as discussed above in the New Brunswick example

## Appeals

The decision of the professional conduct committee as to the finding of guilt, the penalty handed down, or both may be appealed to the board of directors or the council of the association by notification in writing within a specified time. If the decision on the appeal is still unfavourable, the nurse may appeal, in most provinces, to the provincial superior court (in Alberta, to the Alberta Court of Appeal, which may order a new hearing before the Alberta Court of Queen's Bench). Prince Edward Island, Nova Scotia, and Yukon do not allow further appeals to the courts, although an application for judicial review can always be brought to challenge the decision on the basis of the denial of natural justice, fraud, or the committee's having exceeded its jurisdiction. In the Northwest Territories and Newfoundland and Labrador, the decision of the Trial Division of the Supreme Court on an appeal from a disciplinary committee's decision is final and may not be appealed further to their respective Courts of Appeal. In Ontario, appeals are taken to the Health Professions Appeal and Review Board (see *Ministry of Health Appeal and Review Boards Act*, 1998). In Quebec, they are taken to the **Professions Tribunal** (see *Professional Code*, Quebec).

The penalties that may be levied against the guilty professional include:

- Revocation or suspension of the certificate of registration
- Imposition of terms, conditions, or limitations on the certificate for a specified period of time, including criteria that must be satisfied before the restrictions, terms, or conditions may be lifted
- A reprimand by the panel
- A fine

All provincial and territorial regulatory bodies may impose penalties, and those penalties vary across the country. In Ontario, for example, a professional who has been found guilty of sexual misconduct can be ordered to reimburse the College for expenses incurred in providing a program for therapy and counselling for patients who were sexually abused by professionals (*Health Professions Procedural Code* [*HPPC*], 1991, s. 51(2), para. 5.1). The guilty professional may also be reprimanded, and his or her licence may be revoked if the sexual abuse consisted of certain specified acts (*HPPC*, 1991, s. 51(5)). In such a case, the patient is allowed to make, and the panel must consider, a statement describing the impact that the abuse has had on him or her.

If a nurse's professional care demonstrates a lack of knowledge, skill, or judgement, or exhibits disregard for the welfare of a patient, the professional may be deemed incompetent.

If the professional's conduct demonstrates that he or she is unfit to continue to practise, or that his or her practice should be restricted, the committee may also find that professional incompetent to practise. This is different from a finding of professional misconduct.

Regardless of the nature of the finding, the panel must render its decision in writing and give it to all parties. The College is required to publish its decisions and the reasons for these, including the member's name if he or she requests it, in its annual report and in any other of its publications. (A member might make such a request, for example, if he or she has been cleared of any wrongdoing and wishes to make this known to colleagues and patients.)

## The Fitness to Practise Committee

It should be noted that not all provincial and territorial regulatory bodies have a fitness to practise committee. In British Columbia, for example, the inquiry committee is charged with reviewing, among other issues, the competence of a nurse member to engage in the practice of nursing. In Manitoba, this task is the responsibility of the investigation committee.

This section will specifically discuss the Ontario College of Nurse's fitness to practise committee as an example of the workings of a particular structure within the regulatory body responsible for reviewing a nurse's competence. As noted above, the process and particular regulatory sub-body responsible for carrying out such a function will vary by province or territory; however, many of the essential considerations and features described in this section will be similar among all provinces and territories.

The investigation of a nurse's fitness and capacity to practise does not necessarily raise questions of professional misconduct. The member's behaviour may be such that there is concern about his or her physical or mental abilities.

Inquiries as to a professional's capacity will usually be commenced by the registrar, using the extensive investigatory powers granted under the *Health Professions Procedural Code* (1991). If the registrar has reason to believe that the member in question may be incapacitated, the registrar must report the supporting findings to the executive committee for further action (*HPPC*, 1991, s. 57). If further action is warranted, and it has received the registrar's report or a referral from a panel of the complaints committee, the fitness to practise committee may appoint a board of inquiry to determine whether the professional is incapacitated. Some of that committee's members must be drawn from among the College's general membership. In this way, the professional's fitness to practise is evaluated by his or her peers.

As part of its inquiry, the board may order the member to undergo physical or psychological examinations conducted or ordered by a health professional (i.e., a physician or psychiatrist). Further, the member's licence may be suspended until he or she agrees to be examined or until the inquiry is complete (*HPPC*, 1991, s. 59). Upon conclusion of the inquiry, the board is required to submit its report to the executive committee, which, in turn, may refer it to the fitness to practise committee if it decides that further proceedings are necessary.

If the executive committee refers the report to the fitness to practise committee, the latter then selects a panel of at least three of its members to hold a hearing into the fitness of the professional to practise nursing. Unless the professional requests otherwise, the hearing must be closed (i.e., not public). The professional's request for a public hearing may be refused if this would compromise public security or any person's safety or privacy (*HPPC*, 1991, s. 68(2)). The professional is entitled to be represented by legal counsel at the hearing, as are any witnesses who will testify, including any person who may have suffered harm or have been otherwise affected by the member's conduct. Evidence at the hearing may include testimony by medical or psychiatric experts. However, the professional who is the subject of the hearing must be given a copy of the expert's report or a summary of the evidence before it is presented at the hearing.

If the panel concludes that the professional is incapacitated, his or her certificate of registration may be revoked or suspended, or conditions, terms, or restrictions may be imposed on it. If a certificate is revoked, the professional may apply to the registrar to have a new certificate issued or the suspension removed no earlier than one year after the suspension or revocation (*HPPC,* 1991, s. 72(1)).

## The Quality Assurance Committee

Several provinces' and territories' regulatory bodies, including those of Ontario (which will be discussed below) and British Columbia, have a quality assurance committee. In other provinces and territories, quality assurance is carried out by an investigations committee or the disciplinary committee itself. In Manitoba, this work is carried out by a continuing competence committee.

In Ontario, every health professions college is required under the *Regulated Health Professions Act* (*RHPA*) (1991) to establish a quality assurance committee whose task is to review and examine individual members' practices to identify incompetence, incapacity, professional misconduct, and, in particular, the sexual abuse of patients by health professionals. For example, if the executive committee, the complaints committee, or the Health Professions Board receives from the registrar a report of sexual remarks or behaviour directed toward a patient following an investigation into a member's conduct, it may refer the matter to the quality assurance committee.

The *HPPC* defines sexual abuse of a patient as "sexual intercourse or other forms of sexual relations between the member and the patient, touching of a sexual nature of the patient by the member, or behaviour or remarks of a sexual nature by the member towards the patient" (*HPPC*, 1991, s. 1(3)), unless it is touching, behaviour, or remarks of a clinical nature that are appropriate in the context of the treatment being provided by the member.

The quality assurance committee will conduct its own investigation into the professional's practice, not only to identify incompetence or incapacity but also to pinpoint inadequacies in their practice's operations and facilities. If the quality assurance committee believes that, based on its assessment, the professional may have committed an act of misconduct or may be incompetent or incapacitated, it may disclose the professional's name and the allegations against him or her to the executive committee. On receipt of such information, the committee would refer the matter to the discipline committee or to the fitness to practise committee, as required (*HPPC*, 1991, s. 79.1, 80.2, and 83).

## Controlled Acts

One of the distinctive features of several provinces' and territories' health professions regulation systems is that the law specifically defines which medical actions and procedures may be performed and who may perform and delegate them. In some provinces, such as British Columbia, these are known as "reserved acts" (*Nurses (Registered) and Nurse Practitioners Regulation*, 2005, s. 8.) In Ontario, they are called "controlled acts." In Saskatchewan, the specific acts that nurses are authorized to perform are set out in the bylaws of the Saskatchewan Registered Nurses' Association (*Saskatchewan Registered Nurses' Association Bylaws*, Bylaw VI, s. 3), made pursuant to the *Nursing Profession Act* of Saskatchewan. Rather than licensing nurses in areas of practice, its system focuses instead on specific acts. Thus, a registered nurse is not granted a blanket authorization to perform controlled procedures that the nurse believes to be a part of the profession. He or she may perform only those controlled acts that nurses are specifically authorized to perform given the nurse's specific qualifications and professional education. Needless to say, any act within the scope of nursing practice may be performed by a registered nurse or practical nurse unless it is specifically designated as a **controlled act** (or a **restricted act** in Manitoba or a *reserved act* in some other provinces), in which case that act may be performed by the nurse only if he or she is authorized by the *Regulated Health Professions Act*, the *HPPC*, or the *Nursing Act*, for example, to perform it.

In Ontario, the *RHPA* strictly regulates health care controlled acts (*RHPA*, 1991, s. 27) and states who may perform and delegate them. In addition, the registration committee or the registrar may impose restrictions or limitations upon a specific nurse's right to practise nursing.

The *RHPA* sets out 13 controlled acts that may be performed only by members of a professional college who are authorized by the college's governing statute and regulations (see *Nursing Act*, 1991, s. 4) to perform the controlled act (*RHPA*, 1991, s. 27(1)(a)). Of these 13, three acts may be performed by nurses in accordance with the *Nursing Act*, 1991. These are specifically referred to as "authorized acts." If the particular act is to be delegated, it may be delegated only by a member so authorized and only in conformity with the regulations made under the statute governing the member's profession. For example, if a registered nurse is authorized to administer a particular substance by injection (a controlled act under *RHPA*, s. 27(2), para. 5), then he or she may delegate the act to a registered practical nurse, provided that the regulations under the *Nursing Act* allow such a **delegation** and that all procedures for delegation set out in the regulations are followed.

The three authorized acts are:

- Performing a procedure below the dermis, surface of the mucous membrane, the cornea, or in or below the surface of the teeth (including scaling teeth)
- Administering a substance by injection or inhalation
- Putting an instrument, hand, or finger beyond the external ear canal, the point in the nasal passages where they normally narrow, the larynx, the urethral opening, the labia majora, the anal verge, or into an artificial opening into the body (*Nursing Act*, 1991, s. 4)

In addition, nurses with an extended certificate of registration may perform additional acts, provided they have met certain standards of education:

(1) Communicating to a patient or to his or her representative a diagnosis as to the cause of the patient's symptoms, a disease or disorder that can be identified from,
    i.    the patient's health history,
    ii.   the findings of a comprehensive health examination, or
    iii.  the results of any laboratory tests or other tests and investigations that the nurse is authorized to order or perform.
(2) Ordering the application of a form of energy prescribed by the regulations under this Act.
(3) Prescribing a drug designated in the regulations.
(4) Administering, by injection or inhalation, a drug that the member may prescribe under paragraph 3. (*Nursing Act*, 1991, s. 5.1)

## Exemptions

In Ontario, a nonregulated person may also perform certain of the 13 controlled acts if he or she is assisting someone with routine activities of daily living. This would apply, for example, in the case of a home care worker or family member who is assisting a handicapped person in certain daily tasks that the person cannot do unassisted. There has been some concern with this particular exemption. It is felt that persons involved in providing attendant care to the disabled will fall outside the regulatory scheme of the *RHPA*, thereby defeating the purpose of regulation. On the other hand, advocates for the disabled argued prior to passage of this legislation that they did not want activities of daily life of the disabled to be subject to governmental regulation and potential interference, which would have occurred had this exemption not been included.

Acts that are not controlled that are done in the context of treating a person by spiritual means in accordance with the tenets of the religion of the person giving the treatment are permitted (*RHPA*, 1991, s. 29(1)(c)). It is difficult, however, to envision a situation in which some of these enumerated acts would be performed in a spiritual or religious ceremony, especially procedures below the dermis or the administration of substances by injection or inhalation. Certain acts, such as religious circumcision, which is typically performed by a moil, are expressly permitted (*RHPA*, 1991, s. 29(1)(c)).

The *RHPA* also allows certain communication when it is made in the course of counselling a person about emotional, social, educational, or spiritual matters, provided that the communication is not one that a health profession act authorizes a member to make (*RHPA*, 1991, s. 29(2)). Equally significant, the *RHPA* does not apply to Aboriginal healers or midwives when they are providing their services to members of an Aboriginal community (*RHPA*, 1991, s. 35(1)). This would, for example, exempt Aboriginal healers providing services to residents of a First Nations reserve or members of a First Nations band. However, if the Aboriginal healer is a member of a college, he or she is subject to its jurisdiction, regulations, and bylaws.

## Delegation

The Ontario *RHPA* allows nurses to delegate the performance of specific controlled acts to nonqualified persons. This allows a greater degree of flexibility in the provision of health care services.

The fact that persons are permitted to perform certain acts (e.g., administering a drug, communicating a diagnosis, or putting an instrument or hand in natural or artificial body openings) in the context of treating a member of their household can give rise to some interesting situations. For example, suppose a registered nurse in charge of and responsible for the care of a terminally ill patient is asked by a member of the family to be permitted to administer morphine by injection to the patient to control pain. The *RHPA* would allow this provided that the nurse, having delegated a controlled act, ensured that the family member had been adequately instructed in the administration of injections and that all necessary procedures had been followed.

## Other Offences

Nursing statutes of virtually all provinces and territories set out various offences that are designed to prevent unauthorized practice and contravention of the laws and regulations. In B.C., for example, these include a provision that forbids a person from providing a health service when that person is not registered with the regulatory body that regulates the service (e.g., nursing) unless the person provides the service under the supervision of a registered member (see *Health Professions Act*, R.S.B.C., 1996, c. 183, s. 13).

An important distinction should be drawn at this point. The term *competent* is usually used to mean that a professional has the necessary skills, experience, and knowledge to carry out the duties of the particular position. But saying such a professional is "competent" is quite different from saying that the professional is "registered" or "authorized" to perform those duties. The latter expressions convey the notion that an official regulatory agency has assessed and passed judgement upon that person's skills and knowledge and has found these to meet the requirements of regulations. For example, an employment agency that found a position for a private nurse who was not a member or was not properly qualified in B.C., and that knew that that person was unable to perform any of the controlled acts that nurses are permitted to perform, has contravened the law.

To illustrate, offences in Ontario include:

- Obtaining a registration certificate from any one of the colleges by false pretences or knowingly assisting a person to do this (*HPPC*, 1991, s. 92)
- Obstructing an investigator appointed by the registrar of the College in an investigation into professional misconduct, incompetency, or incapacity of a member (*HPPC*, 1991, s. 93(2))
- Disclosing any information revealed at a hearing or inquiry that is closed to the public (*HPPC*, 1991, s. 93(1))
- Failing to permit an assessor of the quality assurance committee of a college to inspect a member's records or premises (*HPPC*, 1991, s. 93(3))
- Failing to report a member (of the same or any other college) when there are reasonable grounds to believe that that member has sexually abused a patient (*HPPC*, 1991, s. 93(4))

Finally, no professional may treat a person if it is reasonably foreseeable that serious physical harm may result from the treatment or advice, or from an omission of such treatment or advice (*RHPA*, 1991, s. 30(1)). Counselling about emotional, social, educational, or spiritual matters, however, is not prohibited by the *RHPA*. Despite this, it would certainly be unethical to counsel someone if psychological harm might foreseeably result. Perhaps including psychological or mental harm in this prohibition would have placed too onerous a burden on health professionals, as the mind, its workings, and the genesis of mental disorders are still imperfectly understood. Others would argue that this gap in the law is a further example that what is legal is not necessarily ethical.

## Standards of Practice

Nursing regulatory bodies and legislation establish standards of nursing practice and professional behaviours, which serve as yardsticks to measure the actions and competence of nurses in Canada and to clarify expectations for the delivery of safe, effective, and ethical nursing care. Provincial regulatory bodies adopt these standards but may choose to adapt them to their setting. Professional and clinical standards make explicit nurses' accountability to the regulatory bodies, their employers, patients and clients, and the public (see, for example, the Web sites of the College of Registered Nurses of British Columbia, the Ontario College of Nurses, and the College & Association of Registered Nurses of Alberta). These standards, which are considered minimum, are used to evaluate the actions of any nurse who is the subject of a complaint or disciplinary process within the regulatory body or of a legal proceeding. Further, these standards are considered a component of the performance appraisal of nurses and serve as a guide for ongoing professional development and education.

It is important to note that these practice and professional standards are of great relevance in terms of negligence and malpractice issues, as is discussed in Chapter 7. The practice standards are directly relevant evidence of the standard of care a nurse is expected to meet and against which his or her actual conduct will be judged in a professional negligence law suit. The standards include details on proper documentation and charting in the course of patient care, and failure to meet these standards may result in a finding that a nurse has breached the standard. Where that breach has resulted in harm or injury to a patient, a nurse may be found legally responsible in an action of negligence brought against him or her by the patient. In any court proceedings, testimony from a qualified nursing professional as to the appropriate and relevant standard in a given clinical setting or treatment situation would suffice to prove the standard. Thus, these standards are useful, not only to ensure patient care of the highest quality but also as a measure against which negligent nursing practice is judged.

Nursing standards reflect the values of the nursing profession and hold nurses accountable to the public with respect to the delivery of safe, competent nursing care. In general, most standards of practice:

- Provide a guide for safe practice
- Describe the responsibilities and accountabilities of the nurse
- Provide performance criteria
- Ensure continuing competence
- Interpret nursing's scope of practice
- Provide direction for nursing education
- Facilitate peer review
- Provide a foundation for research-based practice
- Provide benchmarks for quality improvement (College of Nurses of Ontario, 2002)

For example, the College of Nurses of Ontario (CNO) defines "standards of practice" as "the provincial legislation, regulations, standards, policies and guidelines which establish CNO's expectations in relation to member practice and conduct." Examples of the standards produced by the College include CNO's *Guidelines for Professional Behaviour*, the professional misconduct regulations; *Nursing Documentation Standards*; and the *Professional Standards for Registered Nurses and Registered Practical Nurses in Ontario* (College of Nurses of Ontario, 2002).

The College of Registered Nurses of British Columbia has identified, for example, six professional standards that establish the level of performance nurses are required to meet. These include:

- Responsibility and accountability
- Specialized body of knowledge
- Competent application of knowledge
- Code of ethics
- Provision of service in the public interest
- Self-regulation

Professional standards are established by all regulatory bodies across the country. They reflect the philosophy of nursing practice and ethical standards and codes. Professional standards focus on accountability to the public, knowledge, application of knowledge, ethics, continued competence, and professional behaviour. For each standard, there are usually indicators or descriptors, which assist in clarifying the standard's application to practice and professional behaviour. The College of Nurses of Ontario has identified key indicators, which include the concepts of "communication, leadership, critical thinking and legal professional requirements." They are a guide to the evaluation of the nurse and serve as a benchmark with respect to the extent that the standard is achieved.

## The Responsibility of Regulatory Bodies for the Ongoing Competence of Nurses

Colleges are also responsible for introducing and maintaining mechanisms or processes to evaluate the ongoing competence of nurses.

In Ontario, a quality improvement program, called the CNO Quality Assurance Program, is in place, and all nurses who are registered with the College are expected to participate in it. The program has three parts: reflective practice, competence assessment, and practice setting consultation. Each nurse must participate in one of these components. Full details and documentation concerning the program can be found on the CNO's Web site.

The reflective practice component of this quality improvement program is intended to identify strengths and improvement opportunities. The process involves a self-assessment based on the standards and guidelines for practice, feedback from peers, the development of a learning plan, implementation of the plan, and evaluation.

Other means of evaluation of a nurse's competence to practise include formal processes, such as exams, and observation in the clinical setting. On a regular basis, the College randomly selects nurses from the registrant list to be assessed. Also, an individual nurse or a practice setting may choose to volunteer for an assessment, or the College may initiate an assessment based on a referral from a statutory committee (e.g., as part of a complaint or disciplinary process) (CNO, 2002, p. 1).

In Nova Scotia, the College's Continuing Competence Program (CCP) is a mandatory requirement for licensing as a registered nurse. Continuing competence is defined by this college as "the ongoing ability of a registered nurse to integrate and apply the knowledge, skills, judgment, and interpersonal attributes required to practise safely and ethically in a designated role and setting" (College of Registered Nurses of Nova Scotia, 2007).

The College recognized that registered nurses use a variety of approaches to maintaining competence, including formal education programs and consultation with colleagues. The Continuing Competence Program (CCP) is a formal mechanism to further develop and record these processes, and is based on the philosophy that registered nurses are competent and committed to lifelong learning. A tool called Building Your Profile™, developed with the input of hundreds of registered nurses in Nova Scotia, is "designed to maintain and enhance the continuing competence of registered nurses by engaging them in the processes of reflective practice, lifelong learning and the integration of learning into practice."

The tool formalizes processes most registered nurses already engage in: reflecting on the standards and code of ethics; identifying strengths and learning opportunities; developing learning plans; and implementing and evaluating learning plans (College of Registered Nurses of Nova Scotia, 2007). Those applying for or renewing their licence must complete the tool or an equivalent to meet the requirements of the College.

In Alberta, the CARNA Continuing Competence Program is also based on a reflective practice model. It involves the nurse using the CARNA Nursing Practice Standards to review his or her nursing practice to determine and address learning needs. Its Web site, https://www.nurses.ab.ca/Carna/Login.aspx, provides online guidelines for nurses to meet their Continuing Competence Program requirements.

As in other provinces, in British Columbia, the same requirement exists for nurses to meet continuing competence requirements annually. These include minimum practice hours and completion of a personal practice review. The *Registration Standard of Continuing Competence for Registered Nurses* sets out the expectations for nurses, including the "continuing competence requirements (practice hours and personal practice review) that registered nurses must meet to be eligible to renew practising registration in B.C." (College of Registered Nurses of British Columbia, 2007, p. 1).

All colleges across Canada have mechanisms to evaluate the continuing competence of nurses, and most involve a component of reflective practice and an alignment with established professional and clinical standards. Consult the Web sites of the provincial and territorial colleges for a more comprehensive review of their programs.

Though legislation and regulatory bodies establish broad standards of professional practice, standards are developed more specifically in particular organizations or institutions to represent nursing practice in that setting. Nurses are required to meet these standards, and their actions are evaluated accordingly. Standards of practice also exist for specialty areas within nursing. For example, standards of practice for a nurse in critical care will differ from those for a nurse in a community or psychiatric setting.

## Criminal Background Checks

There has been an increased focus in recent years upon the obligations of professional nursing regulatory bodies to perform adequate criminal background checks on new candidates for admission to nursing. There is a corresponding obligation on employers of nurses to undertake similar checks on nursing candidates. Many jurisdictions, including those of Canada, the United States, and the United Kingdom, have enacted laws to provide for such mandatory checks for both nursing students and nurses seeking employment. The primary aim of any system of criminal background checks is ideally to exclude people one would wish to while not excluding people one would wish to employ (Devitt, 2004). The intent of such criminal check procedures is, ultimately, to exclude potential nursing candidates, both students and prospective nurse employees, from the practice of nursing in such cases as, owing to a prior criminal record, such persons would pose a threat to the safety of vulnerable patients.

In 1996, for instance, British Columbia passed the *Criminal Records Review Act* (*CRRA*). This law provides a scheme for initiating criminal record checks by a variety of persons and bodies from a number of professions, including social workers, health professionals, and teachers (*CRRA*, sched. 2). The main purpose of the Act is to "help prevent the physical and sexual abuse of children by requiring individuals to whom this Act applies to undergo criminal record checks" (*CRRA*, s. 2(1)). It requires governing bodies to do criminal record checks on all members applying for registration (*CRRA*, s. 13). Those who wish to become registered, licensed practical, or psychiatric nurses in British Columbia must authorize the governing body to initiate a criminal record search (*CRRA*, s. 15(1)). If such authorization is not provided, the member cannot be cleared to work with children. Furthermore, if a nurse (or other professional) refuses to authorize a criminal record check, the board of directors of the governing body must take that refusal into account in deciding whether to register the nurse or to set conditions on his or her practice (*Health Professions Act*, 1996, s. 20(3)). A person who seeks registration as a member of a professional governing body and has a criminal record including a "relevant offence" will be subject to further examination by that professional body. The regulatory body will have to determine the nature of the offence; the time that has elapsed since the offence took place; the circumstances of the offence, including the age of the applicant at the time of the offence; and any other relevant factors, including any indications that the applicant might attempt a similar offence in the future and any attempts at rehabilitation. The main purpose of such an enquiry is to determine whether the conviction or outstanding charge indicates that the individual presents a risk of physical or sexual abuse to children. In this way, policymakers in British Columbia have provided the nursing (and other professional) bodies the means to attempt to ensure the health and safety of children and to stem the flood of cases involving the physical and sexual abuse of children by persons entrusted with their care and education.

In Ontario, the general regulation made under the *Nursing Act* (1994) provides that a person applying for a certificate of registration of any class (i.e., temporary, general, special assignment, etc.) must be able to show that he or she has not "been found guilty of a criminal offence or an offence under the *Controlled Drugs and Substances Act* (Canada) or the *Food and Drugs Act* (Canada)" and that he or she has not been subject to a finding of professional misconduct or disciplinary proceedings in another jurisdiction (i.e., another province, territory, state, or country). This is essentially a mandatory self-reporting obligation. Since January 1, 2005, the Ontario College of Nurses has required all applicants for registration or reinstatement to provide a recent Canadian Police Information Centre Criminal Record Synopsis (known as a "CPIC check").

The requirement of criminal background checks for nursing students and prospective nursing employees raises many ethical and legal issues. If a potential candidate for employment as a nurse denies having a criminal record but a subsequent check by a prospective employer health care institution reveals one, the employer may decide that the candidate's denial demonstrates that he or she is untrustworthy and deny employment on this basis (Devitt, 2004, p. 38). But what should such an employer do in cases in which the candidate has, in fact, disclosed a criminal record? Of course, the nature of the offence should be carefully considered because not all offences lead to the conclusion that the candidate may pose a threat to the safety of patients. This is a difficult area for prospective employers, and there are no clear-cut answers. One noteworthy pitfall of a criminal record check that should be borne in mind is that it reveals a record of a criminal act committed at a past point in time. It may not reveal ongoing issues, such as substance abuse or trustworthiness. It might also note criminal activity that occurred a very long time ago during an applicant's youth, which may not be relevant to his or her nursing practice (for example, possession of a controlled substance such as marijuana or underaged drinking).

## Some Disciplinary Decisions

The following decisions illustrate some of the disciplinary matters heard by regulatory bodies across Canada and are provided as examples for further discussion.

### Decision 1—Ontario

A registered practical nurse member of the Ontario College of Nurses was found guilty of three counts of professional misconduct in that on three separate occasions, with respect to three separate patients, the nurse failed to take a blood sugar reading pursuant to a physician's order. In each of the three cases, the nurse subsequently documented that she had taken such readings when, in fact, she had not. She was found guilty, not only of having failed to take the readings but also of having falsified records relating to her practice by claiming to have taken the readings when she had not done so. The nurse pleaded guilty to all three counts. She had been an RPN since 1977 and was a part-time employee of the health care institution where she worked at the time the acts of misconduct were committed. She had also just ended a full-time shift at another institution when her part-time shift began. Her part-time employment had been terminated when her employer discovered the acts. During the disciplinary hearings, she admitted that she was tired on the day that these acts were committed and that her judgement had been impaired as a result. She fully cooperated with the College, was forthright, and took full responsibility for her actions. The disciplinary committee, after finding her guilty on all counts, ordered that she appear before the committee at a later date to be reprimanded; that her registration be suspended for 60 days; that on return to practice, she inform the director of Investigations and Hearings of her new place of employment; that she supply any prospective new employer with a copy of the committee's decision; and that her new employer advise the committee that he or she is aware of the decision and has received a copy of the proceedings.

### Decision 2—Manitoba

A registered nurse was found guilty of professional misconduct for:

- Having obtained medications for patients without a physician's orders
- Having given a security guard at the health care institution where she worked keys to the narcotics cupboard

- Collecting sick benefits at the same time she was receiving overtime pay
- Continuing to practise after receiving doses of narcotics
- Failing to follow warnings and cautions in the Compendium of Pharmaceuticals and Specialties (CPS) prior to prescribing narcotics and controlled substances to patients
- Diagnosing a condition for which she was not familiar with the Clinical Practice Guidelines
- Failing to follow the Clinical Practice Guidelines when prescribing medications
- Failing to report significant findings to the physician
- Making numerous errors and failing to document these on patients' charts and records

She pleaded guilty to all the charges and had the following conditions imposed on her nursing practice entitlement:

1. For the duration of the order, the nurse was to provide to the College written notification within 30 days of each and every change in place of nursing employment or move to another jurisdiction and was to provide the name and address of her employer and the nature of employment.
2. Following a return to nursing practice, the nurse was required to inform her nursing employer(s) of the College's order in its entirety and provide written proof that she had so informed the employer to the College within 30 days.
3. For the duration of the order, the nurse was further required to request any nursing employer(s) to immediately report to the College any suspension or termination of her employment.
4. For the duration of the order, the nurse was to provide to the College written notification of each and every change in her address or telephone number within 30 days.
5. She was to undergo a competence assessment within three months of the date of the order, by a facility agreeable to the College, to determine her competence in pharmacology, documentation, and physical assessment. She was also required to pay all costs for the competence assessment.
6. Following the competence assessment, the nurse was to successfully complete and pay all costs for the courses recommended by the competence assessment.
7. She was not to engage in sole practice until she had successfully completed the courses recommended in the competence assessment.
8. Until the nurse had successfully completed the courses recommended in the competence assessment, she was to limit her practice to a setting where another registered nurse was physically present at all times.
9. Within one month of the date of the order, the nurse was to develop a professional mentor relationship with a nursing colleague in a similar nursing role to enable ongoing professional dialogue regarding professional nursing practice and issues, and she had to advise the College of the name of the mentor.

10. The nurse was to ensure that reports concerning the topics and issues discussed during the professional interactions with her mentor were sent to the College every three months for a period of one year and then every six months for the duration of the order.

11. For the duration of the order, the nurse was required to authorize her nursing employer(s) to report in writing to the College every four months regarding her practice in relation to the *Standards of Practice for Registered Nurses*. The reports were to continue for a period of one year following completion of the courses recommended in the competence assessment. The reports were to address the member's practice with respect to client assessment; appropriate interventions including medication administration; documentation; and communication. These reports had to address all of the standards set out in the *Standards of Practice for Registered Nurses* and indicate that the nurse was meeting all standards at an acceptable level.

12. Within four months of the date of the order, the nurse was to complete and submit a paper to demonstrate learning and insight, which was to contain:

    a.  A description of the incidents that prompted the investigation, as well as practice issues raised in the investigation. This description would include but was not limited to issues with medication administration, medication record keeping, documentation, physical assessment, and nursing interventions.

    b.  Using the *Standards of Practice for Registered Nurses* and the *Code of Ethics for Registered Nurses*, the nurse was to discuss and evaluate how, in these instances, professional conduct such as critical thinking, judgement, documentation, and ethical conduct including responsibility and accountability deviated from the established standards and ethics of nursing practice.

    c.  She was also to discuss the impact of these incidents on future practice.

    d.  Following completion of the paper, she was to review the paper with the Coordinator, Complaints, of the College by no later than one month after the completion date.

13. She was to give all necessary consents to the College for reports contained within the order.

14. She was to pay all costs incurred by the College in monitoring compliance with the agreement.

15. The onus would be on the nurse to provide evidence satisfactory to the College that the conditions set out in the order were completed.

16. Any breach of any term or terms of the order would be deemed to be professional misconduct and grounds for disciplinary action against the nurse.

17. The order was to remain in effect for three years, and if the nurse, at any time during the term of the order was not employed as a registered nurse, then the obligations under Sections 7, 9, and 11, of the order were to be continued until such time as the nurse had completed three years of employment as a registered nurse.

## Summary

This chapter has reviewed the basic structures, roles, and workings of the various professional regulatory nursing bodies in Canada. An overview of common approaches was provided with some specific examples of the function of regulatory bodies in various provinces and territories. It is important for the student to review the regulations in his or her province or territory. It is essential that nurses understand the expectations associated with being a member of a regulated profession and the responsibilities and obligations that come with that privilege. Regulatory bodies identify standards of professional and clinical practice, which provide clarity to the public with regard to what they can expect from nurses. Hence, these standards are significant not only in the ongoing evaluation of nurses with respect to safe, competent, and ethical care but also in measuring the nurse's behaviour with respect to legal and professional expectations. The public interest to ensure the integrity of nurses is demonstrated through an evolving requirement to determine whether a person entering the profession has a criminal record. Though there are challenges with respect to this process and the rights of those who have been rehabilitated, this practice demonstrates the high standards to which nurses are held in Canadian society.

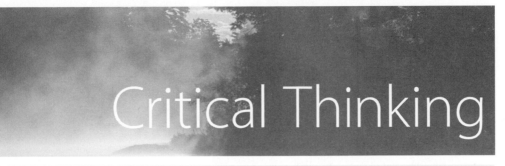

Critical Thinking

## Discussion Points

1. Discuss the structure and purpose of the professional nursing body in your province.
2. How does your provincial nursing governing body handle complaints against nurses? Describe the steps in its disciplinary process. Suggest ways in which the process might be improved or be made more accountable to nurses and to the public.
3. What role do governing bodies play in educating nursing professionals?
4. What role should such bodies play in shaping legislation affecting nursing?
5. How do the standards of practice of the regulatory body in your province compare with the standards within the organization where you are presently employed or receiving clinical experience? How do these standards relate to your curriculum as a student nurse?
6. How are the standards of practice in your setting measured? What mechanisms are in place to ensure these standards are maintained? Can you think of ways to improve this process?

## References

### Statutes

*Criminal Records Review Act*, R.S.B.C. 1996, c. 86 (British Columbia).
*Fair Access to Regulated Professions Act, 2006,* S.O. 2006, c. 31 (Ontario).
*Health Professions Act*, R.S.B.C. 1996, c. 183 (British Columbia).
*Health Professions Act*, R.S.A. 2000, c. H-7 (Alberta).
*Health Professions Procedural Code*, 1991, S.O. 1991, c. 18., Sched. 2 (Ontario).
*Human Rights Code*, R.S.B.C. 1996, c. 210 (British Columbia).
*Ministry of Health Appeal and Review Boards Act*, 1998, S.O. 1998, c. 18, Sched. H (Ontario).
*Nurses Act*, S.N.B. 1984, c. 71, as amended. (New Brunswick).
*Nurses Act*, R.S.Q. c. I-8 (Quebec).
*Nursing Act*, 1991, S.O. 1991, c. 32 (Ontario).
*Nursing Profession Act*, S.N.W.T. 2003, c. 15 (Northwest Territories and Nunavut).
*Pharmaceutical Profession Act*, R.S.A. 2000, c. P-12 (Alberta).
*Professional Code*, R.S.Q., c. C-26 (Quebec).
*Registered Nurses Act*, C.C.S.M., c. R40 (Manitoba).

*Registered Nurses Act*, R.S.N. 1990, c. R-9 (Newfoundland).

*Registered Nurses Act*, S.N.S. 2001, c. 10 (Nova Scotia).

*Registered Nurses Act*, S.P.E.I., 2004, c. 15 (Prince Edward Island).

*Registered Nurses Act*, R.S.P.E.I., 1988, c. R-8.1, s.1(s) (Prince Edward Island).

*The Registered Nurses Act, 1988*, S.S. 1988–89, c. R-12.2 (Saskatchewan).

*Registered Nurses Profession Act*, R.S.Y. 2002, c. 194 (Yukon).

*Regulated Health Professions Act*, 1991, S.O. 1991, c. 18 (Ontario).

## Regulations

*General Regulation Under the Nursing Act,* 1991, O. Reg 275/94 (Ontario).

*Nurses (Registered) and Nurse Practitioners Regulation*, B.C. Reg. 233/2005 (British Columbia).

*Registered Nurses Profession Regulation*, Alta. Reg. 232/2005 (Alberta).

*Registration and Licensing of Nurses Regulations*, P.E.I. Reg. E.C. 93/06 (Prince Edward Island).

## Regulatory Body Bylaws

*Saskatchewan Registered Nurses' Association Bylaws*, Bylaw VI (Saskatchewan).

## Court Decisions

*Mans v. Council of Licensed Practical Nurses* (1990), 14 C.H.R.R. D/221; aff'd. (1993), 77 B.C.L.R. (2d) 47 (C.A.).

## Texts and Articles

Canadian Nurses Association. (2007). *Framework for the practice of registered nurses in Canada.* Ottawa: Author. Retrieved from http://www.cna-aiic.ca/CNA/documents/pdf/publications/RN_Framework_Practice_2007_e.pdf.

College of Nurses of Ontario. (2002). *Professional standards for registered nurses and registered practical nurses in Ontario.* Retrieved from http://www.cno.org/docs/prac/41006_ProfStds.pdf.

College of Registered Nurses of British Columbia. (2007). Registration standard of continuing competence for registered nurses. Vancouver, BC: Author. Retrieved from http://www.crnbc.ca/downloads/458.pdf.

College of Registered Nurses of Nova Scotia. (2007). Continuing competence program. Retrieved from http://www.crnns.ca/default.asp?mn=414.1116.1124.1472.

Devitt, P. (2004, November). Safeguarding children through police checks: A discussion. *Paediatric Nursing, 16*(9), 36–38.

# Chapter 6

## Consent to Treatment

### Learning Objectives

The purpose of this chapter is to enable you to understand:

- The foundation of consent in law and ethics
- The concept of informed consent
- The principle of autonomy and its relationship to informed consent
- The concept of competence and capacity
- The relationship of consent to the tort of battery
- The various types of, and approaches to, consent
- The rights of patients to refuse consent to medical or health care
- The nurse's role in ensuring that informed consent takes place
- How legal rules and ethical theory apply to hypothetical case studies and actual case law
- Consent challenges with respect to the incompetent adult and to children
- Professional responsibilities in emergency situations
- The concept of proxy or substitute consent
- Consent legislation in various provinces

## Introduction

NURSES INTERACT DIRECTLY WITH the mind, body, and spirit of those they care for. Many nursing actions require physical touch. Though intended to promote recovery or to relieve pain and suffering, such actions are not without risk and could result in pain or harm to a person.

Legally, to touch another person without permission constitutes battery. Individuals in Canadian society have the right to determine the course of their lives (so long as they cause no harm to themselves or others), as well as the right to privacy.

The intimacy and integrity of the nurse–client relationship demand that nurses ensure protection of and respect for the rights of their patients and clients. This is achieved through standards, policies, guidelines, legislation, and rules regarding **consent**, which is the subject of this chapter.

## Consent in Law and Ethics

As discussed in Chapter 3, the *Code of Ethics for Registered Nurses* requires that nurses respect and promote the autonomy of clients. Nurses ensure that autonomy is respected by supporting patients or clients in expressing their values and health needs, and by ensuring that they have the right information, guidance, and support to make informed decisions and choices. The Code makes clear that it is the nurse's ethical responsibility to:

- Provide patients or clients with the information they need to make informed decisions about their health and well-being, while respecting the wishes of those who are capable yet do not want such information
- Try to ensure that clear and accurate health information is provided to individuals, families, groups, and populations
- Respect the choices of individuals who make decisions based on family or community values or who choose lifestyles or health treatment plans with which you do not agree
- Ensure he or she has informed consent to provide care, and cease treatment if consent is withdrawn
- Be aware of the powerful position he or she may have in the view of patients or clients, and show caution not to abuse that power
- Stand up for people in his or her care if their health is being compromised by factors beyond their control
- Help families to comprehend a patient's or client's decisions when they disagree with the decisions made
- Assist persons whose capacity for making informed decisions becomes impaired by including them in making choices insofar as they are able
- Adhere to the provincial or territorial law on capacity assessment and substitute decision making if a patient is clearly *incapable* of consent

- Consider the best interests and any known wishes or advance directives of the patient or client (Canadian Nurses Association, 2008)

Founded on the principle of autonomy, these responsibilities stress the significance of informed choice. Consent may be given in writing or verbally, or simply implied (e.g., by holding out an arm to have blood drawn), but to be valid, it must be based on the relevant information required by the patient or client to make that choice. Consent must be free from coercion, and it must be made by someone capable of that level of decision.

The following case scenario highlights the legal and ethical challenges associated with consent.

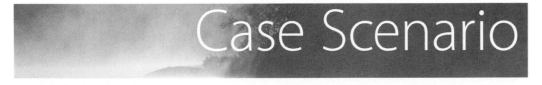

## WHOSE DECISION?

Doris, a widow 75 years of age, lives alone in a suburban bungalow that she and her late husband owned for 30 years. Her few close friends have died in the past few years. She has two grown children, a son and a daughter, both of whom live in another city. Over the past six or seven months, Doris's general health has declined. She has lost weight, has grown weak, and finds it difficult to leave home to go about her daily activities.

One particular week, Sam, her postman, notices that Doris's mail has not been taken in for two days. Sam is concerned; he knows Doris's daily routine, and she always informs him when she plans to go out of town. He knocks on the door but receives no answer. Alarmed, Sam calls the police, who, upon arrival at Doris's home, discover her lying semiconscious on the kitchen floor.

Doris is rushed to hospital. The attending physician makes a preliminary diagnosis of gastrointestinal bleeding and, since it is an emergency, orders a blood transfusion to stabilize her. A few days later, Doris is alert and apparently competent, but the nurses caring for her have noted some occasions when she seems confused as to her surroundings and does not know what day it is.

The physician tells Doris that her condition urgently warrants further tests. She becomes agitated and upset, fearing that the doctors will discover cancer and that she will soon die. Consequently, she refuses to authorize the tests. The members of the team know that any number of easily treatable factors could be causing the bleeding, and they are concerned that Doris's refusal of further investigation and treatment is not in her best interests. Some nurses question whether Doris, in her present state of mind, is capable of making such a decision.

The team wishes to involve her children, but Doris refuses to give any information that would enable contact. She does not want her family involved; she feels she has always been able to take care of herself and does not wish to worry her children.

continued on following page >>

Over the next few days, the team finds evidence that Doris's bleeding is recurring. Something must be done soon or she may die.

### Issues

1. Does Doris have the mental (and hence legal) capacity to make the decision to accept or refuse treatment?
2. Has Doris been given adequate opportunity to make an informed decision with respect to consent to treatment?
3. May the nurses or other team members legally and ethically disclose information pertaining to Doris's condition to her children, assuming they are able to contact them through their own efforts?
4. What are the competing ethical interests in this situation, and how can they be resolved?
5. May the team proceed with the investigation of Doris's condition on the assumption that she is not capable of giving or withholding consent?

### Discussion

In this case scenario, it is clear that the health care team cannot legally proceed without Doris's consent. If they do so, they may be liable for battery, as there is absolutely no consent here, let alone an informed one. Although the nurses and physicians are genuinely motivated by good faith and have Doris's best interests at heart, they are not free to substitute their own judgement and proceed on their own authority. Even if Doris is not mentally competent to consent (which is unclear, based on the details given), the team would not be authorized to proceed of its own accord.

Legal and ethical practice in this area require that, as a first step, a nurse or physician explain to Doris the procedures and their importance, as well as the risks of forgoing them. Also, Doris needs to be given enough time to make her decision. The team needs to respond to her questions and clarify any misconceptions. Nurses can play a role in exploring with patients the factors that might motivate their decisions (e.g., fear, past experiences, misconceptions). If Doris does consent, any subsequent withdrawal of that consent must be respected by the team members.

## Rights

The rights of patients extend to personal autonomy and the right to be informed of all risks material to a particular medical procedure, including the risks, both real and probable, in forgoing such treatment. (A material risk is one that a reasonable person would wish to know in deciding whether to consent to or forgo a given medical procedure.) These rights include the right of a patient not to be subjected to any treatment to which he or she has not given a free and informed consent, if mentally capable, and the moral right to be treated with respect, dignity, and courtesy by all health professionals. Legal rights are enforceable by the courts via the lawsuit. Moral rights are guaranteed by professionals who deem these part of their ethical and professional duty.

## Autonomy

As described in Chapter 2, the principle of autonomy supports the capable and competent patient's right to determine and act on a self-chosen plan. However, autonomy can be meaningful only when patients are given full and complete information as to their medical condition, the risks that the condition poses, and the benefits and drawbacks of any proposed treatment. The risks, material facts, and alternatives, including the consequences of nontreatment, must be explained to the competent patient. For example, if a patient refuses to ambulate or to practise deep breathing and coughing exercises following surgery, the nurse must explain the benefits and risks of such procedures and the consequences of not doing them. The explanation must be respectful and courteous, and the nurse must give the patient an opportunity to change his or her mind.

Competent persons have the right to refuse consent to treatment, regardless of whether that treatment is in their best interests. In some situations, nurses may face a conflict between respect for the individual's wishes and their obligation to help their patients and protect them from harm. But it is the duty of the nurse to support patients through such decisions and to respect their choices. It is also the nurse's responsibility to ensure that the patient has the information required to make such choices, as well as sufficient time to reflect on the alternatives available. Whether or not the nurse is part of an informed consent process, he or she is obligated to advocate for the patient if the patient has not been duly informed or if the patient's wishes have not been respected.

Free and informed consent to treatment is the hallmark of patient autonomy. It is recognized in both civil law and common law throughout Canada. Article 3 of the *Civil Code of Quebec*, for example, declares that every person possesses personality rights, which include the right to life, the right to personal integrity and inviolability, and respect of name, reputation, and privacy. This last-mentioned right of privacy is interesting in that it implies that individuals have the right to make decisions about their life and affairs free of governmental scrutiny and interference (except as permitted by law). This right to privacy is likewise implied in the United States Constitution and has been used to strike down laws restricting abortion rights in that country.

Suppose a patient is in the final phases of metastatic cancer: The cancer has spread to her bones, and she is in severe pain. The care plan is to turn her every two hours to prevent pressure sores and to minimize the likelihood of pneumonia. Turning causes her so much pain that she requires additional sedation, which results in extended drowsiness. Should the nurses give this patient the choice of being turned or not? Are there alternatives? As long as the patient understands, and is willing to accept, the consequences of not being turned, her decision is valid. She may choose to refuse turning in order to avoid the pain and the need for increased sedation.

If the patient is ill informed, or is misled by the information provided, any consent given is, in law, no consent at all. He or she may have decided differently if informed fully and properly. Since he or she has not been able to make a free and *informed* decision as to whether to undergo or forgo treatment, that patient's right to autonomy has been infringed.

Respect for the patient's autonomy is likewise compromised when, in the absence of consent, the health care professional presumes to decide whether treatment should proceed or decides what is and is not a material risk, all of which should be disclosed to the patient. (There are exceptions to the need for such consent in emergencies, as we will see later in this chapter.)

## Features of Consent

### Lack of Consent (Battery)

As discussed in Chapter 7, battery, a category of intentional tort, is legally defined as the touching of another, however slight, without that person's consent. Thus, it is an unwanted intrusion on the physical person. In a health care context, the administration of any medical treatment, surgical procedure, nursing action, diagnostic test, or other such intervention, no matter how necessary or beneficial to the patient's health and well-being in the health care professional's opinion, is forbidden unless the professional who is administering the treatment has obtained the patient's prior consent, or unless the patient has suffered a serious injury that renders him or her unable to give consent, and a lack of prompt medical attention would result in serious bodily harm or death.

It is a fundamental principle of ethics and the law that people who are mentally competent have the right to their bodily integrity and personal autonomy respecting health care treatment. This right applies even to mentally incompetent persons to the extent that their wishes, when they were competent, are known. If the patient is not competent, his or her prior wishes, as expressed to others or in an **advance directive** (discussed in Chapter 8), must be respected to the greatest extent possible. The final decision as to whether any nursing care, medical treatment, or plan of care should or should not proceed rests with the patient. The nurse or other health practitioner who proceeds without the patient's consent runs the risk of being found liable in a civil lawsuit for battery or, if he or she has carelessly informed the patient and harm results, for negligence.

The required conditions of a truly informed consent are as follows:

- The consent must be given voluntarily. There must be no coercion or undue pressure from another person to obtain that consent.
- The patient must be told of all material risks inherent in a proposed procedure, together with its benefits and drawbacks, as well as the risks of forgoing the treatment. The patient must understand the treatment options and benefits.
- The consent given must be specific to the proposed treatment or procedure. For example, a consent to an appendectomy does not authorize the removal of other infected or diseased tissues unrelated to that condition.

- The consent must specify who will perform the procedure or treatment. If a patient has consented to its performance by a particular specialist, this would not authorize the substitution of another, less qualified, or different type of health care practitioner.
- The patient must be legally capable. A minor under a certain age may not be legally qualified to consent, depending on the province.
- Similarly, in most provinces, mental incompetence renders persons legally incapable of consenting unless they are capable of understanding the nature and consequences of the procedure, notwithstanding their mental condition.

## Considerations for Nursing Practice

It is extremely stressful to be placed in a situation in which one has to make very difficult choices—for example, whether to accept treatment that in itself may be life-threatening or may have serious side effects, or when making a decision that may influence the well-being of a child. Nurses have the responsibility to do all they can to enable a decision-making process that is thoughtful and reflective. The following strategies serve as a guide for nurses in ensuring not only respect for one's autonomy and right to informed consent but also that the process itself is ethical.

- If possible, ensure the environment is suitable to the interaction between the patient and the provider obtaining consent. It is important to take into consideration issues of privacy, comfort, and equality. The perceived balance of power may be mitigated when both patient and provider are facing each other at eye level. This is especially important when interacting with children.
- Appreciate that some people may need more time than others to consider the information they have received and to reflect on their choices. In some circumstances, the person is receiving difficult news for the first time and may need to assimilate this information. More than one session or discussion may be required.
- It is important that nurses ensure the patient understands the information and options presented to him or her. The discussion may need to be repeated a number of times in order for some people to fully comprehend the choices available to them. It is also appropriate to communicate with patients at the level of simplicity or sophistication they are familiar with. Nurses may ask probing questions to ensure the patient is comprehending what is being communicated. They must also encourage questions from the patient and his or her family.
- The patient may have had many experiences with health care, or this may be the first. Past experience, or lack thereof, may affect responses.
- It helps to supplement verbal information with written material, Web-based education, videos, pictures, and so on. This is especially important when the client is a child; nurses also have to take into account the stages of child development.
- It is the patient's choice whether to have a friend or family member present not only to provide support but to help interpret or clarify the information being presented.

- It is important to be sensitive to cultural and language issues and the influence these may have not only on comprehension but on how the patient's values may influence their reactions and choices. Professional health care interpreters may be required. They can retain the true meaning of the health care professional's message and ensure the patient fully understands his or her condition and options for treatment.
- It is most important for nurses to be active listeners and to be aware of the patient's emotional and physiological responses to his or her situation.

## Types of Consent

There are two basic types of consent: expressed and implied. *Expressed consent* is a clear statement of consent from the patient. This may not be any specific wording; an expression such as, "Okay, nurse, go ahead" is sufficient. Many provinces require that a written consent also be obtained as evidence that the patient has consented to a medical procedure or treatment. It is important to remember that the patient has the right to withdraw consent or revoke (cancel) a previously given consent at any time, even orally, provided he or she is mentally competent to do so.

*Implied consent* is inferred from a patient's conduct. For example, a nurse advises a patient whose hand has just been punctured by a rusty nail that she will be administering a tetanus vaccine as a precaution to prevent "lockjaw." The patient then holds out his arm to receive the injection. Clearly, through this action, he has consented to the treatment without written or verbal means.

## Record and Timing of Consent

Many nurses may be concerned when no expressed written consent is found in the patient's chart and the patient is ready for surgery and perhaps already sedated. Must a written consent be obtained in this instance? The written consent form itself cannot stand alone; it is documentary evidence of consent, but the mentally competent client can withdraw consent at any time despite the existence of such a document. What matters is that an *informed* consent has been given. If the physician has documented somewhere in the patient's chart the fact of the patient's consent and the disclosure relating to the risks, consequences, and benefits of the procedure, this will usually be sufficient.

Some organizations may continue to use a general consent form, but this is being eliminated since it cannot be solely relied upon and is not specific to a particular procedure or treatment. After obtaining consent, the health care professional should document the fact that the procedure was explained to the patient, along with its risks and consequences, and that the patient verbally consented. Moreover, the nurse in such a situation must be competent to provide the patient or client with information about the risks of the procedure; that is, the nurse cannot go beyond the scope of authorized nursing practice in explaining such procedures and risks. In some situations, it may be more appropriate for another professional in the health care team to provide such explanations.

In many cases, the gravity of the situation or the risks in delaying treatment may preclude the obtaining of a signed consent; thus, documenting the fact of an informed consent is very important. Any such note should be signed and dated by the physician. It can also be signed by any other health care professional who is present at the time when such disclosure is made to the patient.

## Case Law on Consent

### INFORMED CONSENT

The most important case dealing with battery and the requirement of informed consent to medical treatment is *Reibl v. Hughes* (1980). In the Reibl decision, the plaintiff suffered from a blocked left carotid artery. Accordingly, he was booked for an elective internal carotid endarterectomy, which was performed by the defendant, a neurosurgeon. During the surgery, or immediately thereafter, the plaintiff suffered a stroke, which resulted in unilateral paralysis, impotence, and permanent disability. The plaintiff sued the neurosurgeon for negligently performing the operation and for the surgeon's failure to inform him adequately of the risks of the surgery.

The case ultimately reached the Supreme Court of Canada, where the Court held that the surgeon was liable in that he had indeed failed to inform the plaintiff of all material risks attending the surgery. In this case, although there was a real risk of stroke, paralysis, and possible death, the surgeon had told the patient only that it would be better for him to have the surgery. Furthermore, as the plaintiff had difficulty with the English language, it was incumbent upon the surgeon to ensure that the information conveyed was fully understood.

If such disclosure is not made, the health practitioner risks being found liable for negligence. The complete failure to obtain any consent at all, or the obtaining of consent through fraud, would leave the practitioner open to a civil suit for battery.

### REFUSAL OF CONSENT FOR RELIGIOUS OR OTHER REASONS

Along with the issue of informed consent is that of refusal of consent to certain procedures or treatment on moral or religious grounds. The Ontario Court of Appeal dealt with such a case in its decision in *Malette v. Shulman* (1990). In that case, the plaintiff had been seriously injured in a motor vehicle accident and rushed to a nearby hospital. She had sustained serious injuries to her head and face and was bleeding profusely. The physician on duty in Emergency, who attended her upon her arrival, determined that she would need blood transfusions to maintain her blood volume and pressure lest she succumb to irreversible shock. The surgeon who examined her prior to X-rays being taken made the same determination. She was barely conscious at the time.

Meanwhile, shortly after the patient's arrival at the hospital, a nurse discovered a card in the patient's purse printed in French, signed by the patient, identifying her as a Jehovah's Witness. The card read:

## NO BLOOD TRANSFUSION!

As one of Jehovah's Witnesses with firm religious convictions, I request that no blood or blood products be administered to me under any circumstances. I fully realize the implications of this position, but I have resolutely decided to obey the Bible command: "Keep abstaining ... from blood." (Acts 15:28, 29) However, I have no religious objections to use [sic] the non-blood alternatives, such as Dextran, Haemaccel [sic], PVP, Ringer's Lactate, or saline solution. (*Malette v. Shulman*, 1990, p. 419)

The nurse brought the card to the attention of the physician who had first seen the patient.

Before X-rays could be completed, the patient's blood pressure dropped markedly, her respiration became increasingly distressed, and her level of consciousness dropped. She continued to bleed profusely. At that moment, the physician determined that a blood transfusion was necessary to preserve her life. He decided to administer the transfusion to her personally and on his own responsibility, notwithstanding the card that had been brought to his attention.

Usually, nurses would administer a blood transfusion pursuant to an order drawn up by a physician. The question then becomes: What is the legal obligation of a nurse to follow a physician's order when he or she knows that order to be contrary to the patient's wishes and that the patient has not consented to such treatment? In such a case, the law would apply equally to the nurse as to the physician. Both must respect the patient's wishes, and neither may administer treatment for which consent has been withheld, no matter how necessary that treatment or how irrational the patient's decision may seem.

Returning to the Malette case, shortly after the physician administered the transfusion, the patient's daughter arrived at the hospital and became furious when told that a blood transfusion had been administered to her mother. She affirmed her mother's instructions that no blood be given to her and signed a document specifically prohibiting the giving of further blood to the patient, saying that her mother's faith forbade blood transfusions and that she would not wish them.

Despite these objections, the physician refused to follow the daughter's instructions. In his professional opinion, transfusions were absolutely necessary to save the patient's life, and it was his professional duty to ensure that she receive them. He did not believe that the card signed by the patient expressed her current wishes. He could not be sure that she had not changed her religious beliefs or that she had been fully informed of all the risks of forgoing a blood transfusion. (Again, if a nurse were carrying out an order for a blood transfusion under similar circumstances, despite the fact that he or she may have similar misgivings about the instructions, that nurse would be bound by the patient's limitations on consent to treatment.)

After making a full recovery from her injuries, the woman brought a lawsuit for battery, negligence, and religious discrimination against the physician and the hospital. Her action was allowed, and she was awarded damages on the grounds that blood transfusions had been administered against her specific wishes and that this constituted a battery upon her. The physician appealed this judgement in the Ontario Court of Appeal.

The Court of Appeal reviewed the law dealing with informed consent. It found that the common law recognized the right of a patient to refuse consent to medical treatment, and that this right was paramount to the health practitioner's professional opinion about what might be best for that patient. The Court stated that, while it is true that informed consent is not required in emergencies when the patient is unable to give consent (and the physician has no reason to believe that the patient would refuse consent if conscious or able to do so), in the presence of clear instructions such as those contained in the Jehovah's Witness card in this case, the physician was not free to disregard the patient's instructions. There is no corresponding doctrine of "informed refusal" requiring or authorizing a health practitioner to proceed with emergency treatment when the practitioner has not been able to inform the patient of all the consequences and risks of refusing treatment (*Malette v. Shulman*, 1990, p. 432).

The Court upheld the trial judge's finding that there was no rational basis or evidence upon which the physician could found a belief that the card was not valid or that the patient's religious views had changed. Hence, there was no justification for the doctor's refusal to adhere to the patient's advance instructions. The treatment having thus been administered without the patient's consent, the Court of Appeal upheld the finding of liability for battery against the physician (*Malette v. Shulman*, 1990, p. 434).

Of course, the Court made clear the fact that, in this case, it was not deciding the enforceability of advance directives regarding euthanasia or withdrawal of treatment. The patient here asked only that her spiritual beliefs be respected, and she was willing to risk death for them. She did not wish to die, as she consented to the use of nonblood alternatives. This case illustrates a limit on the doctrine of emergency treatment wherein the requirement for consent is waived. It further reinforces the principle that a patient's wishes are the final say on whether treatment shall be administered, no matter how necessary to life that treatment may be.

WITHDRAWAL OF CONSENT

The Supreme Court of Canada reviewed the law of informed consent in a situation in which the patient withdrew consent during a medical procedure to which she had previously consented. Although this case involved an action for battery and negligence against the attending physicians, the principles contained in this decision and developed by the Supreme Court are equally applicable to nursing professionals.

In *Ciarlariello v. Schacter* (1993), the Court was asked to consider whether a doctor still owed to a patient a duty of disclosure of all material risks inherent in a medical procedure if the patient withdraws a previously given informed consent during that procedure (*Ciarlariello v. Schacter*, 1993; per Cory J., p. 123). The plaintiff was asked to be at a hospital for the purpose of undergoing the first of two angiograms meant to determine the exact location of a suspected aneurysm. On the patient's arrival at the hospital, the physician who was to administer the test explained the risks inherent in the procedure, including possible blindness, paralysis, and death. Although the plaintiff's first language was Italian and her English was poor, she claimed at that time to have understood the doctor's explanation.

The plaintiff's daughter acted as interpreter during these explanations. The patient thereupon signed a consent to the tests. Despite this, the doctor had misgivings as to the free and informed nature of the consent.

The doctor therefore destroyed the patient's consent and asked her to go back to her family to consult with them. This she did and later returned with a consent signed by her daughter. The patient took the test; it failed to reveal the aneurysm's location conclusively but indicated a possible site. The doctors in charge of her case decided that a second angiogram would likely pinpoint the site of the aneurysm.

In the meantime, the plaintiff suffered a second severe headache indicating a "rebleed" of the aneurysm, and it was decided that a second angiogram was needed. The patient consented to this second test. Beforehand, a second radiologist (who had worked with the radiologist who administered the first test) carefully explained the test to her, including all possible material risks (skin rash and, on rare occasions, blindness, stroke, paralysis, or both, or death). He stated that the patient appeared to understand, so he proceeded with the angiogram.

During the procedure, the plaintiff began moaning and yelling. She started to hyperventilate and flex her legs. She calmed down sufficiently to tell the doctor, "Enough, no more, stop the test." The test was stopped, and both radiologists proceeded to examine her complaint that her right hand was numb. She was unable to move it or grasp with it. Her left hand was also slightly weak. Gradually, the strength returned to her right hand and both arms, though her left hand remained weak. Her sensory perception was normal. Both radiologists concluded that the residual weakness in her left hand was due to her hyperventilating. Both expected the weakness to be temporary. The rest of her motor function appeared to return to normal.

At this point, the plaintiff became quiet and cooperative. The first radiologist took over the test and explained to her that one more area needed investigation and that this procedure would take five more minutes. She asked the plaintiff if she wished to continue the test, to which the plaintiff replied, "Please go ahead." The final injection of dye was administered, during which the plaintiff suffered an immediate reaction, rendering her a quadriplegic. She sued all the doctors involved in treating her for damages for negligence and battery. She died soon after her lawsuit came to trial, and her family and estate continued the suit.

This case is of some relevance to nursing in that it illustrates that a patient has the right at any time to withdraw consent to treatment. Such withdrawal may occur in difficult circumstances, as in the Ciarlariello case, and it is important for the health practitioner to ascertain whether the consent has been withdrawn. This may not always be clear. A professional who continues to administer treatment, regardless of a patient's instructions to stop, risks being found liable to the patient for battery. In the Ciarlariello case, at a point during the procedure, the patient clearly withdrew her consent. She had given an informed consent that met the requirements laid down in *Reibl v. Hughes* (1980). Thus, the doctors had not been negligent in explaining the risks of the procedure to her.

A further crucial issue with respect to resumption of treatment after consent to it has been withdrawn was addressed in the suit. The criteria laid down by the Court governing the health care professional's actions in such a case include a consideration of whether the risks have changed materially during the procedure and whether a reasonable patient would wish to know of such changes (*Ciarlariello v. Schacter*, 1993, p. 139). In the Ciarlariello case, there was no evidence that the patient's condition had deteriorated to the point that she could not properly consent to the resumption of the treatment. Thus, her consent to resume the tests was valid.

As discussed in Chapter 7, one of the elements that must be proven in a negligence action is that the plaintiff's injury is a result of the defendant's breach of duty toward the plaintiff. In an action for negligence such as that in *Reibl v. Hughes* or *Ciarlariello v. Schacter*, the question becomes whether a reasonable person in the plaintiff's position would still have consented to the procedure if he or she had known the information and risks that the health practitioner failed to disclose.

In *Ciarlariello v. Schacter* (1993), the court found that the plaintiff's consent was an informed one and that there was no negligence on the doctors' part. It also found that, as the risk of quadriplegia resulting from an angiogram was far less than the risks of not locating the aneurysm, a reasonable patient in the plaintiff's position would still have consented to the procedure.

## Competency, Consent, and Substitute Decision Makers

### Incompetent Adults

To return to our case scenario, before her children can be consulted, Doris's attending physicians must determine whether she is mentally competent to make an informed decision respecting the diagnostic tests. If Doris is competent, her wishes that her children not be contacted must be respected.

In cases involving older patients, the initial and seemingly irrational refusal to consent may not necessarily be evidence of mental incompetence. The nurse or other practitioner must remain patient (if the situation is not urgent or life-threatening). Older clients are often fearful of impending illness. Many may have friends or relatives, even a spouse, who have recently succumbed to a serious illness. For example, a patient whose brother has died of cancer may fear that he himself will be stricken with the disease. This fear may paralyze some people's thinking. They may be in a state of denial and may rationalize their refusal to consent on the basis that "if cancer is not detected, then that means I don't have it." This may be what is going on in a patient's mind when he or she says: "No! I don't want to go through those tests. Leave me alone; I'm all right!"

The law allows any mentally competent adult to refuse consent to medical treatment. How, then, can the mental capacity of a patient be determined? Some have suggested the following test: "… can the patient appreciate the nature and consequences of the proposed treatment so as to be capable of rendering an informed judgement?" (This is a formulation suggested by Sharpe (1986), p. 77.) A method of testing for this appreciation is to explain to the patient, carefully and in detail, the risks and nature of the proposed procedure and then to ask the patient to repeat his or her understanding of the risks and treatment, while carefully noting the responses and words used (Sharpe, 1986). On this basis, the health practitioner is then able to form an opinion of the patient's ability to appreciate the nature, risks, and consequences of the proposed procedure.

Of course, patients may be capable of making decisions concerning some matters yet not others, and their mental capacity may fluctuate over time. If the patient has stated an intention that the procedure commence but has displayed an irrational or confused understanding of that procedure or an incapacity to comprehend its nature or its risks, the health practitioner should be reluctant to proceed without the consent of an authorized substitute decision maker.

In some provinces, any health care professional faced with a question of administering treatment to a mentally incompetent patient must obtain the consent of the patient's spouse, parent, a person in lawful custody of that patient, or the patient's next of kin (*Substitute Decisions Act*, 1992; *Health Care Consent Act*, 1996). If no such persons are available, and the situation is not an emergency, a physician may have to obtain the consent of the patient's guardian, appointed under statute (e.g., Ontario's *Health Care Consent Act*, 1996) or a substitute decision maker designated by the patient pursuant to the *Substitute Decisions Act* (1992). Under such a law, a court may be asked by any interested party, usually a spouse or relative, to appoint a person to act in the patient's best interests, including the giving or withholding of consent to medical treatment. This person then has the authority to consent to any medical treatment on behalf of the patient, who will legally have been found incompetent by the court. In such a case, the physician may obtain the necessary consent from the guardian of the person.

For example, the *Civil Code of Quebec* provides that if a person is incapable of giving consent, such consent may be given by a *curator* (or tutor, in the case of a child). He or she (or they) is appointed by the court to act in the incapable person's best interests and to ensure proper care for that person. In the absence of a curator, the person's spouse or, if there is no spouse or the spouse cannot consent due to incapacity, a close relative or adult showing a special interest in the patient may give consent (*Civil Code of Quebec*, article 15). If neither the patient nor the curator can consent, or if the patient or curator refuses consent, a health care professional in Quebec cannot proceed with treatment until and unless he or she obtains an order from the court authorizing the procedure (*Civil Code of Quebec*, art. 16, para. 1).

For example, suppose a patient in the later stages of Alzheimer's disease is rushed to the emergency department suffering from sharp abdominal pain. The patient's son is with him and has been appointed **committee of the person** of his father. The father exhibits classic symptoms of Alzheimer's: He is confused and incoherent and at times does not recognize his son. The emergency team will have to obtain the son's consent to tests and treatment for the father. In such a consultation, health care professionals should encourage the son to make decisions as his father would have made them when he was competent.

## Children

There are likewise competency issues with respect to children. In some provinces, a child who is old enough and mature enough to understand the nature and risks inherent in a medical procedure is given the right to consent to such treatment of his or her own accord.

Ontario's *Health Care Consent Act* (1996), for example, provides that the wishes with respect to medical treatment of any mentally capable person 16 years of age or older must be adhered to (*Health Care Consent Act,* 1996, section 1(c)(iii)). It is important to note that even in the case of a child under the age of 16, such a child's wishes with respect to the granting or withholding of consent to treatment must be respected where the child is "able to understand the information that is relevant to making a decision about the treatment, admission or personal assistance service, as the case may be, and able to appreciate the reasonably foreseeable consequences of a decision or lack of decision" (*Health Care Consent Act*, 1996, section 4(1)). A person (including a child) is presumed to be capable, and a health practitioner is entitled to rely on such a presumption unless the practitioner has reasonable grounds to believe that the person is not in fact capable (*Health Care Consent Act*, 1996, ss. 4(2), (3)). The capacity of the child will depend on each child's age, intelligence, maturity, experience, and other such factors. The information that the child must understand in giving or refusing consent will be provided by the health care practitioner and includes information about:

- The nature of the treatment
- The expected benefits of the treatment
- The material risks of the treatment
- The material side effects of the treatment
- Alternative courses of action
- The likely consequences of not having the treatment (*Health Care Consent Act*, 1996, s. 11(3))

This is the same information as must be provided to any patient, regardless of age, when obtaining the person's informed consent.

In Quebec, any child over the age of 14 may give consent freely without need for recourse to his or her parent or guardian (*Civil Code of Quebec*, art. 14, para. 2). However, if such a child refuses consent, a court order is necessary before treatment may proceed, even if the health care professional has obtained the consent of that child's parent or guardian (*Civil Code of Quebec*, article 16, paragraph 2).

A Children's Aid Society (CAS) may apply to a court to have a child in need of protection made its ward so that it can make treatment decisions on that child's behalf. This would usually occur in situations in which the health care professional and children's aid workers had reasonable grounds to believe that a child was not capable of giving an informed consent because of the child's lack of maturity, young age, and so forth. This procedure has been followed in numerous cases involving parents who had refused medical treatment for their children on religious grounds. If their refusal places the child's life at risk by denying life-saving treatment, the court can deem the child a "child in need of protection" and can authorize the CAS or other such body (in some provinces, the director of child welfare) to give the required consent if it is in the child's best interests. A recent Alberta case provides an example of an intervention by child welfare authorities in the consent to treatment process involving a seriously ill 16-year-old girl. In *Alberta (Director of Child Welfare) v. B.H.* (2002), the teenage girl had been diagnosed with acute myeloid leukemia (AML). With the full support of her parents, she advised the medical professionals at the hospital that she would not consent to the prescribed treatment (a blood transfusion or the administration of blood products) because she, like her parents, was a devout member of the Jehovah's Witnesses church. The health care professionals refused to proceed with treatment in the face of her refusal of consent. They felt that she was sufficiently mature to make such a decision. A few days later, a judge attended a hearing at the hospital on the application of the Alberta director of child welfare for an apprehension order and a medical treatment order directing that the treatment be administered to the girl. The girl's father then gave a written consent and the court proceeding was suspended. A few days later, the girl was still refusing consent, and the director of child welfare renewed his application. The court subsequently granted the order that she be apprehended from the custody of her parents and that the medical treatment be administered to her.

It was clear from the evidence of the medical experts consulted by the treating physician that a blood transfusion was the best treatment option under the circumstances, that the survival rates the physician had relied on were accurate, that the treatment could not be administered without blood products, and that the physician had not missed any reasonable treatment options. The child's lawyer argued that the court had no right to make the order because she was a mature minor who had made a decision to refuse treatment. She was, therefore, not a child in need of protection under Alberta child welfare laws, and hence the director had no grounds to support his application. The court ruled that despite the opinion of the hospital's bioethics committee that she was sufficiently mature to refuse treatment, the father's opinion that she was not was most compelling. The girl had in effect made a decision, not only to refuse medical treatment that would likely prolong her life, but to die. Moreover, an expert physician involved in the child's treatment was of the view that while the child was intelligent and had a sophisticated understanding of what she was facing, she was in no way concerned or fearful of the very likely consequences of her refusal, had no real understanding of the imminent physical death of her body, and was really childlike in many ways. She lacked the maturity to truly appreciate the nature and finality of death. Accordingly, the court granted the order requiring that the treatment be administered to her. Moreover, the court ruled that while the Charter rights to life, liberty, and security of her person had been infringed by the granting of the order, such an infringement was justified under section 1 of the Charter and a reasonable limit demonstrably justified in a free and democratic society. The state had a valid interest in intervening to save the life of a child who had refused treatment. The court's decision was upheld on appeal to the Alberta Court of Queen's Bench (*Alberta (Director of Child Welfare) v. B.H.*, 2002).

## Emergency Treatment

In all cases, the law in all the common law provinces and territories and in Quebec allows physicians and other health care professionals to administer treatment in an emergency even if the patient's consent cannot be obtained. Such a situation might arise because of the nature of the injuries or illness, or because no time can be spared in administering treatment. Health care professionals acting in extreme emergencies will be absolved of any liability for administering treatment, provided there is no gross negligence on their part.

## Proxy Consent

Traditionally, common law did not allow **proxy consent** to treatment—that is, a consent granted by a third party designated by the incapable person (when capable) to make decisions on his or her behalf. The only situations in which third-party consent was recognized was in the case of parents consenting on behalf of minors and committees appointed over mentally incompetent persons. However, situations may arise in which the patient is unable to consent, not because of some current or progressive mental infirmity but owing to a physical condition, for example, coma. A proxy decision maker is clearly desirable in such situations.

In our case scenario, the medical team would have to resort to a proxy if Doris were not competent to give or withhold consent.

The following discussion of recent legislative reform of common law in this area focuses on Ontario's legislation, as it is presently the most detailed such legislation in Canada.

## Legislative Reform of Common Law Respecting Consent to Treatment

The main components of the Ontario legislation affecting consent to treatment are contained in the *Health Care Consent Act* (1996) and the *Substitute Decisions Act* (1992).

The *Health Care Consent Act* (1996) enshrines into statute law the existing common law requirements for an informed consent to treatment, as discussed above. It preserves the right and duty of health care professionals to restrain or confine persons when necessary to prevent serious bodily harm either to themselves or to others (*Health Care Consent Act*, 1996, s. 7). The Act requires all health care professionals (including nurses) to ensure, firstly, that the patient to be treated is capable of consenting and, secondly, that the patient, in fact, consents. If the patient is not capable, the health care professional must obtain the consent from another person authorized to give consent under the Act (*Health Care Consent Act*, 1996, s. 10(1)). The Act also provides for other consents by patients to admission to a care facility, such as a nursing home, or to personal assistance services, such as assistance with dressing, hygiene, eating, grooming, and so forth (*Health Care Consent Act*, 1996, ss. 2(1), "personal assistance service," 4(1)).

Ontario's statute defines informed consent in much the same way as discussed earlier in this chapter: That is, it allows the consent to be expressed or implied, provided that (a) an informed consent has been given, (b) it relates to the treatment proposed, (c) it is voluntary, and (d) it has not been obtained through fraud or misrepresentation (*Health Care Consent Act*, 1996, s. 11). Consent is informed if, before giving it, a patient received information about the nature of the treatment, its expected benefits, material risks, material side effects, alternative courses of action, and the consequences of not having the treatment (*Health Care Consent Act*, 1996, s. 11(3)). A health care professional (which under this Act includes nurses) is entitled to presume that consent to a treatment includes consent to variations or adjustments in the treatment or the continuation of the treatment in a different setting, provided the benefits, risks, and material side effects of such alterations do not differ significantly from those of the original treatment.

This provision has a practical purpose. It would be quite impractical to require the health care professional to obtain renewed consent, along with having to restate all the information required, every time a course of treatment was altered in even the slightest way. This legislative provision also addresses the issue that arose in *Ciarlariello v. Schacter* (discussed above), in which there were few or no significant changes to the risks and side effects from one angiogram to the next.

The legislation also defines when a person is capable of giving consent. A person is capable if he or she understands the information given that is relevant to making a decision concerning the treatment, and can appreciate the reasonably foreseeable consequences of a decision or lack thereof. A person is always presumed to be capable unless a health care professional has reasonable grounds to believe that he or she is not (*Health Care Consent Act*, 1996, s. 4). For example, a health care professional could not assume that a patient was capable if he or she were to observe erratic or confused behaviour in the patient, or a lack of lucidity or rationality. Although such an observation would not necessarily mean the patient was incapable to give consent, a health care professional could not legally proceed on such basis. The statute provides that persons can be capable with respect to certain treatments and incapable for others, and capable and incapable at different times (*Health Care Consent Act*, 1996, s. 15). This provision addresses concerns that arise when a capable person has not yet given consent and then later may no longer be capable, for example, while under heavy sedation. It also addresses such situations as Alzheimer's patients who have periods of lucidity, only to relapse into a confused state moments later.

The health care professional in charge of the patient's care is responsible for determining whether the patient is capable or incapable of consenting to a proposed treatment. If the patient's capacity to consent returns after another person has made a decision with respect to the patient's treatment, the patient's own decision to give or refuse consent will govern (*Health Care Consent Act*, 1996, s. 16).

If the physician examining the patient determines that he or she is not capable of consenting to treatment, the patient must be informed of that fact and of the consequences of such a finding in accordance with the guidelines laid out by the governing body of the health care practitioner's profession. For nurses in Ontario, this would be the guidelines set out by the College of Nurses of Ontario (*Health Care Consent Act*, 1996, s. 17). Once the health care professional has determined that the patient is incapable (or, if before the treatment is begun, the professional is informed that the person intends to apply to the Consent and Capacity Board for review of the finding of incapacity or has applied for appointment of a representative to give consent to treatment), the professional must not begin treatment or must take steps to prevent such treatment being given until the matter is decided by the Board (*Health Care Consent Act*, 1996, s. 18).

The Consent and Capacity Board is an administrative tribunal. Its role is to hear appeals from findings of incapacity by health care professionals. It also hears applications brought on behalf of incapable persons for the appointment of representatives who can give consent to treatment in specific situations. In the event that the health care professional has found a patient incapable of giving consent, the patient has recourse to this tribunal if he or she still believes himself or herself capable of giving consent. This mechanism protects patients' autonomy and prevents abuses of patients' rights—for example, in a case in which a nonconsenting patient might be subjected to treatment that is not in his or her best interests or is unnecessary. Without such review, a person might be incorrectly deemed incapable of giving consent and may then be subjected to treatment to which he or she would not consent, simply because a health care professional was of the opinion that the patient lacked capacity.

If an incapable person has appointed an attorney who is acting under a validated **power of attorney** for personal care or a court-appointed guardian of the person (see next two sections), such an agent can give the required consent, but only in accordance with the instructions, limitations, and authority contained in the power of attorney or court order (*Health Care Consent Act*, 1996, s. 20).

If a substitute decision maker has been chosen, the known wishes of the patient must be taken into account and must govern the substitute's decision to give or refuse consent to treatment. The wishes may be contained in the power of attorney itself or any other document, or may be known orally. Such documents are commonly known as **living wills** because they provide directions on behalf of the maker that take effect after that person has lost the ability to make those decisions on his or her own behalf. If there are no known wishes requiring the giving or refusal of consent to a given treatment, the substitute decision maker must make the decision in the patient's best interests and in accordance with the incapable person's values and beliefs. In particular, the substitute must consider whether:

- The proposed treatment will likely improve the patient's condition or well-being
- The proposed treatment would prevent the patient's condition or well-being from deteriorating
- The proposed treatment would reduce the extent to which (or the rate at which) the patient's condition or well-being is likely to deteriorate

- The patient's well-being or condition would likely improve, remain the same, or deteriorate without the treatment
- The benefits of treatment outweigh the risks
- A less intrusive or restrictive treatment would be as beneficial as the one proposed (*Health Care Consent Act*, 1996, s. 21(2))

The Act establishes a hierarchy of alternative substitute decision makers (*Health Care Consent Act*, 1996, ss. 20(1), (3)). The persons set out in this list may give or refuse consent only if no person described in the next higher ranking (in descending order of priority, from one to eight) is available and meets the requirements of the Act:

1. A guardian appointed by the court under the *Substitute Decisions Act*, 1992
2. An attorney for personal care acting under a validated power of attorney for personal care that confers that authority
3. The incapable person's representative, appointed by the Board, if the representative has authority to give or refuse consent
4. The incapable person's spouse or partner (a "partner" is defined in section 20(9) of the *Health Care Consent Act* [1996] as one with whom the incapable person has lived for at least one year and with whom he or she has a close personal relationship of primary importance to both their lives; this would apply to same-sex couples. Section 20 also provides recognition for same-sex married couples.)
5. The incapable person's child, or parent, or a Children's Aid Society or other person lawfully entitled to give or refuse consent in place of the parent (this does not include parents having only a right of access over the child and does not include the child's parents if a Children's Aid Society is lawfully entitled to give or refuse treatment in the parents' place)
6. The person's parent with only a right of access
7. The person's brother or sister
8. Any other relative of the incapable person

For example, in our case scenario, let us assume that Doris has not signed a power of attorney appointing an attorney for personal care, nor has any guardian or representative been designated for her; however, she has a younger brother living across town. Let us further assume that a hospital staff psychiatrist has been asked to examine Doris and that he has determined that she appears to be suffering from some form of senile dementia, possibly Alzheimer's disease. He determines that Doris is not capable of giving or refusing informed consent. In such a situation, Doris's children would clearly be entitled to make the decision provided they can be located and are willing, capable, and available to give such consent and that no higher-ranking person is available. Doris's brother could give consent but only if her children could not be found or were incapable or unwilling to assume responsibility for making such a decision.

Other requirements are that the substitute decision maker be:

- At least 16 years of age
- Capable with respect to the treatment
- Not prohibited by court order or separation agreement from having access to the incapable person or giving or refusing consent
- Available, and willing to assume the responsibility of giving or refusing consent (*Health Care Consent Act*, 1996, s. 20(2))

In the event of a conflict between two or more persons claiming to have authority to give consent, the person who ranks highest in the categories listed above prevails. If two persons of equal ranking disagree about whether to give or refuse consent, the public guardian and trustee (see "Attorneys for Personal Care," below) may give or refuse it (*Health Care Consent Act*, 1996, section 20(6)).

As mentioned above, the Act provides that the wishes of a minor aged 16 or older in giving or refusing consent to treatment must be respected. The *Health Care Consent Act* (1996) does not explicitly set out a minimum age for consent. Rather, the guidelines that would likely govern would be the person's capacity to understand the proposed treatment, its risks, benefits, and consequences. As discussed previously, a child under 16 might be capable of giving an informed consent if he or she were of sufficient intelligence and maturity to appreciate the consequences of his or her decision and all the relevant information surrounding the proposed treatment.

Emergency treatment poses a special challenge for the health care professional, and the Act provides special rules for such situations. If a patient is found incapable, in the health care professional's opinion, with respect to a proposed treatment to alleviate severe suffering, or if the patient is at risk of serious bodily harm if the treatment is not administered promptly, and it is not possible to find a substitute decision maker without delaying such treatment, then the practitioner may administer the treatment. He or she may do so even when an application has been made to the Consent and Capacity Review Board for the appointment of a representative to give such consent on the patient's behalf.

The authority to proceed extends to any examination of the patient or diagnostic procedures (if these are reasonably necessary) to determine whether the patient is at risk of serious bodily harm or is experiencing severe suffering. The emergency treatment can continue for as long as is reasonably required to find someone who can give the necessary consent from among the list of persons authorized to do so. The Act obliges the health care professional to ensure that a continuing search is made for any substitute decision makers willing to assume responsibility to give or refuse consent. In the event that the patient becomes capable once again, his or her wishes govern.

The health care professional is also required to note in the patient's chart the opinions required by the Act to permit treatment without consent in an emergency (*Health Care Consent Act*, 1996, s. 25(5)).

If the health care professional has reasonable grounds to believe that the incapable patient, while capable and after the person reached the age of 16, expressed a wish to refuse treatment in such circumstances, he or she may not administer treatment. Thus, for example, if the patient is unconscious and an attorney for personal care advises the health care professional that this patient once expressed the desire that no blood transfusions be administered in an emergency, the professional may not administer such treatment (*Health Care Consent Act*, 1996, s. 26).

Despite a refusal of consent by someone in the above list, the health care professional may proceed if he or she believes that the treatment is necessary to alleviate suffering or to avoid serious bodily harm, and that the person refusing the consent has done so against the patient's previous wishes or has not acted in the patient's best interests in accordance with the guidelines and considerations enumerated in the Act. The authority to proceed as discussed above extends to having the person admitted to a hospital or psychiatric facility for treatment. However, a health care professional must respect the wishes of a patient who objects to such admission primarily for treatment of a mental disorder. This provision was included to cover situations in which a person might be forced to undergo psychiatric treatment against his or her will. There are separate procedures for admission of mental patients to psychiatric facilities set out in the *Mental Health Act* (1990). These include legal safeguards to ensure that otherwise mentally healthy persons are not detained against their will in psychiatric institutions.

## Attorneys for Personal Care

With respect to substitute decision makers or attorneys for personal care, Ontario's *Substitute Decisions Act* (1992) provides that a person over the age of 16 may exercise power of decision on behalf of an incapacitated person who is also at least 16 years old (*Substitute Decisions Act*, 1992, ss. 43 and 44). In most cases, the parents of an incapacitated adolescent would presumably continue to make treatment decisions and give the necessary consents. The determining factor under this statute for incapacity (thus the need for a substitute decision maker) is similar to that under the *Health Care Consent Act* (1996), but, in this case, the patient must be unable to understand information regarding his or her health care, nutrition, shelter, clothing, hygiene, or safety, or be unable to appreciate the reasonably foreseeable consequences of a decision (or lack of decision) respecting these matters (*Substitute Decisions Act*, 1992, s. 45).

Under the *Substitute Decisions Act* (1992), there are two methods of providing a substitute decision maker for an incapable person. The first is an appointment of a person or persons in a written document (called a **power of attorney for personal care**) in advance of the person (usually referred to as the **grantor**) becoming incapable. Those named in the power of attorney are authorized by the grantor to make decisions concerning personal care on his or her behalf (*Substitute Decisions Act*, 1992, s. 46(1)). The person named in the power of attorney (the attorney need not be a lawyer) for personal care may be the grantor's spouse, partner, a relative, or another. It cannot be anyone who provides health care to the grantor for compensation or who provides residential, social, training, or support services to the grantor for compensation (*Substitute Decisions Act*, 1992, s. 46(3)). This provision is important since in some situations the grantor may be tempted to name his or her physician, or a respected and trusted nurse, as an attorney. The legislation prevents any such conflict of interest from arising. However, critics point out that a nurse may be one of the persons more knowledgeable about care and treatment issues, particularly in respect to the incapable patient, and thus a practical and beneficial choice for attorney. This provision may therefore be viewed as a questionable limitation on the incapable patient's right to choose and appoint an attorney.

The attorney may act only in accordance with this statute and the limitations stipulated by the grantor in the power of attorney. A person who does not have a trusted friend, partner, spouse, nor relative to name as attorney can name the public guardian and trustee of Ontario (with the public guardian's permission, obtained prior to signing the power of attorney) (*Substitute Decisions Act*, 1992, s. 46(2)). This is a government official charged with ensuring that mentally incompetent persons, orphaned children having no legal guardians, and their property are cared for and their legal rights protected when there is no one else available to act in their interest.

Powers of attorney for personal care in Ontario no longer need to be validated, as was the case before amendments to the *Substitute Decisions Act*, which came into force in 1996. A power of attorney for personal care is a fully and legally valid document from the moment the grantor becomes incapable to make treatment decisions and give consent to treatment within the requirements of the *Health Care Consent Act* (1996) and the *Substitute Decisions Act* (1992).

Of course, the grantor making the power of attorney must be mentally capable of giving it. The test for determining this capacity is: Does the grantor understand whether the proposed attorney has a genuine concern for his or her welfare, and does the grantor appreciate that he or she may need to rely on the attorney to make decisions (*Substitute Decisions Act*, 1992, s. 47(1))? The power of attorney for personal care can be revoked at any time, provided the grantor is mentally capable when he or she does so. The grantor must also have had the capacity to make decisions with respect to any instructions contained in the power of attorney for personal care.

The formalities for making a legally valid power of attorney for personal care in Ontario are not complicated but should be carefully observed. Otherwise, there is a risk that the power of attorney might be declared invalid by a court. The power of attorney for personal care must be signed by the grantor in the presence of two witnesses, who cannot be:

- The proposed attorney or that person's spouse or partner
- The grantor's spouse or partner
- A child of the grantor or a person that the grantor has treated as if that person were his or her child
- Someone whose own property is under a guardianship (this prevents a potentially incompetent person from being a witness)
- A person under 18 years of age (*Substitute Decisions Act*, 1992, ss. 10(1), (2), 48(2)).

The power of attorney for personal care takes effect to provide the attorney with full authority to make a decision respecting the grantor's personal care if the *Health Care Consent Act* (1996) authorizes the attorney to make the decision or if the attorney has reasonable grounds to believe that the grantor is incapable of making the decision. This is subject to any condition in the document "that prevents the attorney from making the decision unless the fact that the grantor is incapable of personal care has been confirmed" (*Substitute Decisions Act*, 1992, s. 49(1)(b)). For such a condition to be legally effective, an assessor must certify, within 30 days of the signing of the document, that the grantor was capable when he or she signed it. In addition, the grantor must also sign a statement certifying that he or she understood the effect of these provisions and that he or she can revoke (cancel) the power of attorney only if, in the 30 days before the revocation, an assessor has made a statement that the grantor was capable when the revocation was signed and that sets out the facts on which the assessor has based that opinion.

The legislation allows maximum protection for the grantor against having decisions made without his or her consent. For example, the grantor has the right to request the attorney's assistance in arranging an assessment by an assessor, who may be a physician, a psychologist, or a psychiatrist, as designated by government regulation to make such an assessment. The grantor may place conditions on the authority of the substitute decision maker and can specify the manner in which his or her capacity is to be assessed (*Substitute Decisions Act*, 1992, s. 49(2)). The assessor is responsible for determining whether the grantor is in fact incapable with respect to making some, if not all, treatment decisions. The attorney is not required to make such arrangements, however, if the person was assessed within six months prior to the request for an assessment (*Substitute Decisions Act*, 1992, s. 55(1)).

In addition, the *Substitute Decisions Act* (1992) provides the attorney with the authority to use such reasonable force as is necessary to determine the grantor's capacity, to confirm whether the grantor is incapable of personal care, to take the grantor to any place of treatment, or to admit the grantor to such place and detain and restrain him or her there for the duration of the treatment (*Substitute Decisions Act*, 1992, s. 59(3)).

## Court-Appointed Guardians of the Person

The second method of providing a substitute decision maker under the *Substitute Decisions Act* in Ontario is through an application to the court for the appointment of a guardian of the person (*Substitute Decisions Act*, 1992, s. 55(1)). This route is more difficult. The court must consider whether there is an alternative course of action (e.g., one that is less restrictive of the patient's decision-making rights) for making decisions that does not require it to declare the applicant incapable of his or her own personal care (*Substitute Decisions Act*, 1992, s. 55(2)). Thus, the legislation is aimed at encouraging alternatives to court proceedings in these matters.

Any person (i.e., a physician, close friend, relative, spouse, partner, or any person who has an interest in the applicant's care) may apply for the appointment of a guardian. In any event, the appointed guardian cannot be someone who provides health care for compensation (*Substitute Decisions Act*, 1992, s. 57(1)) but may be the applicant's attorney for personal care. An exception may be made if there is no other suitable person who can act as guardian (*Substitute Decisions Act*, 1992, s. 57(2.1)). The appointment of an attorney could expand his or her decision-making power over and above the authorization contained in the power of attorney for personal care. If it is made in a court order for full guardianship, it might include the power to:

- Determine the person's living arrangements, shelter, and safety
- Take charge of any lawsuits by or against the applicant
- Gain access to personal information about the applicant
- Make decisions about the applicant's health care, nutrition, and hygiene
- Give or refuse consent to medical treatment on the person's behalf pursuant to the *Health Care Consent Act* (1996)
- Make decisions about the applicant's employment, education, training, clothing, and recreation, and any other duties and powers specified in the order

In short, a full guardianship may (depending on the exact provisions of the court order) grant power to the guardian over all facets of the incapable person's life.

Before appointing a guardian, the court must find that the patient is, in fact, incapable according to the definition outlined above (see page 172). The appointment of the guardian may be for a limited time or may have other conditions attached to it as the court considers appropriate. In deciding the application, the court must consider (a) whether the proposed guardian is the attorney under a power of attorney, (b) the incapable person's wishes, to the extent that these can be ascertained, and (c) the closeness of the relationship between the person applying for the guardianship and the incapable person.

A partial guardianship order may be made when the court considers the patient incapable with respect to some, but not all, aspects of personal care and health. In such a case, the guardianship order will specify those matters in which the guardian has the power to make decisions, leaving other matters to the patient's own discretion. In this way, any court order can be tailored to be as unobtrusive as possible to the incapable patient's life while still affording the protection of a competent guardian to make crucial decisions on his or her behalf.

## Duties of Guardians and Attorneys for Personal Care

The philosophy behind the law is to involve the incapable person in the process of consent to the greatest extent possible under the circumstances. This accords with the basic principle of autonomy, discussed in Chapter 2. Thus, both guardians and attorneys are required to exercise their powers diligently and in good faith, and to explain their powers and duties to the incapable person. As mentioned, his or her wishes, made while capable, must guide the guardian or attorney when faced with decisions relevant to these wishes; the guardian or attorney must make diligent efforts to ascertain the existence and substance of prior wishes; and the most recent wish made while the person was capable must prevail over an earlier related wish. To determine these prior wishes, the guardian or attorney must take the incapable person's values and beliefs into account. In addition, the guardian must consider whether his or her decision is likely to improve the quality of the incapable person's life, prevent that quality of life from deteriorating, and reduce the extent to which (or rate at which) the person's quality of life is likely to deteriorate. Further, he or she must weigh the relative risks and benefits the person is expected to derive from the decision against those that may arise from an alternative decision.

If it is not possible to make a decision in accordance with an incapable person's wish, or if such wishes or instructions cannot be determined, the guardian or attorney must make the decision in the person's best interests. The least restrictive and least intrusive course of action under the circumstances must be chosen, and, in making any decision, the guardian should foster the incapable person's independence as far as possible. The guardian should consult with the person's family, friends, and health care professionals. Here, nurses caring for such patients have an opportunity to make their perspectives and views known and to contribute to the quality of care. Unlike attorneys for personal care, however, court-appointed guardians of the person must have written guardianship plans (usually written by lawyers, with the assistance of the health care professionals involved) to which they must adhere. Guardians and attorneys are also required to maintain records of all decisions affecting the incapable person.

## Manitoba and British Columbia

Manitoba's substitute decision maker legislation, the *Health Care Directives Act*, is fairly similar to that of Ontario. In Manitoba, the document signed by the grantor is called a **directive**, and the grantor is referred to as the *maker of the directive*. The person who is appointed to be the substitute decision maker is the **proxy**.

The Manitoba Act is silent on court-appointed guardians; however, this area is covered through other legislation. The directive need not be witnessed so long as the maker has signed it. However, the Manitoba Act does permit another person to sign for the maker in the maker's presence and in the presence of a witness. Neither the person who signs for the maker nor the witness may be nominated as proxies in the directive. This is intended to cover directives made by blind persons or others who, though mentally competent, are physically unable to sign the document.

British Columbia has enacted the *Representation Agreement Act* (1996), which establishes procedures respecting agreements with substitute decision makers, similar to Ontario's and Manitoba's. Under the *Representation Agreement Act*, a competent adult also has the right to appoint a substitute decision maker (called a *representative*) to make treatment and care decisions on his or her behalf. The document making the appointment is called a representation agreement, which must be signed by the patient's representative (unlike Ontario's or Manitoba's legislation). The signatures of each party to the agreement must be witnessed by two persons. The representative of the incapable person is also supervised by a monitor whose duty it is to ensure that the representative carries out all of his or her obligations under the agreement and in accordance with the wishes of the incapable person (as expressed when he or she was capable). British Columbia has also recently passed the *Health Care (Consent) and Care Facility (Admission) Act* (1996), which codifies much of the law on informed consent and is broadly similar to Ontario's *Health Care Consent Act* (1996).

## Other Provinces and Territories

Several other Canadian jurisdictions, notably Newfoundland and Labrador, Prince Edward Island, Nova Scotia, Saskatchewan, and Yukon, have also recently passed legislation respecting the power of persons to make advance directives or allowing for substitute decision makers. See:

- Newfoundland and Labrador: *Advanced Health Care Directives Act* (1995)
- Prince Edward Island: *Consent to Treatment and Health Care Directives Act* (1988)
- Nova Scotia: *Medical Consent Act* (1989)
- Saskatchewan: *Health Care Directives and Substitute Health Care Decision Makers Act* (1997)
- Yukon: *Enduring Power of Attorney Act* (2002)

Of these other jurisdictions, only P.E.I.'s legislation actually codifies the law requiring a patient to give consent to treatment as does Ontario's *Health Care Consent Act* (1996). The statutes of the other four jurisdictions purport to deal with the powers of substitute decision makers and advance directives to make treatment decisions for incapable persons. The P.E.I. statute, interestingly, makes legal any advance directive made before the law was passed (*Consent to Treatment and Health Care Directives Act*, 1988, s. 1(e), "directive"), acknowledging that the practice of making so-called living wills arose before the law had a chance to respond to this societal change. The directive in P.E.I. may set out the maker's wishes with respect to treatment, may be limited simply to appointing a proxy, or may both set out wishes and appoint a proxy.

The P.E.I. statute, like Ontario's, sets out what does and does not constitute treatment. Included in this list are:

- An examination or assessment conducted under P.E.I.'s *Adult Protection Act*, *Mental Health Act*, *Public Health Act*, *Public Trustee Act*, or any other statute respecting capacity or guardianship of the person
- The assessment or examination of a person to determine his or her general health and condition
- The taking of a person's health history
- The communication of an assessment or diagnosis
- The admission of a person to a hospital or other facility
- A personal assistance service
- A treatment posing little or no risk of harm

- Counselling that is primarily in the nature of advice, education, or motivation
- Any other act prescribed by regulation

The provisions in this statute are subject to any contrary provisions in the *Mental Health Act* and the *Public Health Act* of P.E.I.

P.E.I.'s statute sets out specific "consent rights," including the right of the patient to give or refuse treatment on any grounds, including moral and religious grounds, even if his or her death results as a consequence (*Consent to Treatment and Health Care Directives Act*, 1988, s. 4). A patient is also permitted to have a trusted advisor, referred to as an "associate," to assist him or her and has the right to select the health care professional and form of treatment on any grounds. The provisions respecting the giving of consent and prohibitions on administering treatment without consent are similar to Ontario's. The requirements for determining capacity and whether consent is informed are also similar; however, a person may waive the right in writing to receive information as to the nature of the proposed treatment (*Consent to Treatment and Health Care Directives Act*, 1988, s. 6). In determining capacity, a health care professional must inform the patient of his or her right to the assistance of an associate but must also take into account the associate's assistance.

As in Ontario, P.E.I. provides for specific persons to act as substitute decision makers in decreasing order of priority (*Consent to Treatment and Health Care Directives Act*, 1988, s. 11(1)). The order is quite similar to that outlined in Ontario's legislation. A substitute decision maker is not authorized by the Act to give consent to electric shock therapy, the removal of nonregenerative tissue, an abortion (except in cases in which there is likely immediate danger to the life or health of the patient), sterilization not medically necessary for the protection of the patient's health, or a procedure whose primary purpose is research except where the research is for the patient's own benefit. This is somewhat different from Ontario's legislation, which does allow consent to electric shock therapy if consent is given in accordance with the *Health Care Consent Act* (1996).

Unlike in Ontario, P.E.I.'s legislation does not provide for a Consent Capacity Board. In both Ontario and P.E.I., health care professionals acting on the basis of an apparently valid consent are shielded from legal liability for their actions. Neither is a substitute decision maker, or proxy in P.E.I., liable for a decision made while acting in good faith and in accordance with the law. "Good faith" means that the substitute decision maker must have an honestly held belief that the patient is either capable of giving an informed consent or incapable of doing so, and acts appropriately.

While in Ontario two persons must witness the making of a power of attorney for personal care, only one witness is required in P.E.I. In P.E.I., any interestsed person may file a complaint about a proxy with a public official designated by the Minister of Health and Social Services (*Consent to Treatment and Health Care Directives Act*, 1988, s. 27). A proxy cannot delegate the authority to make decisions to anyone else. Further, a decision by a proxy under an advance directive takes precedence over a decision made by a court or any other person, including a guardian, unless the directive provides otherwise. A directive made outside P.E.I. is valid in that province if it meets the requirements of the P.E.I. legislation or accords with the laws of the province (or country) where it was made and if the maker was habitually resident in that other province or country.

Saskatchewan's *Health Care Directives and Substitute Health Care Decision Makers Act* (1997) is fairly similar to the acts described above but does not codify completely the common law relating to informed consent. It provides for the making of health care directives in a similar manner. Saskatchewan's law is notable in that it does not authorize the use of a directive to consent to anything that is prohibited by the *Criminal Code*, active euthanasia, or assisted suicide (*Health Care Directives and Substitute Health Care Decision Makers Act*, 1997, s. 2(2)). Given the decision involving Robert Latimer in Saskatchewan (*R. v. Latimer*, 1997), discussed in detail in Chapter 8, this provision in the law sends a strong message about that province's policy on assisted suicide and euthanasia.

In Saskatchewan, the proxy must be an adult—that is, a person over the age of 18 years. However, the maker of a health care directive may be anyone who is capable and over 16 years of age. As in P.E.I., only one witness is required to the making of a health care directive.

Yukon's legislation (*Enduring Power of Attorney Act*, 2002) is similar to that of the provinces. It provides that a regular power of attorney becomes an "enduring power of attorney" if it is in writing, signed by its "donor," dated, and contains a provision that it is to continue to be in force after the donor's incapacity or is to take effect at such time (*Enduring Power of Attorney Act*, 2002 s. 3(1)). The Yukon statute also requires that certain notes on the enduring power of attorney be included in it. These notes relate to the donor's appreciation of the nature of the document, the powers it grants to the attorney, when it takes effect, and when (and under what circumstances) it can be cancelled. A lawyer must attest in writing that the donor understands the document, was competent when he or she signed it, and was an adult, and that the power was given freely and voluntarily. The legislation does not explicitly set out what powers or restrictions may be contained in the enduring power of attorney. The attorney is prohibited from renouncing his or her appointment once it has taken effect without the permission of the court. Consent to treatment in Yukon is dealt with under that territory's health act, insofar as the attorney as substitute decision maker is concerned.

## Summary

This chapter has focussed on the ethical and legal foundations of consent and has given examples to clarify their application in practice. Many challenges exist for nurses seeking to protect their clients' autonomy: advances in technology, the complexities within the health care system, increasing emphasis on individual choice, questions regarding whether a person has the capacity to provide consent, and concerns regarding potential litigation, to name but a few. Further, legislation pertaining to consent is constantly being revised to achieve a balance between respecting client choice and protecting people from harm.

Consent policies, rules, and legislation are very much based on the principle of autonomy, which recognizes that a capable and competent individual is free to determine and act in accordance with a self-chosen plan. Other equally important ethical principles, such as beneficence and nonmaleficence, that nurses must consider, at times may compete with this principle.

Each clinical environment or institution in which nurses work needs to establish nursing guidelines relative to consent. Ethics committees to assist nurses and other members of the team to deal with challenging situations should be in place. Ongoing education, peer review, and continuous quality improvement are necessary to ensure that standards are consistently high.

There are many complex dynamics involved in dealing with ill, vulnerable patients whose capacity to make informed choices may be challenged. Nurses must take seriously their role in caring for and supporting these clients, ensuring their rights are respected, and protecting them from harm.

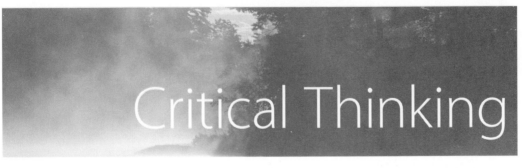

Critical Thinking

The following case scenarios are for further reflection, discussion, and analysis.

## OLD ENOUGH TO CHOOSE?

Ronnie, a 13-year-old girl with acute lymphocytic leukemia, is presently in the pediatric unit of a large tertiary cancer centre. Her leukemia was diagnosed when she was eight, at which time she had several rounds of chemotherapy. The cancer went into remission, but since her form of leukemia is severe, the team asked her parents to consider a bone marrow transplant. Her brother, Robert, 2 years older than she, was a perfect match. The bone marrow retrieval was scary for Robert, as it required a general anesthetic and he experienced much pain afterward. However, his pain and suffering was nothing like Ronnie's. In preparation for the transplant, she received high doses of chemotherapy and underwent total body radiation. A short time after the transplant, the new marrow started to reject her body (graft versus host disease).

Ronnie recovered, and the past 5 years have been great for her. Now, however, she has relapsed. The team is proposing more chemo and possibly another bone marrow transplant.

Francine is Ronnie's primary nurse; they have known each other since the beginning of Ronnie's illness. Ronnie tells Francine that, although she knows her parents favour more treatment, she herself is tired and has "had enough." Further, two friends whom she met in the hospital underwent similar treatments and ultimately died anyway. Although Ronnie wants only to go home and spend time with her family and friends, she plans to go ahead with the treatment because she does not wish to upset her parents.

## AN INFORMED DECISION?

Elizabeth is an 86-year-old Hungarian woman who is visited regularly by a nurse practitioner, Nori, who works within a family practice unit. Elizabeth came to Canada with her husband in 1956, after being unsettled during the Second World War and the subsequent revolution in Hungary. They looked forward to a new life in Canada and ultimately became very successful. Elizabeth's husband died about 10 years ago; she now lives alone in a condominium but is visited regularly by her children and grandchildren.

continued on following page >>

Elizabeth has just shared with Nori reports from recent studies undertaken on her gallbladder. Elizabeth has some narrowing of her bile duct, and the surgeons are recommending dilatation under laparoscopy. Elizabeth has declined. She has survived for 86 years without surgery and doesn't want to break her "record." She would prefer to "take her chances."

Nori is concerned. She knows the procedure is straightforward and that without it, Elizabeth will experience more pain and may possibly become septic and die. Elizabeth is otherwise healthy, and this decision could affect the quality of her life.

### Discussion Points

1. Identify 10 nursing interventions in which the patient's or client's consent is implied.
2. In what circumstances should nursing interventions require a more explicit consent?
3. Provide some examples of when the principle of beneficence is in conflict with the person's right to choose. How might this dilemma be resolved?
4. Your patient is about to go for an exploratory laparotomy. He has received his preoperative teaching and was seen by the surgeon the evening before. The family has come a long distance to be with him the morning of his surgery. It is only after you give him the preoperative sedation that you notice the consent form has not been signed. What would you do? What would be the practice in your facility if this were to occur?
5. Should parents be permitted to give or refuse consent for their young children regardless of the circumstances? Why or why not? Should the child's best interests govern? Are there any legal avenues open to ensuring that the child's best interests are considered?
6. It is a busy evening, and one of your confused older patients is restless and keeps trying to climb over the bed rails. You believe your only option to protect this patient is to restrain her. As you prepare to do this, the patient—appearing lucid for the moment—states she wishes simply to sit up in the chair. She says she doesn't want to be tied down. What do you do?
7. You are a nurse in the obstetrical wing of a busy teaching hospital. A woman comes in for a pelvic examination under general anesthetic a few days prior to her due date. A young nursing student asks you whether he can observe the examination. What do you tell the patient? Can you assume the patient knows that students will observe procedures as part of their training? What are the risks of proceeding without properly informing the patient and obtaining her consent?

### References

#### Statutes

*Advanced Health Care Directives Act*, S.N.L. 1995, c. A-4.1 (Newfoundland and Labrador).
*Civil Code of Quebec*, C.c.Q. (Quebec).
*Consent to Treatment and Health Care Directives Act*, R.S.P.E.I. 1988, c. C-17.2 (Prince Edward Island).

*Enduring Power of Attorney Act*, R.S.Y. 2002, c. 73 (Yukon).

*Health Care (Consent) and Care Facility (Admission) Act*, R.S.B.C. 1996, c. 181 (British Columbia).

*Health Care Consent Act, 1996*, S.O. 1996, c. 2, Sched. A (Ontario).

*Health Care Directives Act*, C.C.S.M., c. H27 (Manitoba).

*Health Care Directives and Substitute Health Care Decision Makers Act*, S.S. 1997, c. H-0.001 (Saskatchewan).

*Medical Consent Act*, R.S.N.S. 1989, c. 279 (Nova Scotia).

*Mental Health Act*, R.S.O. 1990, c. M.7 (Ontario).

*Representation Agreement Act*, R.S.B.C. 1996, c. 405 (British Columbia).

*Substitute Decisions Act, 1992*, S.O. 1992, c. 30 (Ontario).

## Case Law

*Alberta (Director of Child Welfare) v. B.H.*, [2002] 11 W.W.R. 752, (2002), 31 R.F.L. (5th) 16, (2002), 6 Alta. L.R. (4th) 34, 2002 ABPC 39 (CanLii), affirmed *B.H. v. Alberta (Director of Child Welfare)*, 2002 ABQB 371, [2002] 302 A.R. 201, [2002] 7 W.W.R. 616, (2002), 28 R.F.L. (5th) 334, (2002), 95 C.R.R. (2d) 333, (2002), 3 Alta. L.R. (4th) 16) (Alta. Q.B.).

*Ciarlariello v. Schacter*, [1993] 2 SCR 119, aff'g. (1991), 44 OAC 385; 76 DLR (4th) 449; 5 CCLT (2d) 221 (CA), aff'g. (1987), 7 ACWS (3d) 51 (Ont. HCJ).

*Malette v. Shulman* (1990), 72 OR (2d) 417 (CA), aff'g. 63 OR (3d) 243; 47 DLR (4th) 18; 43 CCLT (2d) 62 (HCJ).

*R. v. Latimer* (1997), 121 CCC (3d) 226 (Sask. QB), aff'd (1998), 131 C.C.C. (3d) 191, 172 Sask. R. 161, 185 W.A.C. 161, 22 C.R. (5th) 380, [1999] 6 W.W.R. 118, [1998] S.J. No. 731 (QL); aff'd. [2001] 1 S.C.R. 3; (2001), 193 D.L.R. (4th) 577; [2001] 6 W.W.R. 409; (2001), 150 C.C.C. (3d) 129; (2001), 39 C.R. (5th) 1; (2001), 80 C.R.R. (2d) 189; (2001), 203 Sask. R. 1.

*Reibl v. Hughes*, [1980] 2 SCR 880; (1980) 14 CCLT 1; 114 DLR (3d) 1; 33 NR 361.

## Texts and Articles

Canadian Nurses Association (CNA). (2008). *Code of ethics for registered nurses*. Ottawa, ON: Author.

Canadian Nurses Protective Society. (2004). Consent of the incapable adult. *InfoLaw,* 13(3), 1–2.

Sharpe, G. (1986). *The law and medicine in Canada* (2nd ed.). Toronto, ON: Butterworths.

# Chapter 7

## The Nurse's Legal Accountabilities: Professional Competence, Misconduct, Malpractice, and Nursing Documentation

### Learning Objectives

The purpose of this chapter is to enable you to understand:

- The professional responsibilities and accountabilities of the nurse
- The ethical and legal aspects of professional competence, negligence, torts, misconduct, and malpractice
- The nurse's ethical and legal responsibilities to the patient and to other health care professionals
- The challenges associated with "whistle-blowing"
- The legal concepts of negligence, duty of care, vicarious liability, standard of care, and causation
- The criminal law with respect to standard of care and negligence
- The role of the coroner's office and the implications of a coroner's inquest
- The legal requirements of proper nursing documentation, its significance, and how it is used in legal proceedings
- The importance of meeting standards for timely, accurate, and complete documentation in ensuring safe and effective nursing care
- The role of expert witnesses in interpreting nursing documentation

## Introduction

As DISCUSSED IN PREVIOUS chapters, society holds nurses, as professionals, to high standards. Nurses are accountable to the public for meeting the standards of practice for their profession, for following professional codes of ethics, and for engaging in ongoing professional development and acquiring new knowledge to ensure competence is maintained. Under the value of accountability, the *Code of Ethics for Registered Nurses* requires that:

> Nurses, as members of a self-regulating profession, practise according to the values and responsibilities in the Code of Ethics for Registered Nurses and in keeping with the professional standards, laws and regulations supporting ethical practice. (Canadian Nurses Association, 2008, p. 15)

Hence, the Code makes clear the nurse's responsibility to practise ethically and to maintain both professional and legal standards and rules.

Society places its trust in nurses and is clear about its expectations. The legal system measures the performance and behaviour of nurses against professional and ethical standards, such as those stated in the Code, and imposes significant consequences when nurses fail to meet them. An awareness of the processes and legal analysis that make up a negligence action in a professional nursing setting helps nurses gain a better understanding of those consequences.

This chapter describes the legal consequences that nurses may face when failure to meet professional standards results in harm to patients, clients, or others entrusted to their care. It also reviews practice standards and the significance of documentation when issues such as negligence are before the legal system.

## Professional Competence, Misconduct, and Malpractice

### The Difference Between Professional Misconduct and Malpractice

When examining the disciplinary and professional competence responsibilities and obligations of nursing's regulatory bodies, one must understand the distinction between **professional misconduct** and **malpractice**.

Many provincial and territorial statutes regulating nursing and other health care professions provide a legal definition of *professional misconduct*. Though examples from only some provinces are presented, the same principles apply across the country. Readers are encouraged to read their own provincial or territorial statutes. A regulation of Ontario's *Nursing Act* (1991) specifically sets out 37 acts of professional misconduct (*Professional Misconduct Regulation*, O. Reg. 799/93, s. 1). These include such acts as:

- Contravening or failing to meet a standard of practice of the profession
- Improperly or unlawfully delegating a controlled act
- Directing a nurse or nursing student to perform a nursing function for which he or she is not prepared or competent to perform

- Improperly discontinuing professional services for a patient
- Practising nursing while one's ability to do so is impaired by drugs or alcohol
- Verbally, physically, emotionally, or sexually abusing a patient
- Failing to keep records as required

One of the most noteworthy of such acts is: "Engaging in conduct or performing an act, relevant to the practice of nursing, that, having regard to all the circumstances, would reasonably be regarded by members as disgraceful, dishonourable or unprofessional" (*Professional Misconduct Regulation*, s. 1).

*Malpractice*, however, does not necessarily involve any such misconduct but, rather (as is discussed in more detail below), involves performing lawful acts in a careless manner or in a manner that does not conform with a generally recognized practice standard or standard of care in the nursing profession. Thus, a nurse can perform a lawful act in a way that does not involve any misconduct, but he or she might perform such an act or function in a way that is careless or lacking in skill and that could lead to harm or injury to a patient or otherwise compromise a patient's course of treatment or health.

One interesting provision in the Ontario Act (similar provisions exist in the acts of other provinces and territories) with important consequences for nurses states that it is professional misconduct to do anything to a client for a therapeutic, preventive, palliative, diagnostic, cosmetic, or other health-related purpose for which consent is required by law without first obtaining such consent (*Professional Misconduct Regulation*, s. 1, para. 9). This is significant in light of Ontario's *Health Care Consent Act* (1996) (discussed in Chapter 6), which contains provisions for informed consent and disclosure of material risks.

The ethical and legal aspects of professional competence, misconduct, and malpractice are interrelated. Two means by which the skills and conduct of nurses are gauged are the civil law (as in the civil lawsuit) and the complaints procedures related to the disciplinary powers of the nursing regulatory bodies (as discussed in Chapter 5). Through these regulatory and self-governing mechanisms, nurses are made accountable to their patients, clients, the community, and society.

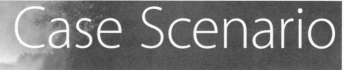

# Case Scenario

## SHARED ACCOUNTABILITY?

Several nurses in a nursing team rotate through the same schedule in a busy Intensive Care Unit (ICU) of a major hospital. One of the nurses, Kathy, has recently been under extreme personal stress owing to the breakup of a relationship and the death of a close family member.

continued on following page >>

Over the past four to five weeks, her colleagues have noticed occasions on which Kathy has arrived for the night shift smelling of alcohol. When the other nurses have raised their concerns with her, Kathy has explained that she had a glass or two of wine over dinner with some friends. As the weeks go by, these incidents increase in frequency. At times, Kathy's speech seems slurred. The other nurses on the team hesitate to report these incidents to the nurse manager, as they do not wish to add to Kathy's stress. They hope that as she deals with her personal problems, this issue will resolve itself. To protect Kathy and to minimize the risks to her patients, the nurses in charge give her easy assignments and send her on a break whenever the night supervisor visits the unit.

In this ICU, nurses are expected to have and to use specialized skills and to perform certain delegated medical acts. As well, under the hospital's nursing standards policy, each nurse is subject to an annual review of knowledge and skills. Kathy is three months overdue for hers. The unit educator has scheduled it three times, but on each occasion, Kathy has cancelled, citing illness or heavy workload. It is unclear when her review can be rescheduled, since, as a result of budget cuts, the number of educators has been reduced.

One night, when Kathy again arrives smelling of alcohol, she is assigned a patient who is experiencing cardiac arrhythmias. During her shift, Kathy notes an arrhythmia on the patient's monitor, which she identifies as runs of ventricular tachycardia. In this unit, nurses have been delegated the act of administering lidocaine, a drug that treats such an arrhythmia. Kathy prepares and administers the intravenous bolus of lidocaine. A few minutes later, the patient has a respiratory and cardiac arrest. Fortunately, he is easily resuscitated.

Upon review of the patient's status, it is noted that he had, in fact, experienced supraventricular tachycardia, for which lidocaine is not indicated. Furthermore, one of the other nurses noticed that the empty drug ampoule contained pancuronium, not lidocaine. These drugs are contained in similar-sized ampoules, and the labelling is the same colour. Pancuronium causes paralysis and is used during general anesthesia or, sometimes, for patients who are being mechanically ventilated in an ICU. Clearly, the drug led to the patient's cardiac arrest. Subsequently it was discovered that the pancuronium ampoules had been placed in the wrong container. The container was labelled *lidocaine*.

## Issues

1. Do the nurses in the unit have an obligation to "blow the whistle" on Kathy (i.e., report her alcohol use)? Are they able to evaluate Kathy's risk to her patients?
2. What are Kathy's responsibilities for reviewing her knowledge and skills? What are the hospital's responsibilities?
3. Does the educator have any responsibility for ensuring that Kathy's review takes place?
4. What responsibility, if any, does the second nurse have to report that the incorrect drug was given?
5. Does the charge nurse have any specific accountability or duty that is distinct from that of Kathy's colleagues?

continued on following page >>

6. Does the hospital have any obligation to disclose the occurrence to the family of the patient (and the patient himself, if living)?
7. Are Kathy, the hospital, and the nursing team at risk of any legal, civil, or criminal actions against them?
8. Should any disciplinary action be taken with Kathy and her colleagues?
9. Is the fact that the pancuronium ampoules were placed in the wrong container a factor from the perspective of either Kathy or the hospital?
10. How accountable are hospitals for making resource allocation decisions that ensure the provision of safe patient care?

## Discussion

This scenario highlights a number of significant ethical and legal challenges. What is a nurse's ethical and legal responsibility when a colleague demonstrates incompetence? What is the individual professional's responsibility to maintain competence, and what is the organization's responsibility to ensure the overall competence of staff? Further, what are nurses' responsibilities regarding colleagues who are in need of help?

As noted in the Canadian Nurses Association's *Code of Ethics for Registered Nurses*, nurses have a responsibility to safeguard the quality of nursing care that clients receive. The Code states that:

> Nurses question and intervene to address unsafe, non-compassionate, unethical or incompetent practice or conditions that interfere with their ability to provide safe, compassionate, competent and ethical care to those to whom they are providing care, and they support those who do the same. (Canadian Nurses Association, 2008, p. 9)

Therefore, nurses must take preventive and corrective action to protect clients from unsafe, incompetent, or unethical care. They must ensure that they have the skills and knowledge to remain competent. When they suspect unethical, incompetent, or unsafe care, or doubt the safety of conditions in the care setting, they must take the appropriate steps to resolve the problem.

It is clear, then, that when we become aware of incompetence on the part of another nurse or other health care professional, we are obligated to take action to ensure the safety of patients. When a nurse fails to take such action, he or she shares responsibility for any subsequent consequences of that incompetence.

Delegation of added responsibilities to nurses should be appropriate, and processes must be in place to ensure ongoing competence with respect to these responsibilities. In this scenario, Kathy, her colleagues, and the educator had a shared professional responsibility to ensure that patients continually received competent care.

Nurses have a responsibility to maintain their professional competence by meeting at least the minimum standards required by their regulatory body. When the health facilities that

continued on following page >>

employ them, such as hospitals or community agencies, impose a higher standard, then these higher standards must be met. In this case, both Kathy and the hospital bear responsibility for ensuring her competence. The leadership within any organization must take steps to ensure the competence of its employees. If the employee does not respond to a requirement for reassessment or **recertification**, then reminders, counselling, and (if required) disciplinary action must take place.

Nurses are required to collaborate with one another to ensure the care environment is consistent with safe and ethical practice and to provide mentoring and guidance to ensure the continued competency and professional development of not only students but also practising nurses. This is of particular import in highly technological critical care environments, where patients are vulnerable and at risk of serious harm if not cared for by highly competent professionals.

What was happening to Kathy in this situation? Did her colleagues understand the significance of her behaviour? Were they aware of the warning signs that Kathy was in crisis and needed help? Kathy's colleagues, concerned about her personal situation, thought they were protecting her. They seemed to be hoping that Kathy's crisis would resolve itself and made efforts to shield her from further harm. Though one might sympathize with their concern, their strategy was counterproductive to Kathy's needs, placed the lives of patients in jeopardy, and compromised their own professional integrity.

Nurses function within a highly stressful work environment. (In Chapter 11, the importance of a healthy work environment is discussed in detail.) When personal problems add to this stress, some nurses, like others in society, may become vulnerable to the abuse of substances such as alcohol or drugs when seeking short-term relief of their symptoms. In fact, nurses may be even more vulnerable to controlled substances, such as narcotics, since they have ready access to them. Nurses need to be aware that there are programs and support available for colleagues facing these sorts of challenges (Dunn, 2005). Kathy's colleagues, if unsuccessful in dealing with her directly, have a responsibility both to Kathy and to her patients to take their concerns to the manager, a staff counsellor, or another professional. A concerned and astute manager should also recognize Kathy's need for help.

Early intervention in such situations is necessary. It is better for the nurse involved to get counselling and therapy early on rather than to wait until patient care is compromised and his or her career is in jeopardy.

This scenario raises additional issues regarding the organization's accountability. The institution is responsible for assessing the competence of staff and also for ensuring regular staff development is undertaken. Further, though it appears Kathy failed to read the label accurately, the hospital should have processes in place to ensure these drugs are placed in the correct containers. When high-risk medications have a similar "look," additional steps should be taken (e.g., storing medications in different locations, posting signs to alert nurses to the risk).

## Negligence and the Duty of Care

## Torts

A **tort** is a civil wrong committed by one person against another causing that other some injury or damage, either to person or property. Torts may be *intentional* or *nonintentional*. An assault is an example of an intentional tort, in that the person who commits it intends the action that causes harm to the victim. Nonintentional torts generally constitute negligence. In the scenario above, Kathy obviously did not intend to cause harm to the patient but was negligent in making the wrong assessment and in giving the wrong medication.

In civil law, as applies in Quebec, torts are called **delicts** and come within the *Civil Code* provisions dealing with obligations. Specific provisions of the *Civil Code* define and govern the concept of delicts and the elements that must be proved in court for the plaintiff to recover damages. Under civil law, anyone under a duty not to cause harm to another is at fault if he or she fails in that duty by not acting according to the expected standard of care.

### INTENTIONAL TORTS

*Battery and Assault*

Of particular importance to the nursing profession are the concepts of battery and assault. Since much of a nurse's work involves the physical touching of patients—for example, administering injections, suturing wounds, establishing intravenous lines, physically moving patients, and other invasive measures—nurses must understand that such procedures may be done only upon a consenting patient. Consent, explained more fully below, may be expressed orally, obtained in writing, or simply implied and inferred from the patient's conduct and the circumstances.

**Battery** in common law is defined as the intentional bringing about of a harmful or offensive and nonconsensual contact upon another (Fleming, 1983, p. 23; see also Linden, 1993, p. 40). An obvious example of battery would be one person striking another. The harmful or offensive contact may be either direct, such as a slap in the face, or indirect, such as pulling on a person's chair, causing him or her to fall to the ground (Linden, 1993, pp. 40–41). In either case, there has been an *intentional* interference with the bodily integrity and security of another. Moreover, these acts are seen as potential inducements to further violence, because the victim may be provoked into retaliation. The chief aim of tort law is to prevent violence by making perpetrators of such acts civilly liable to their victims for damages. The law is also concerned with the need to restore the victim of the tort, as much as is possible through the award of monetary damages, to the situation he or she was in prior to the battery or assault.

The offensive or intrusive conduct need not be violent, as even seemingly insignificant unwanted touching may amount to battery. The perpetrator need not intend any harmful result. Thus, even a kiss on the cheek may amount to battery if it is not consented to by the recipient.

However, certain common, everyday acts will not usually amount to battery. For instance, the Western custom of shaking hands is not considered battery. One need not ask another's permission prior to shaking hands; consent would be implied by the holding out of one's hand. It must be noted, however, that in a diverse society such as Canada's, nurses must be sensitive to patients whose cultural background might not recognize or welcome such conduct, especially if the patient is of a different gender than the nurse. There is also the special consideration of nurses who care for children. Cuddling and holding, appropriate to the child's developmental age, is often essential to their care and well-being.

**Assault** is the "intentional creation of the apprehension of imminent harmful or offensive contact" (Linden, 1993, p. 42). For example, if one person lunges threateningly at another who is close by but does not actually strike, that person is still liable to damages for assault. A court would likely conclude that the victim was reasonably concerned about being harmed in this situation and that the threat was imminent. However, there would be no assault if the victim could not reasonably conclude from the circumstances that the perpetrator was actually able to carry out the threat. The reasonableness of the victim's state of mind is the key factor in such an analysis. There is no requirement that the perpetrator actually be able to carry out the threat; it is sufficient that the evidence of the circumstances in which the threat was made led to a reasonable conclusion that the defendant was able to carry it out.

*Consent*

Consent to treatment is discussed fully in Chapter 6, but since its relevance in the discussion of torts is significant, we will revisit it briefly here.

Generally, if the aggrieved person has consented to the conduct being visited upon him or her, the perpetrator may escape liability for such conduct in some cases. **Consent**, which can be defined as permission given by a person for someone else to perform an act upon him or her, can be *explicit* (expressed) or *implied* by the circumstances or by the conduct of the aggrieved person. Expressed consent may be given orally or in writing. The written consent is not consent in and of itself but, rather, is evidence that the party giving it has consented to an act.

Implied consent is agreement to an act inferred from the actions of the recipient. An example of implied consent in a medical setting might be a patient's holding out an arm to a nurse to have his blood pressure checked. The patient cannot then say that he did not consent to the touching since a reasonable person would infer from his conduct that he had consented. This illustrates another aspect of implied consent—that is, the existence of consent is measured against an **objective standard**.

For consent to be valid in law, the person giving it must be capable of doing so. In the case of a mentally ill patient, consent to treatment may or may not be valid, depending on whether the mental illness makes that patient unable to appreciate the nature, quality, and consequences of the proposed treatment. Children under the age of majority (or under 16, in some provinces) usually cannot consent to medical treatment, in which case their parents or legal guardians would be called upon to give consent. However, if the child is mature enough to understand the nature and risks of the proposed treatment, the caregiver or institution may rely upon that consent or assent (agreement by the child that treatment may proceed based on the informed consent of the parent).

Consent will be invalidated if it was obtained by force or fraud. Duress or the use of force invalidates any consent because the recipient is obviously not making a decision of his or her own free will. Only a freely given and voluntary consent is valid in law.

In the context of health care, it is important to remember that no medical treatment, no matter how crucial to the health or survival of the patient, may be administered without that patient's consent, unless the situation is life-threatening and the patient is unconscious or mentally incompetent (e.g., see Saskatchewan's *Emergency Medical Aid Act*, 1978, ss. 2(b), 3). Statutes such as the *Emergency Medical Aid Act* permit a registered nurse to administer emergency medical treatment to an unconscious person involved in an accident without incurring liability for negligence as a result of an act or omission on his or her part. It does not, however, excuse the nurse from *gross negligence*—that is, conduct that drastically departs from the standard of the reasonably competent nurse.

In a clinical setting, only that specific treatment that is consented to may be administered, and in most cases, only those health professionals specified in the patient's consent may administer the consented-to treatment. The patient's consent must also be informed. This means that the nature of the treatment to be administered, its benefits and attendant risks, and any and all material information must be given to the patient for the consent to be valid.

The issue of consent, and its many ethical and legal pitfalls, is as relevant to the nursing profession as it is to physicians. Many fine lines are drawn, and it is not always easy to determine the extent and scope of the consent.

## NONINTENTIONAL TORTS

### Negligence

As previously suggested, in common law, negligence falls under the nonintentional category of torts. A defendant may still be liable for a tort while not having intended any harm or injury. For a defendant to be liable for negligence, three elements must be present (Linden, 1993, p. 92). These are summarized in Table 7.1. First, the defendant must owe a duty of care in law toward the plaintiff. Second, the defendant must have breached that duty and failed to discharge the standard of care required by law in the particular situation. Third, the plaintiff must have suffered damage or harm caused by the defendant's breach of the duty of care. Another related legal principle is that if the plaintiff was in any way partly responsible for his or her injuries as a result of negligence, the defendant will be absolved of liability to the extent of the plaintiff's own negligence. This principle is called **contributory negligence**.

To use a nursing example, a nurse owes a duty of care to a patient when administering a medication. Suppose the nurse misreads the label on a bottle containing a certain medication. What if the medication administered is in fact one to which the patient is highly allergic? In reading the medication label incorrectly and failing to notice that the patient is allergic to the medication, legally, the nurse has breached the duty owed to that patient. As a result of that breach, the patient receives a harmful substance and suffers a severe allergic reaction that, in turn, causes brain damage. His brain damage is a direct and foreseeable result of that breach.

### Table 7.1: The Elements of Negligence

1   Duty of care owed to the plaintiff (e.g., a patient or client).

2   Breach of duty of care by the defendant (e.g., a nurse or physician) by failure to administer treatment or provide health care in accordance with a particular standard of care.

3   Patient suffers damage as a direct result of the breach of the duty of care.

Factors that help determine whether a defendant will be held liable (responsible) in a case of negligence include duty of care, standard of care, proximate cause, and contributory negligence. We will now discuss each of these factors in detail.

## Duty of Care and the Standard of Care

To be liable in tort, a defendant must owe a **duty of care** to the plaintiff, either personally or as a member of a class of persons such as, for example, patients seeking medical care or perhaps schoolchildren being transported to school on school buses (where the bus manufacturer would owe a duty to them). The law imposes a duty of care in many but not all situations. If there is no duty of care in law, the defendant will not be liable to the plaintiff, even if the defendant's conduct was the immediate cause of the plaintiff's injuries.

Common law holds that one owes a duty of care to those people who are close to, or closely connected with, one's conduct or activities. Professionals such as nurses owe a duty of care to those who retain their services or are placed in their care to act in a competent and diligent manner according to the standard of the reasonably competent nurse. This includes a responsibility for the nurse, as with any other professional, to keep abreast of current developments and techniques within the profession and to undertake retraining as necessary.

The classic definition of the duty of care can be found in an old case that originated in Scotland in the early 1930s. In the decision in *Donoghue v. Stevenson* (1932), Lord Atkin, one of the Lord Justices of the House of Lords to which the case had been appealed, spoke of the duty thus:

> The rule that you are to love your neighbour becomes in law, you must not injure your neighbour; and the lawyer's question, Who is my neighbour? receives a restricted reply. You must take reasonable care to avoid acts or omissions which you can reasonably foresee would be likely to injure your neighbour. Who, then, in law is my neighbour? The answer seems to be persons who are so closely and directly affected by my act that I ought reasonably to have them in contemplation as being so affected when I am directing my mind to the acts or omissions which are called in question. (*Donoghue v. Stevenson*, 1932, p. 580; 101 LJPC 119, at p. 127; 147 LT 281 (HL); see also Linden, 1993, p. 258)

A case from Ontario will serve to illustrate these concepts in a medical setting. In *Latin v. Hospital for Sick Children et al.* (2007), a 14-month-old girl was admitted to a pediatric hospital in late January 1998 with a very high fever. The triage nurse assessed her as an "urgent" patient using the hospital's triage classification system of "emergent," "urgent," and "nonurgent." One hour and 20 minutes after the girl's arrival at the emergency department and before she was brought in for medical assessment, she began a generalized tonic-clonic seizure in the waiting room. She was immediately taken into a treatment room, where medical staff attempted to bring her seizure under control. Despite these efforts, seizure activity continued for a considerable length of time. She was eventually discharged from the hospital some weeks later with profound brain damage and extreme and permanent disabilities. The infant's mother and grandparents brought a lawsuit against the hospital and the triage and charge nurse on duty that day as well as against several other nurses involved in the child's treatment in the emergency department together with the child's family physician and the physicians at the hospital who had been involved in providing care to the child. The lawsuit against the doctors was discontinued before the trial. A diagnosis as to what caused the child's brain damage was never made, but the parties in the lawsuit advanced numerous theories to explain the injury.

It appeared that the child had been suffering from croup since one month prior to her admission. On the day before her admission, the mother had called her family pediatrician about the child's high fever and was given an appointment for the following day. In the evening, the child was restless with fever, was not eating or drinking well and wanted only to be held. The following day, the child's body jerked violently while she was sitting in her grandmother's lap. The mother eventually reached the family physician, who told her he felt the child was experiencing febrile seizures and that the infant might be dehydrated but that it was better for her to be assessed at the hospital. Subsequently, the child was taken to the hospital's emergency department. The girl was seen at triage at 1240 hours and assessed, following which her mother was told to go to registration and advised to bring the child back to the triage nurse if her condition changed.

Some time later, the child began having seizures and was brought back to the emergency department waiting room. She was immediately taken into an acute care room in the emergency department and attended to and treated by physicians and nurses. She continued to experience seizures for more than 90 minutes thereafter. After some five hours, the child was transferred to the pediatric intensive care unit of the hospital. An EEG was performed the following day and showed a result consistent with a diffuse encephalopathy. Three days later:

> she was noted to be generally more awake, moving all four limbs normally, with no abnormal movements or further seizures, but still with an abnormal level of consciousness and activity. She was transferred from the PICU to the ward at 1330 hours on this day. Approximately two hours later, [the child] again began seizure activity of a focal right-sided nature. Between 1540 and approximately 2400 hours on January 24, at least seven seizures were noted, and at approximately 0130 on January 25, [the infant]

was transferred back to the PICU from the ward, where she remained unresponsive, with decreased power on her right side and abnormal movements.

Over the next two days, consultations were obtained, including those from the infectious disease service, metabolics and the neurology service. On January 26, a second CT scan was performed, which showed diffuse cerebral edema, primarily in the frontal regions of the girl's brain. . . .

[The girl] was transferred from the PICU back to the ward on January 28, where she remained until she was discharged to [a rehabilitation institution] for further rehabilitation on February 17. . . .

[She] was a healthy, normally developing infant when she was brought to the Hospital. [At the time of the lawsuit, she was] 9 years of age and very disabled due to her brain injury, particularly on the right side of her body. She was discharged from [the hospital] without a diagnosis as to the cause of her brain injury. (*Latin v. Hospital for Sick Children et al.*, 2007, paras. 19–21).

The child's family's lawsuit against the hospital and the triage nurse and charge nurse who were involved in assessing and treating the child that day proceeded to trial. Their claim was that when they first showed up at the emergency department, the girl was in a state of "early/compensated distributive shock due to sepsis as a result of bacterial pneumonia" (*Latin v. Hospital for Sick Children et al.*, 2007, para. 23). They alleged that this infection was not noticed by the team because the triage nurse had taken an inadequate history of the child at the time. The girl later progressed to a state of shock, and the medical team then tried to manage the shock rather than trying to ensure her brain received an adequate oxygen supply. They alleged that as a result of this, she suffered a hypoxic-ischemic brain injury. They had a number of experts testify at the trial with respect to the level of nursing (among other medical) care the child received during treatment. They alleged that the girl had been incorrectly classified as an urgent rather than emergent case. As an emergent case, they claimed, she would have been seen sooner by a physician who would have recognized that she was in shock (*Latin v. Hospital for Sick Children et al.*, 2007, para. 24).

The defendant hospital, on its own behalf and on behalf of the nurses involved in the girl's treatment, alleged that the girl's brain damage was caused by an infectious process in her brain (in all likelihood, influenza A virus), which was not considered as an explanation for her brain damage at the time of her hospitalization. With subsequent increased knowledge of influenza A in the years since the events in question, it is now known that this was the viral agent that caused the infection, but this would not have been detected with the medical knowledge available at the time. No treatment available then could have reversed this process. The shock theory was not supported by the evidence, and even if the child had been classified as an emergent case and seen immediately by a doctor, no useful treatment could have been administered before the seizures began (*Latin v. Hospital for Sick Children et al.*, 2007, para. 26).

The court first had to determine the appropriate standard of care owed to the child by the nurses and the hospital. The girl's family alleged that the nursing treatment had fallen below the standard of care and that this had resulted in her brain damage. Evidence as to the appropriate standard of care in this situation was to be gleaned from a number of sources, including the testimony of the nursing experts, the hospital's own written policies, information given to members of the public on procedures in the emergency department, nursing manuals and academic literature, and the testimony of physicians who were knowledgeable in emergency medicine (*Latin v. Hospital for Sick Children et al.*, 2007, para. 31).

The court found that the triage nurse (who was one of the nurses being sued) had not failed to meet the standard of care expected of her in assessing the child as urgent rather than emergent. She had conducted an assessment of suitable length (5 minutes), and there was no evidence that the length of the assessment had any bearing on the standard of care. She had not taken the child's blood pressure or respiration rate on triage; however, the child was crying at the time, and the nurse had noted this on the triage form. The child's crying, the court noted from the expert evidence, would have naturally prevented the nurse from being able to obtain a meaningful respiration rate or blood pressure (*Latin v. Hospital for Sick Children et al.*, 2007, para. 67). The court ruled that it was not routine procedure at the time to measure blood pressure in triage unless it was clearly indicated as an issue by history or assessment (*Latin v. Hospital for Sick Children et al.*, 2007, para. 66). It should be noted that in the adult setting, nurses would expect blood pressure to be taken at triage, but in the case of children, this would not normally be done unless the child's history clearly required it (for example, in the case of children with pre-existing cardiac conditions or kidney disease) (*Latin v. Hospital for Sick Children et al.*, 2007, paras. 62, 63).

In terms of the alleged failure of the triage nurse to record the child's respiration rate, the court concluded on the evidence, and a review of the child's medical and emergency department nursing records, that there was nothing at the time to alert that nurse to any difficulties in the child's breathing. Even the child's mother testified that she did not note any difficulty in the child's breathing (*Latin v. Hospital for Sick Children et al.*, 2007, para. 80). The court finally concluded that, with respect to the triage nurse's conduct, she had correctly exercised her clinical judgement in assessing the girl as an urgent case. Determining this classification was a function that fell within a nurse's clinical judgement, and in this case, it was in accordance with the hospital's own triage classification policy and was, on the evidence, a reasonable and appropriate decision (*Latin v. Hospital for Sick Children et al.*, 2007, paras. 100–109). Even if the triage nurse had been wrong, she had appropriately exercised her judgement about the seriousness of the girl's condition. The court concluded that she had met the standard of care of a reasonable and prudent nurse in acting as she did then and in her subsequent reassessment of the child. The court noted in passing that the nurse should have documented the reassessment results but that her failure to do so did not amount to negligence (*Latin v. Hospital for Sick Children et al.*, 2007, para. 109).

The court also considered the conduct of the charge nurse who provided treatment to the child. The child's family alleged that she had failed to meet the standard of care because there were examination rooms available at the time the child arrived in the emergency department yet the child was not sent to one of them; she allowed a more stable patient in the urgent category to be seen before the child; and she permitted a nonurgent patient to be seen ahead of the child (*Latin v. Hospital for Sick Children et al.*, 2007, para. 110). The evidence of the physicians and nursing experts indicated that the charge nurse's evaluation of when it would be appropriate to send patients to an examination room from the waiting room was complex. Availability of rooms was only one factor; other factors included the availability of physicians, support staff including discharge planners to assist patients about to be discharged, and cleaning staff to prepare rooms for new patients (*Latin v. Hospital for Sick Children et al.*, 2007, para. 112). On this point, the court found that while it would be inexcusable to keep patients waiting if there were an available treatment room, there was nothing in the evidence to suggest that the child could have been seen any earlier than 1400 hours. The evidence fell short of establishing that there were appropriate resources available before then such as to indicate that the charge nurse had failed to assign the child to a treatment room at an earlier time (*Latin v. Hospital for Sick Children et al.*, 2007, para. 118). There was also no evidence that the child was critically ill before 1400 hours or that her condition was precarious. The charge nurse reprioritized the patients in the emergency department as situations changed to ensure that available resources were assigned to the most serious cases. The court held that deference had to be shown to the judgement of those who manage the work of an emergency department, in this case, the charge nurse. The court concluded that the charge nurse had met the standard of care of a reasonable and prudent charge nurse that day (*Latin v. Hospital for Sick Children et al.*, 2007, para. 126).

## Duty of Care in Emergencies

A breach of a duty of care will be found to exist when one person has placed others in peril as a result of his or her conduct. Furthermore, a person who creates a hazard, even unwittingly and through no negligence of his or her own, may still be held liable if he or she fails to warn others of the hazard and they are injured.

It is both interesting and troubling to note that under common law, unlike under the civil law of Quebec (see, for example, *Gaudreault v. Drapeau* (1987); Quebec's Charter of Human Rights and Freedoms, arts. 1, 2, 4, 5, 7, 8, 49; and examples from the civil law countries of Europe), there is no general duty to aid someone in peril (Linden, 1993, p. 266). This absence is one illustration of the divergence that can occur between law and ethics. What may clearly be a moral or ethical imperative may not necessarily be a legal requirement.

For example, in common law provinces, a passerby may observe a man in cardiac arrest and not render assistance. There is no positive duty to act in such cases. (See, for example, the *Criminal Code of Canada*, 1985, s. 215 (failing to provide necessities of life to a child), s. 218 (abandoning a child), s. 216 (duty of persons undertaking acts dangerous to life to use reasonable skill and care in so doing), and s. 217, which reads: "Every one who undertakes to do an act is under a legal duty to do so if an omission to do the act is or may be dangerous to life.") However, most people, acting morally, would likely intervene to save a person in obvious danger. If someone does act, the law imposes a duty of care upon him or her not to conduct such rescue negligently. A person who fails in a rescue bid may be civilly liable for any injury or death resulting to the person being rescued (Linden, 1993, pp. 279–281). Usually, however, for the rescuer to be found liable, his or her conduct must amount to gross negligence—that is, a substantial and marked departure from the standard of the reasonably competent and skilled rescuer.

As we saw in the *Latin* case, nurses have a special relationship to those whom they serve, and it is thus desirable to impose on them a duty of care (Linden, 1993, pp. 270–272). They have special training and expertise and are required to exercise a very high degree of care in carrying out their tasks.

## Breach of the Standard of Care

How do courts determine whether or not a defendant's conduct has been negligent? Common law has developed the concept of the **standard of care** as an objective measure of such conduct. If a defendant's conduct is seen as having fallen below the standard of what a competent person, acting reasonably and responsibly in similar circumstances, would have done, a court may find that defendant's conduct to be negligent. In the *Latin* case, the standard was determined by means of the expert testimony of nurses, emergency physicians, and literature and documentation illustrating hospital policies and procedures. The particular standard against which any given conduct is judged will vary depending on the circumstances and people involved. For example, a doctor will be judged by the standard of the reasonably competent physician. Similarly, a nurse's conduct in the treatment of a patient who has suffered harm as a result of his or her acts or omissions will be judged by the standard of the reasonably competent nurse.

The nurses in *Latin* were judged by the average standards of the triage nurse and charge nurse possessed of reasonable knowledge, skill, and ability. These would include minimal standards of competence and knowledge set by the governing body for nurses in the various provinces and any applicable standards prescribed by the health facility in which that nurse is employed. Such standards also include the requirement to keep up to date with the latest professional and technological developments. Additional education should be taken as required to maintain expertise to the appropriate standard. A professional who fails to keep up to date with new knowledge and standards runs the risk of employing methods that have been discredited or proved harmful by the latest studies and thinking in that field. If that professional's conduct were ever called into question, such failure would be evidence of negligence.

## Causation, Proximate Cause, and Remoteness

A defendant will be liable for harm to a plaintiff if that harm was caused by the defendant's negligent conduct. This seems straightforward and logical. However, can a plaintiff be compensated for all possible harm that may occur as a result of the defendant's negligent act? Some results that follow negligent conduct can be so remote (i.e., removed from the foreseeable chain of events and consequences) that they should not be within the purview of what is compensable damage. To qualify as damage for which a plaintiff can recover compensation, that damage must be something that a reasonable person could foresee as resulting from the negligent conduct, meaning that the cause should be reasonably **proximate** to, or the reasonably foreseeable cause of the ensuing damage.

In the *Latin* decision, the court applied the principle that if a defendant's negligence has caused or contributed to the plaintiff's injury and if that injury would not have occurred but for such negligence, the plaintiff has proved **causation**. The child's family in *Latin* alleged that it was a delay in diagnosing and treating the child that essentially caused her brain damage and that that delay was the result of the negligence of the triage nurse, the charge nurse, and other members of the health care team involved on the day the child was brought to Emergency. The court had available before it three alternative possible causes of the child's brain injury: (1) idiopathic status epilepticus, (2) shock, and (3) viral encephalitis (*Latin v. Hospital for Sick Children et al.*, 2007, para. 148). The court rejected the first cause because it was very rare for status epilepticus to cause brain damage in a normal child without the presence of underlying shock (*Latin v. Hospital for Sick Children et al.*, 2007, para. 149). The court further found that there was no evidence of significant fluid loss or dehydration such as would lead to significant circulatory disturbances due to hypovolemia. The child had an elevated heart rate after 1400 hours (as high as 230 bpm at one point), but the expert evidence suggested this could have been caused by the seizures and fever alone. The child's rapid heart rate could have been a sign of shock but also of dehydration and possibly states other than shock, such as fever and stress. The experts stated that such a rapid pulse would be expected in a child experiencing febrile seizures. The evidence was that a pulse as high as 230 bpm would have permitted her cardiac output to provide adequate blood flow to the brain and other vital organs. She was never hypotensive and had adequate blood flow to perfuse the tissues of her body. The evidence further indicated that the physicians were not treating the child for shock, but, rather, fluid boluses were administered to her to counteract the hypotensive effects of the anticonvulsive medication she was given for the seizures (*Latin v. Hospital for Sick Children et al.*, 2007, para. 202). The court accordingly concluded that shock was not the cause of her brain injury.

The court eventually found that the child's very high fever was caused by an underlying infection, but it was unclear as to whether its source was bacterial or viral. The court, in the end, could not conclude that on a balance of probabilities (the civil standard of proof), the child's brain injury was caused by shock, a fever, or infection. Thus, it could safely conclude that if she was in a state of shock at triage, it was highly improbable that an emergent classification by the triage nurse would have resulted in any different treatment prior to 1400 hours. The nurses were therefore found not liable for the girl's injuries since nothing they did could have contributed to or caused those injuries.

## Contributory Negligence

In earlier times under common law, if a plaintiff was found to be partly at fault for the harm he or she suffered, the law would deny him or her the right to recover damages from the defendant (see *Butterfield v. Forrester* (1809)). Today, in all common law provinces and territories, a plaintiff may still recover damages even if partly at fault, but the damages awarded will be reduced by the percentage to which he or she was to blame or contributed to the loss. (See Alberta: *Contributory Negligence Act*, R.S.A. 2000, c. C-27; British Columbia: *Negligence Act*, R.S.B.C. 1996, c. 333; Manitoba: *Tortfeasors and Contributory Negligence Act*, C.C.S.M. c. T90; New Brunswick: *Contributory Negligence Act*, R.S.N.B. 1973, c. C-19; Newfoundland and Labrador: *Contributory Negligence Act*, R.S.N.L. 1990, c. C-33; Northwest Territories and Nunavut: *Contributory Negligence Act*, R.S.N.W.T. 1988, c. C-18; Nova Scotia: *Contributory Negligence Act*, R.S.N.S. 1989, c. 95; Ontario: *Negligence Act*, R.S.O. 1990, c. N.1; Prince Edward Island: *Contributory Negligence Act*, R.S.P.E.I. 1988, c. C-21; Saskatchewan: *Contributory Negligence Act*, R.S.S. 1978, c. C-31; and Yukon: *Contributory Negligence Act*, R.S.Y. 2002, c. 42.) Lawyers say in such situations that the plaintiff was **contributorily negligent**. Of course, if the evidence shows that the plaintiff was completely to blame for the harm that befell him or her, the defendant would escape liability entirely. The court will apportion the liability among the parties—that is, it will determine as best it can the percentage or proportion to which each party is to blame for the loss. In this respect, the law is basically the same in all common law provinces and territories and in the province of Quebec, where it is known as the principle of common fault (*Civil Code of Quebec*, art. 1478; see also Linden, 1993, pp. 440–441).

## Statutory Duty of Care

Most provincial nursing statutes explicitly or implicitly impose certain duties that nurses owe to patients in their care. Among these is the duty to report a fellow nurse whose conduct displays a lack of proper skill, judgement, knowledge, or training. (See, for example, Saskatchewan: *Registered Nurses Act*, 1988–89, S.S. 1988, c. R-12.2, s. 26(2)(k); and Manitoba: *Registered Nurses Act*, R.S.M. 1987, c. R40, C.C.S.M. c. R40, s. 46(1).) This also includes, in many provinces, a duty to report a nurse who is under the influence of alcohol or drugs.

In Nova Scotia, for example, section 2(ag) of the *Registered Nurses Act* (2001) defines professional misconduct as including:

> such conduct or acts relevant to the practice of nursing that, having regard to all the circumstances, would reasonably be regarded as disgraceful, dishonourable or unprofessional which, without limiting the generality of the foregoing, may include
> (i)  failing to maintain the College of Registered Nurses of Nova Scotia Standards for Nursing Practice,
> (ii)  failing to uphold the code of ethics adopted by the College,
> (iii)  abusing a person verbally, physically, emotionally or sexually,
> (iv)  misappropriating personal property, drugs or other property belonging to a client or a registrant's employer,
> (v)  inappropriately influencing a client to change a will,
> (vi)  wrongfully abandoning a client,

(vii) failing to exercise discretion in respect of the disclosure of confidential information,

(viii) falsifying records,

(ix) inappropriately using professional-nursing status for personal gain,

(x) promoting for personal gain any drug, device, treatment, procedure, product or service that is unnecessary, ineffective or unsafe,

(xi) publishing, or causing to be published, any advertisement that is false, fraudulent, deceptive or misleading, [and]

(xii) engaging or assisting in fraud, misrepresentation, deception or concealment of a material fact when applying for or securing registration or a licence to practise nursing or taking any examination provided for in this Act, including using fraudulently procured credentials. (*Registered Nurses Act* (2001), s. 2(ag))

Thus, in our case scenario, Kathy's colleagues clearly have engaged in professional misconduct by failing to report incidents of intoxication (which would be deemed unprofessional conduct under the Nova Scotia statute, for example). In covering up a potentially harmful situation, they are ethically and probably legally culpable for any harm to patients that may arise. Kathy has also breached her duty not to practise when her ability to do so was impaired by alcohol.

## Common Law Duty of Care

As has been discussed above regarding the *Latin* case, common law also imposes a duty of care. In any negligence lawsuit involving a nurse or other health care professional, the trial will essentially amount to an evaluation of the nurse's conduct and the degree to which he or she has met an accepted standard of care. The nurse, as a professional, is legally required to operate and act at a level that meets or exceeds the standard of care of a reasonably prudent caregiver or health care professional. This, of course, implies that the nurse has a duty to maintain a level of expertise through continuing education to ensure that he or she practises in accordance with the latest standards. It would not do, for example, for a nurse trained in the 1970s to continue to operate and practise according to the standards of that decade over 30 years later.

Since Kathy in our case scenario is presenting herself as a qualified health practitioner, she owes a duty of proper care to all her patients. This duty has been described in law as "the duty to exercise a reasonable degree of skill, knowledge and care in the treatment of a patient" (*Thompson Estate v. Byrne et al.* (1993), p. 423). Quite apart from the issue of Kathy's practising her profession while under the influence of alcohol is the issue of her having mistakenly identified the arrhythmia on the patient's monitor as ventricular tachycardia when, in fact, the patient was experiencing supraventricular tachycardia. Kathy has not fulfilled her duty to read and interpret the monitor signs correctly. Has she lived up to the standard of care required of her?

## Application to Kathy's Case Scenario

A similar analytical process as was applied in the *Latin v. Hospital for Sick Children et al.* (2007) decision will apply in assessing Kathy's conduct. Her actions would be re-examined with the aid of expert testimony to determine whether and, if so, how she had breached her duty of care to her patient. As the hospital is likewise under a duty to provide proper and competent medical and nursing staff to patients in its care (*Kolesar v. Jeffries*, 1974, p. 376), it also would likely be named as a defendant in any subsequent lawsuit, assuming the patient had suffered harm.

Kathy and the hospital may be sued by the patient, his family, or his estate, if he subsequently died. The plaintiff might allege that the hospital had breached its duty toward him to provide proper care and to ensure competent nursing and other health care staff. Thus, the hospital could be held directly liable for any damage or injury caused by Kathy as a result of her negligence.

For example, the hospital may be considered negligent for failing to ensure adequate and safe emergency procedures and, in this case scenario, in failing to ensure that drugs were safely and properly stored (e.g., vials of pancuronium may have been placed in the container labelled lidocaine). The finding of liability is possible also because the hospital, through Kathy's supervisor, failed to review Kathy's skills to ensure that she was competent and able to carry out her duties properly and effectively. She was an employee of the hospital, and her actions were under its control. This is known as the *doctrine of vicarious liability*.

Similarly, Kathy is under a duty to ensure that she arrives at work in a fit and proper condition. She clearly breached her duty in arriving at the hospital in an impaired state, and her condition may have placed the patient in jeopardy and contributed to the risks of harm.

Another aspect of **vicarious liability** as it relates to hospitals is that physicians, who provide instructions to nursing staff in the care of their patients, are entitled to rely on the assumption that the hospital has hired duly qualified, competent, and properly trained nurses. The doctors are not responsible for ensuring that nurses carry out their instructions properly unless they have actual knowledge that the nurses are not competent to carry out those instructions. Thus, in cases in which a claim of negligence is brought against the physician and his or her instructions were not properly followed, the doctor may argue as a defence that the nurse was negligent. However, the instructions provided by the physician must not be negligent in and of themselves.

## Professional Liability Insurance

Professionals today are held to rigorous standards of care. An increasingly litigious public will not hesitate to bring negligence lawsuits against accountants, lawyers, architects, physicians, or surgeons for any injury or damages suffered as a consequence of the breach of applicable standards of professional conduct. Many health care professionals who practise independently carry professional liability insurance to shield them from what may often be financially catastrophic negligence claims. Physicians, for instance, carry insurance from the Canadian Medical Protective Association, a professional group insurer that offers liability insurance tailored to each professional's type and scope of practice. For example, there are policies specifically designed for neurosurgeons, obstetricians, and family practitioners. Physicians and surgeons are, for the most part, self-employed and are liable for their own acts of negligence.

Most nurses in Canada are employed by publicly funded health facilities, which carry negligence insurance, some with fairly large policy limits, depending on the institution's size, scope of treatments offered, claims history, and any specialization undertaken by the institution. As mentioned in Chapter 3, health facilities, as employers, are vicariously liable for the negligent acts of their employees. The employer institution's liability is not unlimited, however. It extends only as far as the scope of the negligent nurse's expressed or apparent authority. A nurse who performs acts outside the normal scope of nursing would not attract liability to the employer; the nurse would remain fully liable for his or her own negligence. Nurses who are self-employed need to consider insurance coverage, therefore, to ensure adequate financial protection. The often devastating consequences of personal uninsured liability can include bankruptcy, loss of professional status, and personal upheaval.

Insurance coverage usually includes an obligation by the insurance company (usually referred to as the insurer) to defend the health professional in any ensuing litigation. This means the insurer will retain and pay for the services of a lawyer to represent and defend the professional accused of negligent conduct. In some cases, the insurer will leave the choice of lawyer up to the professional involved. Some policies, however, provide that the choice of lawyer and the source of the lawyer's instructions remain with the insurer. The professional is then required to cooperate fully with the insurer in investigating and defending the claim against him or her, which may require his or her attendance at meetings with insurance adjusters, claims representatives, and the lawyers chosen to defend the claim, as well as at all court appearances and examinations for discovery. (These aspects of the civil justice system are more fully discussed in Chapter 4.) Any insured professional who has knowledge of an actual or potential negligence claim against him or her is required to inform the insurer of the claim immediately and to cooperate fully with the insurer.

Those policies that do not contain an obligation to defend will pay only for any negligence judgement ultimately pronounced against the professional. In the meantime, therefore, the professional must retain (hire) and pay for his or her own lawyer to defend the negligence action, though these costs will be recovered from the plaintiff if the suit is dismissed.

## The Standard of Care and Causation

As seen in *Latin v. Hospital for Sick Children et al.* (2007), in legal proceedings, the nurse's practice is examined and compared to normal, competent, and reasonable standards of nursing practice to determine whether the conduct in question conformed with that expected of a reasonably competent and skilled nurse. Of course, standards change over time as new knowledge and technology are introduced and become widely available. Standards also differ from one institution to another and from one treatment setting to another. For example, the standards and expectations of a nurse in a critical care setting will differ from those of a nurse in a rehabilitation setting. Patients have a right to expect that a nurse employed in an ICU will have the specialized knowledge and skills required to provide the necessary care. In the case scenario, the fact that Kathy administered the wrong drug (and, even if it had been the drug she intended, one that was not indicated for this patient's condition) shows that she did not meet the basic standard of care with respect to the administration of medication (i.e., checking the label carefully prior to administering the drug) and thus breached her common law duty to provide reasonably competent, knowledgeable, and skilled nursing care to her patient. She was therefore negligent.

Many hospitals and other health care facilities that employ nurses have policies and procedures in place for an annual review of the nurses' skills and competencies. This practice would be recognized as a standard of care in any negligence suit brought against such an institution. The institution is responsible for ensuring that these reviews take place, and nurses cannot refuse to participate in them. In *Latin v. Hospital for Sick Children et al.* (2007), for example, the defendant hospital had written policies in place that were admitted into evidence and carefully considered by the trial judge in arriving at the appropriate standard of care with respect to the triage classification of a patient presenting in the emergency department as "emergent," "urgent," or "nonurgent" (*Latin v. Hospital for Sick Children et al.*, 2007, paras. 33 to 35).

In Kathy's situation, the nurses in the Cardiovascular Intensive Care Unit (CVICU) were expected to perform certain specialized medical acts, including the interpretation of arrhythmias and, when required, the administration of lidocaine. Kathy's skills should have been reviewed to ensure that she was competent and knowledgeable in the proper interpretation of arrhythmias. This inability led Kathy to conclude that lidocaine was needed when it was not.

Employers also have a common law duty to take active steps to ensure that nurses falling short of a standard receive the appropriate improvement plan. Such steps may include counselling, additional education, and, in some cases, disciplinary measures. This duty includes ensuring that the nurse's skills are reviewed on a regular basis (although the nurse also has such a duty). In Kathy's case, counselling would be in order, but the hospital may have to resort to disciplinary measures if Kathy persistently fails to meet the standards of practice expected of her. When downsizing and budget cuts happen, institutions must still have in place a process to ensure the competence of staff. Budget cuts are not a defensible excuse for negligence.

In some institutions, the review of skills is completely the responsibility of the nurse, and appropriate action must be taken against the nurse if such expectations are not met. If this is the case, this stipulation should be made explicit at the outset of the nurse's employment with the institution or agency.

Finally, Kathy breached her professional obligation not to work while intoxicated. All provincial and territorial nursing statutes prohibit a nurse from working while impaired.

In fact, in Ontario, Prince Edward Island, and Saskatchewan, practising nursing while one's ability to do so is impaired by any substance constitutes professional misconduct (Ontario: *Professional Misconduct Regulation*, s. 1, para. 6; Saskatchewan: *Registered Nurses Act*, 1988–89, s. 26(2)(n); Prince Edward Island: *Registered Nurses Act*, 1988, s. 1(t)(ii)). It would also likely constitute misconduct under the legislation of the remaining provinces and territories (even though these statutes do not expressly refer to impairment of the nurse while on duty), as it would adversely influence the nurse's ability to practise safely and properly. It may also constitute a threat to the safety of patients.

Furthermore, Kathy's fellow nurses may also be found negligent. Since they know of Kathy's possible impairment when she is caring for the cardiac patient, they may, in permitting her to continue to provide care, be contributing to the risk of injury to that patient. It is clearly their professional and ethical duty to alert Kathy's manager of the fact that Kathy may have a drinking problem and, more important, that she may be under the influence of alcohol as she provides care. In some cases, failure to report improper, negligent, or unethical conduct could in and of itself constitute professional misconduct. The matter, in most cases, will then be taken up according to the disciplinary procedures and mechanisms of the provincial regulatory body (as discussed in Chapter 5).

Standards of care provide a baseline for assessment, planning, decision making, and action. They help to ensure the provision of safe and efficient nursing care within the institution or health care agency. The case scenario illustrates two crucial duties that the nurse must discharge properly: (a) the correct assessment of a patient's condition and (b) the administration of the correct medication if required. Also, it is a critical duty of the institution to ensure nurses are competent to practise and that their competence is reviewed on a regular basis.

## Criminal Law Sources of Liability

Criminal law imposes significant consequences for nurses and other health practitioners who act carelessly or with recklessness. In Chapter 4, the *Criminal Code* provisions concerning the omission to do that which a health care professional has undertaken to do are mentioned. Section 216 of the *Criminal Code of Canada* states:

> Every one who undertakes to administer surgical or medical treatment to another person or to do any other lawful act that may endanger the life of another person is, except in cases of necessity, under a legal duty to have and to use reasonable knowledge, skill and care in so doing.

In specific relation to the practice of nursing, this places an obligation upon people who represent themselves as qualified and competent nurses to ensure that their skills and education are adequate to perform properly the treatment that they are called upon to administer. The section excludes "cases of necessity," which imply emergency or life-threatening situations. However, a nurse would not normally administer such treatment if a more qualified practitioner, such as a physician, were available to perform, for example, emergency surgery. In the absence of a more qualified practitioner, a nurse, acting in good faith, could proceed if he or she performed to the best of his or her ability. The legal policy here is to encourage people to render treatment to those in urgent need of it. In some extreme cases, such treatment could include surgery.

## Criminal Law Standard of Care

A person who represents herself or himself as a duly qualified health care practitioner will, if serious injury or bodily harm ensues, be held to the standard of the reasonably qualified practitioner. The decision of the British Columbia County Court, in the case of *R. v. Sullivan and Lemay* (1986), illustrates this point. Although that case involved two midwives, the principle discussed is equally applicable to nurses. In that case, the midwives were assisting in a home birth. The infant died as a result of their negligent delivery, and they were each charged with criminal negligence causing death (with respect to the infant) and with criminal negligence causing bodily harm (to the mother, as a result of their negligent delivery procedures).

In addressing the standard of expertise to which the defendants would be held, the court said that the midwives' conduct constituted a lawful act that might endanger the life of another person within the meaning of the statute. Therefore, they were under a legal duty to have and use reasonable skill, care, and knowledge in performing the delivery, and their conduct would be held to the standard of a competent childbirth attendant, even though they had no formal training as midwives.

## Criminal Negligence

Section 219 of the *Criminal Code of Canada* defines criminal negligence in this way:

> Every one is criminally negligent who (a) in doing anything, or (b) in omitting to do anything that it is his duty to do, shows wanton or reckless disregard for the lives or safety of other persons.

The "duty" of which this section speaks is a duty imposed by law, either statute law or common law (*R. v. Coyne*, 1958). This section must be read in conjunction with section 217 of the Code, which states:

> Every one who undertakes to do an act is under a legal duty to do it if an omission to do the act is or may be dangerous to life.

Thus, if a nurse fails to perform some act that is part of his or her nursing procedures and duties, and, as a result, someone dies or suffers serious bodily harm, the nurse's omission may constitute a criminal offence of either criminal negligence causing death or criminal negligence causing bodily harm, depending on the impact on the patient. Before the conduct could be characterized as negligent, however, it would have to demonstrate a marked or substantial departure from conduct that one would expect from a reasonable and competent nurse. There would have to be extreme carelessness or recklessness (i.e., a complete disregard for the consequences of one's actions), or such grave and serious omission as to show that the nurse failed to recognize obvious risks or, if aware of those risks, that he or she chose to take them anyway, "reckless" and oblivious to the consequences. Such a formulation in the law shows how extreme and outrageous the carelessness must be in order to be judged criminally negligent.

In the case scenario, Kathy's intoxication and failure to see she was administering the wrong drug might arguably be classified as reckless behaviour.

## Necessity for Causation

By definition, criminal negligence must cause death (*Criminal Code of Canada*, s. 220) or bodily harm (*Criminal Code of Canada*, s. 221) to another. Impairment is often a factor in finding drivers criminally negligent when they have either hurt or killed others in accidents. In such cases, the fact that the accused was intoxicated of his or her own volition is evidence that may lead a court to decide that the driver acted with wanton or reckless disregard for the lives or safety of others (*R. v. Anderson*, 1985, p. 133). Intoxication is therefore a relevant factor in determining whether a person acted wantonly or recklessly.

### Application to Kathy's Case Scenario

In Kathy's case, if the patient had died, the fact that she was impaired would be relevant in a charge of criminal negligence causing death. The fact that her intoxication rendered her incapable of appreciating the probable consequences of her actions would not be a defence. Whether a conviction could be successfully obtained, however, would depend on whether the mistake of administering the wrong drug demonstrated a wanton or reckless disregard for the life or safety of the patient. Even if Kathy's conduct was found to be grossly negligent in a civil law context, that conduct may not be sufficient to show the degree of wanton or reckless disregard required to convict her of criminal negligence. The patient would have to have suffered some harm or have died.

There is a substantial difference between being negligent in a civil lawsuit and being criminally negligent. The latter type of negligence requires conduct that does not meet what one would normally expect of a reasonable person (in this case, a reasonable nurse). The intent of the accused is irrelevant. It is sufficient that the accused acted in such a manner as to demonstrate either that he or she recognized the obvious risk of danger to another and took that risk anyway or that he or she ought reasonably to have foreseen such a risk yet failed to do so (*R. v. Sharpe*, 1984). In other words, the accused was completely indifferent to the risks that his or her actions posed to the life or safety of others who might reasonably be expected to be so affected.

## The Provincial Coroners' and Medical Examiners' Systems

The coroners' and medical examiners' systems merit discussion, as these are integral to both the criminal justice system and the provincial constitutional responsibility for administering justice within the province. In every province, an unexplained death must be investigated with a view to determining its causes and identifying ways to prevent similar occurrences in the future. Thus, if there is any evidence of negligence on the part of nursing or medical staff that contributes to the death of a person, an inquest may be ordered by a coroner or a court to determine the circumstances and all possible causes of the death. It is important for nurses to have a basic understanding of both the coroners' and medical examiners' systems in use across Canada since nurses may be called upon to testify at such inquests.

The **coroner's inquest** is primarily a fact-finding and investigatory endeavour. In earlier times, a coroner's court could also find criminal or civil responsibility; however, the modern coroner's inquest is not a criminal trial. There is no accused person. In some provinces, the coroner has the authority, upon conclusion of an inquest, to order the arrest of anyone who has been found to be responsible for the death investigated. However, none of the evidence and testimony given at an inquest may be used in a criminal trial.

Ontario, Quebec, New Brunswick, Prince Edward Island, Saskatchewan, British Columbia, Yukon, the Northwest Territories, and Nunavut use the traditional coroner's system adopted from English common law. The remaining provinces have moved away from this system to a more modernized medical examiner's system. Both systems, however, operate similarly as a means to investigate suspicious deaths. In the medical examiner's system, the function of holding an inquiry is usually left to a judge, or, in the case of Alberta, the Fatality Review Board (*Fatality Inquiries Act*, 2000).

A detailed review of each province's system is beyond the scope of this book. However, Ontario's system will serve as an example. Under Ontario's *Coroners Act* (1990), a chief coroner for Ontario is appointed to supervise a number of coroners throughout the province. A coroner is appointed for a particular region. He or she must be a resident of that region and be a legally qualified medical practitioner.

Under the Act, a death under any of the following circumstances must be reported either to a coroner or to the police (*Coroners Act*, 1990, s. 10(1)):

- As a result of violence, misadventure (e.g., an accident), negligence, misconduct, or malpractice
- By unfair means
- During pregnancy or following pregnancy in such circumstances to which the death could be attributed to the pregnancy
- Suddenly and unexpectedly
- From disease or sickness for which the person was not treated by a legally qualified medical practitioner
- From any cause other than disease
- Under circumstances that require investigation

Similarly, if a person dies while in a home for the aged, a children's residence, a home for developmentally delayed persons, a mental institution, a nursing home, or a public or private hospital to which the person was transferred from one of those previously mentioned institutions, the person in charge of such institution must notify the coroner in writing of the death (*Coroners Act*, 1990, s. 10(2)). Pending an order from the coroner, no person may in any way alter the condition or interfere with the body of the deceased.

Once notified, the local coroner will issue a warrant to take possession of the body as part of his or her investigation. The investigation and fact-finding into the circumstances of the death begin at this point. The coroner has the power to enter into any place where the death occurred, inspect and extract information from any records or writings relating to the deceased, and seize anything that he or she believes is material to the purposes of the investigation.

In cases in which someone has died under care of a health facility or agency, it is likely that the coroner would seize the deceased's medical records immediately upon being notified of the death. This is a precaution to preserve the character of the evidence and to avoid the possibility of additions being made to such records that might obscure the medical circumstances and condition of the deceased at the moment of death.

It is important, therefore, to ensure that records are made as contemporaneously as possible with the act being recorded. The nurse involved in the care of the deceased is at the very least a potential witness to the circumstances surrounding the treatment, care, and condition of that person immediately prior to the death. At most, the nurse may be called upon to testify at the coroner's inquest, if indeed there is one, and will have to rely upon the records to refresh his or her memory as to the events leading up to the death. Questions asked of witnesses in such cases may be quite specific and require precise and detailed interpretation of the nursing notes and other records. Therefore, as discussed later in this chapter, the necessity of making clear and accurate records as close as possible to the time when the nursing act was performed cannot be overstressed.

A coroner can order that an inquest be held into the circumstances of the deceased's death if he or she deems it advisable. Otherwise, the matter will proceed no further.

If an inquest is held, the coroner will convene a hearing, in some provinces, with the aid of a jury (usually smaller than a criminal trial jury of 12). The jury's function is to determine the cause of death based on the evidence heard at the inquest and to aid in making recommendations as to any improvements to procedures, policies, and standards that may help to prevent similar occurrences in the future.

The inquest will usually proceed along the same lines as a trial. However, as mentioned above, the inquest is not a criminal trial; there is no prosecution and no accused. The Crown attorney may be a participant, and any other parties who are material witnesses or participants in the events leading up to the person's death may be called to testify at the inquest.

A person charged of a criminal offence cannot be compelled to testify at an inquest. Any person called to testify will have the right to the aid of a lawyer. However, the lawyer's involvement may be limited to advising on answers to questions and the rights of the witness. In most provinces, the witness has the right not to have any evidence that he or she gives at an inquest used against him or her in any ensuing criminal proceedings. This is to ensure that the witness's rights (under the *Charter of Rights and Freedoms*) against self-incrimination are maintained. This does not mean, however, that the witness has the right to refuse to answer any proper questions put to him or her. A refusal to answer may place that witness in danger of being found in contempt of court, a judgement that carries with it fines and a possible jail term.

The inquest is more relaxed in terms of the strict rules of evidence normally applied in a court. However, coroners tend to follow such rules, especially in recent years.

In provinces with a medical examiner's system, the medical examiner takes the place of the coroner. Appointed by the provincial government, a medical examiner must be a trained physician, given the medical complexities and technicalities that tend to be the focus of such inquests. Coroners however, historically were laypersons, untrained in medical matters. In the past few decades there has been a trend away from lay coroners, and now all coroners must be duly qualified and licensed physicians. The procedures across the country are fairly similar, except that in some provinces (i.e., Nova Scotia, Manitoba, and Alberta), the inquest may be held by a provincial court judge. The investigative and inquiry functions are thus kept separate.

Once the inquest is concluded, the coroner or judicial officer conducting the hearing may give a decision (taking into consideration any recommendations made by the jury) on the causes of the deceased's death and anything that could have been done to prevent it. For example, if the inquest is into the death of a patient at a hospital, the jury might recommend changes to certain policies or procedures that it feels may have contributed to the death. Further, if the coroner's decision suggests criminal responsibility, it is possible that criminal charges may be laid in the wake of his or her decision. The criminal justice process would then take over to determine the guilt or innocence of any accused person.

## Interaction Between Coroner's Inquests and Criminal Law

A coroner's inquest that took place in Ontario in 2000 illustrates the interface between the criminal law system and the coroner's inquest system. Both systems are distinct and separate from one another and a finding of liability in a coroner's inquest does not necessarily lead to a criminal conviction. In this case, a 10-year-old girl attended a pediatric hospital for treatment of (unusual) pain associated with an earlier fracture of her femur. The girl was experiencing considerable leg pain and a burning sensation as a result of a rare condition known as reflex sympathetic dystrophy syndrome and, at the direction of the treating physicians, was given an injection of morphine for pain control. The girl died a few hours later. The coroner's jury concluded, after an inquest, that the girl had died from respiratory and heart failure due to a severe reaction to the morphine and its interaction with another drug that she had been given. The jury ruled that the death was a "homicide."

**Homicide**, for the purposes of a coroner's inquest, is the death of a person caused by the actions of another person or persons. It is the pure physical act that causes the death of a human being. The verdict in a coroner's jury determines only how the death occurred. There is no assignment of blame or criminal responsibility as in a criminal trial. As stated earlier, coroners' juries do not have the power to assign legal liability—that is, to determine civil (as in a lawsuit) or criminal responsibility on the part of any particular person involved in the death. The inquest's chief purpose is to determine the means by which a person has died when the death is unexpected or the result of an accident or unexplained circumstances.

If criminal charges are later laid by the police against an individual, the ensuing criminal trial will determine whether the act of killing was the result of an intentional act or criminal negligence (discussed above). It is at this juncture that the criminal system is engaged. In the case of the 10-year-old girl, criminal charges were initially laid by the police against the two nurses directly involved in the girl's treatment. Shortly into the preliminary hearing (see Chapter 4 for a discussion of preliminary hearings), the charges were stayed (halted) by the Crown (the prosecution) because Crown counsel believed that there was no evidence that would lead to a conviction.

## Nursing Documentation

### Introduction

Careful and accurate documentation is an important component of professional nursing practice. The nurse's assessment and progress notes monitor, on a continuing basis, the course of treatment and the effect of interventions. From this record, a clear picture emerges of the patient's or client's progress toward the stated goals and outcomes, and any impending complications can be identified before they become problematic.

Failure to document specific acts or treatment accurately and contemporaneously can have serious consequences for the health care professional in a negligence action. Inadequate documentation, or failure to review client information and history, negatively influences the quality of care.

### Use of Documentation in Legal Proceedings

EVIDENTIARY USE

In many cases of medical malpractice, the trial of the actions of health care professionals will occur several years after the events leading up to and including the negligent acts. Memories fade with time, and the evidence given by witnesses, such as nurses and physicians, will often be hazy or incomplete. Therefore, the notes and records prepared by the health care team assume added value and significance, as these are often the only source of information regarding what occurred.

The goal of the courts is to obtain the truth. Often, the truth lies in the health care records. Meticulous, clear, legible, and well-organized records not only help the court (i.e., the judge and, in some cases, the jury) to determine the exact sequence of events and the circumstances of treatment; they also improve the credibility of the witnesses who made them. Thus, with a well-constructed health care record, the nurses and other caregivers who made the notes will be able to impart their testimony more forcefully, and that testimony will be accorded greater weight than would be the case with an inadequate record.

The court will be interested in all aspects of the record, including nursing progress notes, care plan, checklists, flow charts, hospital policies in force at the time, and so forth. These will provide a more complete picture of events. In many cases, the record will also document the thought processes and frame of mind of the health professionals at the time. For example, the patient's chart may reveal that a certain treatment or intervention was or was not warranted under the circumstances and given that patient's condition. This is a further reason for ensuring that records are made and kept according to the highest possible standards.

In the Ontario coroner's case, and in the *Latin v. Hospital for Sick Children et al.* (2007) decision discussed earlier in this chapter, the medical charts, nursing records, and notes surrounding the treatment afforded the patients were essential. They provided the evidence to show the type of care received and served as a means of communication between the various members of the health care teams. In *Latin*, for example, the triage nurse's contemporaneous notes of her observations of the child were carefully considered and her notations studied. Her notes taken in the emergency department that day showed that she noted the vital signs of each patient she examined, including a respiratory rate. In the child's case, she had written the word *cry* in the space where the rate was to be recorded. The court took this, along with evidence from the girl's mother, to mean that the child's crying made it difficult for the nurse to obtain the respiration rate. The following section discusses the uses and importance of proper documentation in nursing practice.

EXPERT WITNESSES

Assessing the conduct of nurses in a particular situation in relation to the appropriate standard of care often requires drawing upon expert testimony. The court calls upon experts because the judges trying a case rarely possess the necessary expertise to make valid conclusions and draw inferences from technical data. A nursing expert, on the other hand, can interpret the health care record and assist the court in reconstructing the events and drawing inferences. Experts can also be used by the parties to a lawsuit either to support the plaintiff's position and interpretation of the evidence or to refute these for the defence and perhaps suggest another cause for the injury. Although such inferences are properly the function of the judge or jury, the expert, because of his or her unique knowledge and experience, is permitted to formulate and express an opinion. This is an exception to the general evidentiary rule that a witness's opinion on a matter at issue is inadmissible. More important, the nurse expert is able to describe the appropriate standard of care in a particular case and, upon review of the health care record and, in particular, the nursing notes, give an opinion on whether proper documentation and nursing procedures were followed.

Prior to the nurse's giving testimony, the lawyer for the party wishing to rely on the nurse's evidence must first ask questions in court about his or her education, experience, nursing background, and continuing education. The purpose here is to establish in the trial record that the witness has the necessary qualifications to give such testimony or opinion.

In some cases, expert testimony may also be elicited as part of the nurse's own involvement in the care of the plaintiff. The nurse may be asked questions about his or her notations in the patient's record. It is important that the nurse answer such questions truthfully and as accurately as possible. As well, it is important that he or she ensure accuracy, clarity, and objectivity when making notes in the first place.

As a rule of evidence, the person who recorded the note or observation will be allowed to use those notes to refresh his or her memory when testifying in court. However, the court must first be satisfied of the following:

1. The notes were indeed made by that person.
2. It was part of that nurse's duty to make such notes.
3. The notes were made contemporaneously (or reasonably so) with the event or act that they record.
4. There have been no alterations, additions, or deletions to those notes since they were made.

Usually, items 1 and 2 pose no problem, as the nurse witness will have been involved in the patient's care and will have been the one who made the notes in the first place as part of his or her normal duty.

Item 3 can pose a problem. For example, in the case of *Kolesar v. Jeffries* (1976, 9 O.R. (2d) 41 (HCJ)), the court commented upon the documentation practices in the surgical unit where the plaintiff was placed postoperatively. The plaintiff was returned to the Recovery Room shortly after 1200 hours, sedated and unconscious, secured in a supine position to a Stryker frame following surgery on his spinal column. Although the standard of care in such a case would include rousing the patient at frequent and regular intervals to cough to keep his lungs clear, the plaintiff was permitted to sleep undisturbed by an overworked staff who made one round at midnight with flashlights. At 0500 hours the next day, one of the nurses discovered the plaintiff dead. He had suffered pulmonary edema and hemorrhage secondary to the aspiration of gastric juices.

The court heard evidence that no nursing notes were made over a period of seven hours. Indeed, it was the practice in that nursing unit to record vital signs and any other observations as to the patients' condition on scraps of paper during the shift. Afterward, the nurses would get together and, with the aid of these scraps of paper, would reconstruct the record for each patient. The nurses would assist "each other to recall and record the events of the evening" (*Kolesar v. Jeffries*, 1974, para. 13). This practice does not fulfill the requirements of contemporaneous recording.

Upon discovering that no entries had been made on the plaintiff between 2200 hours and 0500 hours the next day, the assistant director of nursing asked one of the nurses on duty that night to write up a report of the events. Here, the court noted:

One is always suspicious of records made after the event, and if any credence is to be attached to [the nurse's report], it shows that at all times the patient was quite pale, very pale, and was allowed to sleep soundly to his death. (*Kolesar v. Jeffries*, 1974, p. 48)

Thus, the absence of adequate nursing records served only to reinforce the court's opinion that the standard of nursing practised in this patient's care had been wholly inadequate. If efforts had been made to rouse the patient regularly in order to check and record his condition and vital signs, his death could have been avoided.

As for the fourth item above, problems may also arise with respect to alterations, deletions, or additions made to the nursing notes after the original entries were made. In *Meyer v. Gordon* (1981), the alteration of the records prompted Mr. Justice Legg to remark:

> The hospital chart contains alterations and additions which compel me to view with suspicion the accuracy of many of the observations which are recorded. The chart also contains at least one entry which was discovered during this trial [in May 1980] to have been made after the fact. That also casts suspicion on the reliability of those who made the entries and undermines the accuracy of medical opinions based upon these entries and observations. (*Meyer v. Gordon*, 1981, p. 15)

Thus, any attempt to conceal an alteration of the health care record can effectively cast doubt on the witness's evidence, as well as on any other evidence based on the entries and observations contained in the altered record.

## Legal Requirement to Keep Records

In all provinces, hospitals and other health care facilities are required to keep and maintain records on all the patients they treat. For example, in Ontario, a record of admission, diagnosis, consent forms, treatment, care plan, nursing notes, and so forth must be kept on each patient (see, for example, *Hospital Management Regulation*, 1990, s. 19, made under the *Public Hospitals Act*, 1990). Physicians' orders must be in writing and signed or authenticated by the physician who made the order. All entries in the patient record made by nurses and other health professionals must be initialled or signed and dated, with the exact time of the entry noted. Late entries must also be indicated.

As well, most provinces impose an obligation to obtain and record a diagnosis on an admitted patient within a specified period of time. Also, records must be kept for a specified time—for example, in Ontario, for 10 years (*Hospital Management Regulation*, 1990, s. 19(f)).

# Case Scenario

## DOCUMENTING: IS IT ENOUGH?

An 8-month-old boy is brought into a hospital emergency department late one evening presenting with vomiting and diarrhea and a history of toxoplasmosis. On arrival, his pulse rate is 120; his respiration rate, 24. He is seen by the physician on duty in Emergency and then by the hospital pediatrician, who admits the child and writes treatment orders for an IV, as well as tests for hemoglobin and BUN electrolytes.

While in the hospital, the child's condition deteriorates. The nurses monitoring him over the next 4 to 5 hours note that his heart rate has increased to 164 and that his respiration is 64. Nurse H., who is looking after the boy, is concerned. She speaks to the charge nurse, who echoes her concerns, and then she phones the child's physician at his home even though it is the middle of the night.

Nurse H. informs the physician of the child's condition, pulse rate, respiration rate, and of the results of the tests for hemoglobin and BUN electrolytes, which were also abnormal. In particular, the $CO_2$ level was at 10.9 instead of the normal range of 22 to 32. The physician replies: "That's fine. Just continue doing what you've been doing."

Not satisfied with the doctor's response, Nurse H. again speaks to the charge nurse, who says: "Well, you're not the doctor; he is. Whatever he says is what we do; don't worry about it."

All of the abnormal results and readings, including fluid balances, are duly recorded by Nurse H. in the boy's chart. Also noted are the conversations with the charge nurse and the boy's physician, and the times at which these took place. The boy dies the next morning at 0600 hours.

### Issues

1. What should the charge nurse have done when Nurse H. consulted her after phoning the boy's physician?
2. Should Nurse H. have taken her concerns about the boy's poor test results to a higher authority?
3. What steps should have been taken with respect to documenting the boy's vital signs and fluid intake, both in the emergency department and in Pediatrics?
4. Should Nurse H. have called the physician back to confirm his instructions? In speaking with the doctor, should she have placed greater emphasis on the boy's abnormal vital signs and test results?

continued on following page >>

## Discussion

Nurse H. should have attempted to contact the physician a second time to impress upon him the urgency of the situation, especially since he'd likely been roused from a deep sleep that might have clouded his judgement.

A critical issue in this situation is the charge nurse's responsibility in assisting Nurse H. to obtain the help of the physician. Through her assessment, Nurse H. obviously realized the seriousness of the boy's condition. The standard of care would require that Nurse H. bypass her nonsupportive charge nurse and find a higher authority for instructions. Lack of support from a supervisor, even if accurately documented in the patient's chart, would not protect a nurse from liability. (However, this scenario raises serious concerns regarding the safety and team culture of this unit. The issue of caregiver rights is discussed in Chapter 11.)

Having determined the high risks of inaction, a nurse must act. He or she cannot avoid liability by using the excuse that "the doctor said . . ." or by simply documenting the doctor's instructions. The nurse has the responsibility to protect the patient from harm. In this situation, the appropriate standard of care required that the nurses know and understand the severe consequences of inaction. The conduct of both nurses clearly fell below the required professional and legal standard of care.

In the real-life situation on which this case scenario is based, a coroner's inquest was called to investigate the boy's death. One of the issues that arose at the inquest was the documentation of the fluid balance, particularly in the emergency department. It had not been totalled accurately, and it was difficult to determine how much fluid the patient had been given, both in Emergency and in Pediatrics.

At the inquest, the boy's physician denied that the nurse had reported the patient's vital signs. The doctor further denied that he had been given the results of the electrolyte tests (specifically, the $CO_2$ level). There were no other nurses on the floor that evening who witnessed what was going on, and thus no one to corroborate the nurse's telephone conversation with the physician. The doctor claimed he'd been roused from a deep sleep, that he had been up all the night before, that he was very tired, and that if the nurse had really had such a pressing concern, she should have phoned him back to confirm his instructions and make sure he realized the severity of the situation. In such a case, he said, he certainly would have taken the appropriate action. It was obvious that, regardless of which version of events was the correct one, the child died because of a serious breakdown in communication.

The coroner's jury found, first, that the nurse should have documented her concerns in greater detail and that this record should ideally have been witnessed by another nurse. Second, she should have called the doctor back to repeat her concerns and had another nurse present to attest that she did so. Third, the hospital should have had procedures in place for the nurse to bypass the physician's instructions and to seek another doctor in the hospital to ensure that proper instructions were provided in the treatment of this child.

continued on following page >>

The cause of death, as determined in the autopsy, was dehydration. The IV that had been administered to the child was wholly inadequate. The inquest determined that the boy's fluid intake should have been checked more frequently and recorded systematically. In particular, the levels might have been checked and recorded by nursing staff just prior to the child's leaving the emergency department and then again by the nurses in Pediatrics immediately upon his transfer to that ward.

The jury did not accept the physician's excuse in this case, and he was found negligent for having given improper instructions. He was subsequently reported to the College of Physicians and Surgeons of Ontario and severely disciplined.

## The Need for and Uses of Documentation

In most cases, the patient's chart, nurses' progress notes, and other documentation constitute the only written evidence of what care a patient has received. This record is vital during the course of treatment in that it facilitates communication between nurses and other health care professionals actively involved in the patient's care. Without it, effective, safe, and proper care would be impossible. In this case, as the fluid balance was inaccurately recorded, the standard of accurate and complete documentation was not met.

The record is also a useful tool in planning the course of treatment. It encourages an accurate tracing of the patient's vital signs and condition, which, in turn, promotes quality control of nursing and medical care, and permits caregivers to assess which interventions should be altered and which left in place. Thus, assessments must be complete and comprehensive. The documentation should also reflect the nurse's judgements, including identification of any problems and recommendations on the action to be taken. This permits others to follow through on the recommendations and to follow up on the efficacy of actions taken. Effective communication through documentation is absolutely critical to effective team function and patient safety, as will be discussed in Chapter 10.

Consider a situation in which the assessment of a patient's pain is documented as "severe." How adequate is such a description? It does not indicate whether the pain assessment was reported to the patient's physician, whether any medication was given, or whether another intervention was implemented. It would not, then, indicate the effectiveness of any medication or intervention.

What if a nurse encountered a patient who was extremely agitated? Should previous documentation assist the nurse in understanding the source of the agitation and what was effective in managing the agitation in the past? Accurate documentation is essential to ensuring a safe and consistent standard of care.

A good patient record will contain information on any allergies (especially allergies to medications) and whom to contact in an emergency, which is especially important in cases in which the patient is not capable and a substitute decision maker has been appointed to make treatment decisions on the patient's behalf. Equally important, the record should contain all previous treatment orders for the patient, plus any notes concerning the outcome of these interventions.

The patient record provides evidence of the adequacy of any treatment that is administered, the appropriateness of care, and the quality of care received. This is especially important for audit purposes, in any disciplinary proceedings for alleged improper or unprofessional conduct, and in any negligence actions, criminal proceedings, or coroner's inquests in the event of the patient's death under circumstances requiring investigation.

## Accuracy of Documentation

The documentation must be an accurate record of what was done, what medication was administered, and what the patient's condition was at the time the action was taken and afterward.

In the case of *Meyer v. Gordon* (1981), the parents of a newborn infant who suffered severe brain damage and ensuing cerebral palsy during delivery brought an action of negligence against two of the participating nurses, the hospital, and the attending physician. In all, three nurses were involved in the delivery. The plaintiff had previously had a very fast labour, her first child having been born within four hours of the onset of labour. The plaintiff's doctor knew this but had not advised the nursing or hospital staff when he had his patient admitted to the hospital at approximately 1130 hours on the morning her labour began.

Ascertaining the patient's birth history is a normal and standard part of any labour assessment performed by a nurse; however, the first nurse who examined the plaintiff, Nurse W., did not ascertain whether this was her first or second birth and, in fact, failed to obtain any obstetrical history. It was made clear at the trial that had she done so, the history would have indicated that this patient should have been closely watched. Nurse W.'s failure to determine the obstetrical history of the mother in this case shows a marked departure from acceptable standards of practice in Canada.

As well, there was evidence that the charting done by the two nurses who were named in the suit was inaccurate and incomplete. As a result, their notes were rejected by the trial judge as unreliable. Upon the plaintiff's admission to the hospital, Nurse W. performed the initial examination and established that she was in the early stages of labour. She did not record this, however, and was imprecise as to the position of the fetus at that time, noting the position only as "mid." Neither did the nurse record the duration of the contractions during her first, and only, vaginal examination. At this point, she did ascertain and record that dilation was three centimetres, but the character of the cervix (an important indication of the progress of labour) was not recorded accurately.

A second nurse, Nurse M., assisted Nurse W. in these examinations. Neither nurse appeared to have recognized the danger of leaving the mother lying on her back, the position she remained in until delivery. The court found, among other things, that permitting the plaintiff to remain in this position contributed greatly to the fetal distress and constituted a marked departure from the standard of care at that hospital, which was known for excellence in obstetrics. The mother should clearly have been positioned on her side.

The fetal heart rate was checked at 1150 hours and again at 1200. However, this information did not appear to have been recorded until much later. At noon, the patient's doctor prescribed an injection of Demerol and Gravol to ease her pain and nausea. Although this was not explicitly stated by the court or in the evidence as reported, the giving of Demerol would no doubt have had a sedative effect not only on the mother but also on the fetus and could have contributed to the onset of fetal distress. The physician did not instruct Nurse M. to conduct a vaginal examination prior to administering the Demerol and, in fact, none was conducted before the drug was given at 1205 hours. This was also against generally accepted practice.

From the time the Demerol was administered until the child was born at 1232 hours, the plaintiff was left lying on her back, alone and completely unattended despite her excruciating and rapid labour pains and despite Nurse W.'s opinion that the fetal heart rate ought to have been checked every 15 minutes at that point. The court noted that the obstetrical ward appeared to have been extremely busy that day and that the plaintiff did not appear to have been anyone's patient in particular from that point on.

At 1215 hours, the plaintiff's husband, distressed by his wife's extreme pain, sought out Nurse W. He told her that he believed his wife was about to give birth and needed assistance. The evidence at trial indicates that Nurse W. may have brushed off his concern, dismissing him as a nervous husband. The court found it deplorable that there was no nursing care available to the plaintiff when her husband sought it (*Meyer v. Gordon*, 1981, p. 15).

At approximately 1230 hours, the plaintiff's husband again sought out a nurse, saying that his wife was giving birth. A third nurse (Nurse T.) responded and went to the plaintiff. She found the baby's head already born with a very large amount of meconium around it. She completed the delivery; however, as Nurse M. (who assisted her) had failed to include a suction bulb in the emergency bundle, Nurse T. was unable to suction the meconium from the baby's nose and mouth. The expert physicians who testified at trial deemed this a serious oversight.

The baby was not breathing when she was born. Nurse T. described the baby as "very flaccid and limp." The baby was brought to the case room for resuscitation, where another doctor was involved in her resuscitation using initial suctioning, positive pressure ventilation, and oxygen with endotracheal suctioning. As the court noted later, all these factors contributed to the fetal distress. The resuscitation efforts continued for some time with the assistance of two other physicians and were ultimately successful. The child was moved to the hospital's Intensive Care Nursery. It was soon discovered, however, that she had suffered brain damage as a result of fetal distress and resulting asphyxia in conjunction with meconium aspiration (*Meyer v. Gordon*, 1981, p. 9).

The plaintiffs sued the mother's doctor, the doctors involved in the resuscitation efforts, and, more important, the nurses and hospital that had provided the nursing care. The court dismissed the suit against the doctors (except the plaintiffs' own doctor, whom it found 25% liable on the basis that he had failed to instruct Nurse M. to conduct a vaginal examination of the plaintiff prior to administering the Demerol). The hospital was found 75%

responsible for the baby's brain damage, as a result of its negligence in failing to provide adequate and proper nursing care.

The court noted that both nurses had gone back and altered the chart some hours after the delivery to make the record appear more complete than it actually was, which meant that the court was unable to rely upon the nurses' notes as an accurate account of what had happened. Much was made of the fact that the nurses' notes were inaccurate and inadequate. For example, the time of the plaintiff's arrival at the hospital was not recorded (*Meyer v. Gordon*, 1981, p. 7); upon her initial examination of the patient, Nurse W. noted that the fetal heart rate was "normal," that the plaintiff's labour was "good," that the cervix had dilated three centimetres, and that "strong" contractions were occurring every two minutes (*Meyer v. Gordon*, 1981, p. 7); and the duration of the contractions was not recorded, as it should have been.

The court found that the description of the labour as "good" did not indicate the fact (later brought out in Nurse W.'s testimony) that the plaintiff was in active labour, which would require a fetal heart rate check every 15 minutes (*Meyer v. Gordon*, 1981, p. 12). The court was equally critical of the inexact description of the fetus's position as "mid" and of the lack of record as to the character or effacement of the cervix. Such inaccuracies and inadequacies contributed to a poor appreciation of the advanced stage of the plaintiff's labour.

In most court cases, failure to document a particular act during the course of treatment may mean that the court will assume the act was not done. Such failure seriously undermines how probative the evidence is—that is, how much the testimony proves or how convincing it is that the act was actually done. Records that are sketchy and incomplete may not be accorded much weight by the court.

In assessing the quality and accuracy of Nurse W.'s recorded observations, the court relied on the expert evidence of two nurses (presumably, with obstetrical experience) who stated that an obstetrical nurse, when assessing fetal position, looks for the height of the presenting part of the fetus in relation to the ischial spines of the mother's pelvis. When asked about Nurse W.'s assessment of the fetal position as "mid," one of the experts commented that such a notation was not specific enough to aid in the evaluation of the labour. The other expert stated that the expression "mid" used in the record had no meaning (*Meyer v. Gordon*, 1981, p. 12). This case thus illustrates the importance of accurate and precise observations when documenting details of patient care and treatment.

## Other Standards of Documentation

There are agency and government regulations that govern how records ought to be made and organized. For example, Accreditation Canada (formerly known as the Canadian Council on Health Services Accreditation (CCHSA)) has set standards, as has each provincial regulatory body. As well, nursing departments within health care agencies usually have standards and policies governing proper patient documentation. For example, in the practice of charting by exception, a problem or condition is documented only if it deviates significantly from what one would normally expect in such circumstances. Another practice is that of recording facts by means of defined checklists. For example, nurses may place their initials beside a listed procedure, which may mean (according to the policy manual on documentation) that the procedure was completed with no problems. If problems or changes in the patient's condition had occurred, the policy would require further documentation in the progress notes.

No matter what standards are in use, these will be backed by institutional policies and definitions of those standards. When these standards, definitions, and policies exist, such documentation falls within legally acceptable standards.

## Guidelines for Proper Documentation

Some rules of thumb have evolved to ensure timely and accurate recording, from both a legal and a practice perspective, of details of a patient's care, condition, and treatment from hour to hour.

RECORD CONTEMPORANEOUSLY

Timely reporting makes a record more accurate and reliable, ensures safer care, and affords the record greater weight in any legal proceedings. Therefore, the record should be made at the time of occurrence of the event or action that is recorded. It is not always possible to record items, events, or actions at the time they occur, especially during emergencies. The longer the delay in documenting a fact, however, the more likely it is that the accuracy of the observation or detail will be questioned later, especially in a trial. For example, in *Meyer v. Gordon* (1981, p. 9), the nurses who treated the plaintiff had recorded some of their observations a considerable time after the fact and, further, had altered the record to make it appear that the observations had been recorded contemporaneously. Thus, the nurses' notes were deemed unreliable as an evidentiary source.

Another reason for contemporaneous documentation is that memory fades with time. A fact is more likely to be recorded accurately and completely soonest after the occurrence. Documentation of treatment is vital not only in providing safe and quality patient care but also in court proceedings, as it is often the only source of evidence of what occurred. As a considerable length of time may pass before a trial or hearing is convened, a well-constructed and well-maintained record serves to refresh the memory of the person who made it.

If it was not possible to record the act or event when it occurred (e.g., the nurse had other pressing obligations or simply forgot), the late entry should still be recorded, to the nurse's best recollection, and noted as a late entry, thus:

1230 h, patient regurgitated reddish coffee-ground fluid; recorded at 1330 h because called away on emergency to assist in another patient's resuscitation. [*Signed,* etc.]

A late entry is clearly better than no entry at all. The nurses in the Meyer case attempted to cover up the fact that some of their entries had been made late rather than contemporaneously. This practice is strongly discouraged and potentially fraudulent.

### RECORD ONLY YOUR OWN ACTIONS

The nurse should record only his or her own actions. Since the notes may form the basis of testimony in any ensuing criminal or civil proceedings, the nurse will be permitted to testify only as to his or her own actions.

In particular, care should be taken when documenting a fact or detail on computer. The nurse should use only his or her own password or access card when accessing a computer record. This ensures that the computer log will accurately reflect the fact that a particular nurse made the entry.

### RECORD IN CHRONOLOGICAL ORDER

All entries should be made in chronological order. Otherwise, a confused record would result, which could have serious repercussions in the course of treatment, especially with respect to the administration of medication. It would also make the record of limited use in any litigation and undermine the nurse's testimony.

### RECORD CLEARLY AND CONCISELY

Entries should be clear, concise, factual, and as objective as possible. Any evidence that leads the nurse to draw a particular conclusion should be carefully documented. A subjective entry potentially creates problems in patient care and, in a court proceeding, might leave the nurse's testimony open to challenge.

### MAKE REGULAR ENTRIES

The nurse should make sure that the record contains regular entries throughout. If there are significant gaps in the record, the benefits of continuous monitoring of the patient are lost. Further, a lengthy gap in the record (e.g., a gap of a number of hours prior to a patient's cardiac or respiratory arrest, pulmonary edema, or, in a psychiatric setting, a psychotic event or suicide attempt) would be questioned in court.

### RECORD CORRECTIONS CLEARLY

Any alterations, corrections, or deletions to the record should be carefully documented, dated (including the hour), and initialled by the nurse who makes the change. Otherwise, the nurse's credibility could be undermined in a court proceeding. No attempt should be made to cover up one's mistakes by surreptitiously altering the record to make it look complete.

In cases in which a coroner's investigation is begun, the coroner usually seizes nursing notes and other patient records quickly in order to ascertain the circumstances of the patient's treatment or condition in the moments prior to death. This is especially so with computerized records. An entry in the computer is dated with the computer signature of the person making it. Because in most computer systems this can never be altered, the recorded act is "etched in time." Yet, there have been situations in which nurses have attempted to alter the record upon learning of a coroner's inquest, only to learn later that the coroner had already seized the record and made copies of it. The coroner thus had an accurate version of the record at the moment of the patient's death, as well as evidence that the nurses attempted to alter the record afterward. It is best to avoid such embarrassing situations by making clear that one is documenting a fact some time after its occurrence or that one is correcting a previous inaccuracy.

RECORD ACCURATELY

Vague terms should be avoided. For example, rather than describing the fetal position as "mid," the nurse in the Meyer case should have documented the height of the fetus's presenting part relative to the ischial spines of the mother's pelvis.

Nursing assessments are essential to care planning. The initial assessment of a patient entering the care process is crucial and should therefore be thorough and comprehensive. Most agencies and hospitals require that initial assessments be made within a specified period from the time of admission. Inaccurate or incomplete assessments can affect the outcomes of care and raise serious questions in any ensuing legal proceedings.

The frequency of repeat assessments is based on patient need, complexity of care, and agency protocols. For example, in some settings, the initial assessment determines whether a patient is fall-prone. If the patient is, reassessment on a regular basis would be necessary. If this part of the assessment were omitted and the patient subsequently fell, a negligence suit against the nurse(s) and hospital could result. The court would question why the assessment was incomplete and would likely conclude that hospital staff was negligent in (a) failing to foresee that the plaintiff was prone to falling and (b) failing to take appropriate precautions to prevent this.

Key aspects of the initial assessment that should be recorded in the patient's chart are:

- The name of an emergency contact
- The name of the patient's proxy (if any)
- Any decision made by the patient or proxy regarding CPR (see Chapter 8)
- Whether the patient has made an advance directive

Any reassessment should likewise be documented to ensure a complete record.

A notation in the patient's record such as "Slept well, had a good day" is of limited use. In a court trial, the nurse who made the note could well be asked detailed questions about what he or she meant by "a good day" (e.g., any pain felt by the patient, symptoms, vital signs) in an attempt to pinpoint the patient's condition at the time when the notation was made. The nurse would probably be unable to answer such questions meaningfully, as the original meaning of "had a good day" would have been forgotten. It is far better to document, for example: "Patient reported sharp pains in chest radiating down the left arm of 10 min duration, relieved with rest," rather than: "Patient reported chest pain." The latter notation would not bear scrutiny in a legal proceeding. More important, it would be of limited use in an attempt to diagnose the patient's ailment accurately.

FILE INCIDENT REPORTS

Sometimes a patient falls or an error is made in administering medication. In such cases, an incident or occurrence report should be prepared that documents and describes the incident, all relevant facts, any injuries sustained by the patient, and any remedial action.

These reports do not form a part of the medical record. They are used, firstly, to document occurrences out of the ordinary for investigative or quality-assurance purposes. For example, an insurance company might investigate a claim made against a hospital's general liability insurance policy, or a hospital may monitor or audit the rate of occurrence of certain types of incident over a specified period. Thus, such reports can contribute to the hospital's risk management by identifying possible problem areas in systems or procedures. The information gained can be used to educate staff to prevent similar occurrences in the future.

Finally, in the event that a negligence action is brought against the hospital arising out of an incident, the incident report can form part of the evidentiary record at trial and assist the court in understanding the cause of the incident. Such a report is usually introduced along with the testimony of the health care professional(s) who made it.

RECORD LEGIBLY

The records, and any corrections, should be legible. Given the speed with which nurses sometimes are required to perform their duties, illegibility is a very real issue; however, nurses must be aware that illegible entries may result in misreading, which can have disastrous results.

## Computerized Documentation Systems

Today, many organizations use computerized systems for documentation. The same legal and ethical standards apply as with manual documentation. The benefits of computerized systems include greater legibility, reduction in documentation errors, decreased time spent documenting, improved and timely communication across the team, timely and efficient retrieval of data or information, and greater opportunities for monitoring and improving quality of care. Further, integrated systems allow for shared databases and interfaces among departments, such as Laboratories and Radiology. Computers allow for one-time data capture (e.g., if one enters a laboratory value, it would automatically appear in all the components of the system where that value should be documented) (Fischbach, 1996, pp. 28–29).

Concerns that arise with automated systems relate to security, confidentiality, and the legality of the electronic signature. Health care systems usually identify who is doing the documenting through access cards and passwords or a double-password system, which becomes the caregiver's electronic signature. When nurses share their access information with another caregiver, they are effectively allowing that person to use their signature; this could present legal liability at a future date.

To address the issue of confidentiality, most health care computer systems are designed to restrict access points (for example, a technician in the laboratory may be able to access only information relevant to the test he or she is conducting), limit access through the use of security codes and passwords, and monitor access of information. For example, programs are in place to monitor the extent to which patients' charts are accessed by those not involved in their care (Fischbach, 1996, pp. 535–536). In many facilities, access is monitored on a regular basis. Breaches of confidentiality are taken very seriously. It is up to each facility to ensure that safeguards (e.g., standards, guidelines, quality reviews) are in place to protect clients' and patients' privacy.

Computer documentation systems have the further advantage of ensuring greater accountability for documentation in terms of timeliness and accuracy (Fischbach, 1996, pp. 251–254). For example, in online systems, it is difficult to tamper with or erase previous documentation. It is also impossible to document later and attribute the documentation to an earlier time.

As information technologies emerge, nurses are obligated to keep their computer skills up to date. This will enable them to use their facilities' systems to the standards necessary to achieve all the potential benefits.

## Telephone Advice

As new roles emerge for nurses, especially in the areas of home and community care and case management in Workers' Compensation, insurance, and rehabilitation and ambulatory clinic settings, nurses are increasingly managing clients primarily over the phone. This practice poses particular challenges in conducting assessments, giving appropriate advice, and developing a therapeutic relationship with the client.

A nurse should be very careful when giving advice over the telephone, but this does not mean that they should refrain from giving appropriate information and referrals when necessary. When in doubt about a client's condition or safety, the nurse should refer the client to an appropriate caregiver or meet with the client directly. In such a case, accurate and complete documentation of the patient's name, address, phone number, and symptoms is crucial. As well, any advice given to a patient over the telephone should be carefully noted, as well as the date and time of the call. Patients who seem to be experiencing a serious medical problem should be told to attend at the nearest emergency department without delay.

## Summary

This chapter has demonstrated the complexity of the interrelationship between nursing practice, ethics, and the legal system. The significance of the expectations society has of nurses is documented in the serious consequences nurses may face when these expectations are not met. It is critical for nurses to appreciate the gravity of these responsibilities and the extent to which their performance is measured based on professional, ethical, and legal standards. The professional responsibilities and accountabilities of nurses are made explicit by society in order to safeguard and protect the interests and well-being of vulnerable persons entrusted to their care.

We have also demonstrated in this chapter why comprehensive and accurate documentation is a key component of professional nursing. Nursing notes provide a continuous record of the patient's assessment and treatment, and the effect of interventions. From this record, the patient's progress toward stated goals and outcomes may be evaluated, and any impending complications can be identified before they become problematic.

As the health care system moves toward computerized records, there is greater demand for accurate, timely documentation. Once information is documented online, it cannot be changed, nor can the computerized signature of the caregiver be erased.

Not only does documentation serve as a means of defending the nurse's actions and interventions in legal proceedings; it is, in fact, the main means of ongoing communication about a client's care and progress. Nurses are required not only to meet standards of documentation but also to review this documentation on a regular basis. Thus, they will be in a position to provide safe and competent care to clients.

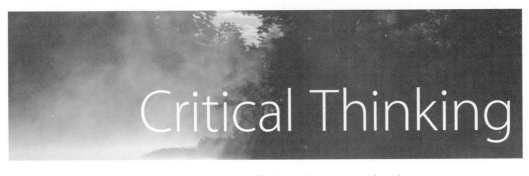

# Critical Thinking

The following case scenarios are for further reflection, discussion, and analysis.

## NO HARM DONE?

Sunita is the only RN on the night shift at a small home for the aged. She is working with Marie, a health care aide. Sunita has worked with Marie on many occasions; she respects her judgement and her caring approach to the patients. One night Sunita asks Marie to clean Mrs. Wakulat, an 80-year-old patient with Alzheimer's, who had just been incontinent. After helping Mrs. Wakulat, Marie leaves the room to dispose of the soiled linen. Unfortunately, Marie forgets to put up the bed rail, and, during her absence, Mrs. Wakulat slips to the floor.

Marie and Sunita check Mrs. Wakulat, who does not appear to have sustained any injury, and return her to bed. Marie is very concerned about the incident and pleads with Sunita not to report it to their manager, Mr. Glove. Mr. Glove recently chastised her over a similar incident, which she did not believe was her fault, in which a patient fell after climbing over the bed rails. Also, Mrs. Wakulat's daughter worries a great deal about her mother's care. Marie is afraid she will be in serious trouble.

Sunita is unsure what to do. She knows how punitive Mr. Glove can be; she also does not want to get Marie into trouble or worry Mrs. Wakulat's daughter unnecessarily.

### Questions
1. Have nurses in this scenario violated any ethical or legal standards?
2. Is there risk of any civil or criminal liability?
3. What do you think Sunita should do?
4. Would Sunita also be accountable for this accident, since she is the registered nurse and Marie is not a regulated health care provider?

## WHO IS RESPONSIBLE?

Mikhaila is a public health nurse (PHN) who has been asked to follow a high-risk mother, Terry, who was just discharged from the hospital only 24 hours after delivery. Terry is single, on welfare, and also has a 2-year-old son. Though Terry had experience with her previous child, the nurse

continued on following page >>

has observed that she is somewhat uncomfortable bathing and feeding the baby. The hospital nurse has suggested that Terry remain in the hospital another day or two since she wants to be assured that Terry is able to provide appropriate care for the baby. As well, in the hospital, Terry could get some rest; her two-year old would stay with neighbours until she comes home.

The unit manager thinks the nurse is overreacting, and the unit is tight for beds. The nurse therefore requests an early visit from the PHN. Although Mikhaila is very busy, she manages a quick visit. Everything seems fine, though Terry is tired and says she is having difficulty feeding the baby.

Mikhaila promises to return the next day; however, the next morning, she phones in ill. The unit is unable to send another nurse until the following day. When this nurse arrives, she finds everything in chaos. The 2-year-old is screaming and seems to have a cold. Terry is very stressed. The new baby has been vomiting and is obviously dehydrated. The nurse calls an ambulance; the baby is taken to the closest emergency department, where she is stabilized.

### Questions

1. Have nurses in this scenario violated any ethical or legal standards?
2. Is there risk of any civil or criminal liability?
3. Who is ethically and legally accountable for the potential harm to the baby: the hospital, the hospital nurse, Mikhaila, the public health unit, the system, or Terry?
4. How could this situation have been prevented?

## SHOULD SHE HAVE STOPPED?

Gail is driving home after a very busy 12-hour shift in the Cardiovascular Intensive Care Unit. She is 5 minutes from home and is looking forward to spending the evening with friends. As she rounds a corner, she sees a multivehicle accident. She slows her car and observes a number of people rushing to help. Reassured that appropriate assistance will be provided, Gail continues home.

The next day, she arrives at work to discover that she is assigned to care for one of the accident victims, a 20-year-old man who sustained serious chest trauma resulting in a tear to his aorta. Delays in the arrival of paramedics resulted in problems with early management of his airway. Now, though surgery has corrected the tear, it is unclear whether inadequate oxygenation to his brain will result in permanent brain damage. Gail feels responsible and wishes she had stopped to help.

### Questions

1. Has the nurse in this scenario violated any ethical or legal standards?
2. Is there risk of any civil or criminal liability?
3. Did Gail have any ethical or legal responsibility to provide assistance to the victims of this accident? Is there a difference between her legal and moral responsibilities?
4. What choice would you have made?

continued on following page >>

## KNOWING THE PATIENT'S STORY

Sylvana was admitted to hospital with anemia and a high fever. Preliminary investigations revealed that she also had a hydronephrosis of the left kidney caused by a stricture of the ureter. This was a result of chronic infection related to an ileal conduit she had had for about 30 years.

Because Sylvana's creatinine was also very high, it was decided that her left ureter must be dilated immediately. This procedure was extremely painful; afterward, Sylvana became septic and was seriously ill for about two weeks. The episode was appropriately documented in the medical record. A few weeks later, just as Sylvana was improving, a nurse accidentally removed the stent (in place to ensure the ureter remained dilated), and the dilation had to be repeated.

Sylvana's daughter Teresa accompanied her during the procedure. Both were concerned that Sylvana would become septic again. Teresa also knew the importance of the monitoring of her mother's vital signs, in particular her temperature, blood pressure, and urine output. The women's concern increased when, 2 hours postprocedure, Sylvana's nurse had not yet come to assess her.

Teresa approached Sylvana's nurse, who told her that this procedure was unusual on this unit (a medical unit) and that she had not known the protocol. Clearly, the nurse had not reviewed Sylvana's file; otherwise, she would have appreciated the risks associated with this procedure.

### Questions
1. Have the nurses in this case violated any ethical or legal standards?
2. Is there risk of any civil or criminal liability?
3. Did Sylvana's nurse after the second dilation meet the standards of practice with respect to documentation? What, if any, professional standards were not fulfilled in this case?
4. Would the facts that this procedure was rarely practised on this unit and that this nurse had never cared for a patient who has had this procedure excuse the nurse's behaviour?

## A MODERN DILEMMA

Keisha works in a busy emergency department. In this hospital, most of the patients' documentation is completed on a computerized system.

One of the residents arrives to assess a patient presenting with severe abdominal pain. This resident has forgotten to bring along the access card that allows him to review his patients' health care information online.

Keisha, aware of the urgency of this review (the patient's condition is rapidly deteriorating), lends the resident her access badge. She knows this is against the confidentiality policy she signed when she received her access card. Nonetheless, while reviewing the data online, the resident notes abnormal findings that require immediate action and, via the system, orders further tests.

continued on following page >>

## Questions

1. Has the nurse in this case violated any ethical or legal standards?
2. Is there risk of any civil or criminal liability?
3. What dilemma was the nurse facing in this scenario?
4. Can Keisha's actions be justified, given the circumstances?
5. What action should Keisha take now?

## Discussion Points

1. What is negligence? How does it compare with, and relate to, tort law? Discuss how concepts of negligence might apply in a nursing practice setting.
2. What systems are in place in your facility to guard against negligence?
3. What standards would the courts use in deciding whether a registered nurse had been negligent?
4. What actions would you take if you realized you had made a mistake? How would your organization respond?
5. Identify the most important reasons for good documentation. Beyond meeting standards, how does good documentation ensure high-quality care?
6. Identify the ethical principles that support good documentation.
7. How are documentation standards evaluated in your facility?
8. Would the quality of your documentation meet the standard during a legal proceeding? Why or why not?
9. What are the key differences between manual and computerized documentation systems? What are the advantages of each?
10. In the case of *Kolesar v. Jeffries* described in the chapter, the nurses assisted one another in reconstructing the record of treatment over their previous shift by means of notes jotted on scraps of paper. How might a nurse's testimony based on such a method be challenged in a subsequent negligence action?
11. What are the risks inherent in using imprecise language when describing and documenting a patient's condition over time? How can you improve the precision of the language you use in your charting?

## References

### Statutes

*Charter of Human Rights and Freedoms*, R.S.Q. c. C-12 (Quebec).
*Civil Code of Quebec*, C.c.Q. (Quebec).
*Contributory Negligence Act*, R.S.A. 2000, c. C-27 (Alberta).
*Contributory Negligence Act*, R.S.N.B. 1973, c. C-19 (New Brunswick).
*Contributory Negligence Act*, R.S.N.L. 1990, c. C-33 (Newfoundland and Labrador).

*Contributory Negligence Act*, R.S.N.W.T. 1988, c. C-18 (Northwest Territories and Nunavut).

*Contributory Negligence Act*, R.S.N.S. 1989, c. 95 (Nova Scotia).

*Contributory Negligence Act*, R.S.P.E.I. 1988, c. C-21 (Prince Edward Island).

*Contributory Negligence Act*, R.S.S. 1978, c. C-31 (Saskatchewan).

*Contributory Negligence Act*, R.S.Y. 2002, c. 42 (Yukon).

*Coroners Act*, R.S.O. 1990, c. C.37 (Ontario).

*Criminal Code of Canada*, R.S.C. 1985, c. C-46 (Canada).

*Emergency Medical Aid Act*, R.S.S. 1978, c. E-8 (Saskatchewan).

*Fatality Inquiries Act*, R.S.A. 2000, c. F-9 (Alberta).

*Health Care Consent Act, 1996*, S.O. 1996, c. 2, Schedule A (Ontario).

*Negligence Act*, R.S.B.C. 1996, c. 333 (British Columbia).

*Negligence Act*, R.S.O. 1990, c. N.1 (Ontario).

*Nursing Act, 1991*, S.O. 1991, c. 32 (Ontario).

*Public Hospitals Act*, R.S.O. 1990, c. P.40. (Ontario).

*Registered Nurses Act*, C.C.S.M., c. R40 (Manitoba).

*Registered Nurses Act*, S.N.S. 2001, c. 10 (Nova Scotia).

*Registered Nurses Act*, R.S.P.E.I. 1988, c. R-8.1 (Prince Edward Island).

*Registered Nurses Act*, S.S. 1988–89, c. R-12.2 (Saskatchewan).

*Tortfeasors and Contributory Negligence Act*, C.C.S.M. c. T90 (Manitoba).

## Regulations

*Professional Misconduct Regulation*, O. Reg. 799/93 (Ontario).

*Hospital Management Regulation*, R.R.O. 1990, Reg. 965 (Ontario).

## Case Law

*Butterfield v. Forrester* (1809), 11 East. 60; 103 ER 926.

*Donoghue v. Stevenson*, [1932] AC 562, at p. 580; 101 LJPC 119, at p. 127; 147 LT 281 (HL).

*Gaudreault v. Drapeau* (1987), 45 CCLT 202 (Que. SC).

*Kolesar v. Jeffries* (1974) 9 O.R. (2d) 41, 59 D.L.R. (3d) 367, varied (1976) 12 O.R. (2d) 142, 68 D.L.R. (3d) 198, affirmed [1978] 1 R.C.S. 491, 2 C.C.L.T. 170, [1978] 1 S.C.R. 491, 15 N.R. 302, 77 D.L.R. (3d) 161.

*Latin v. Hospital for Sick Children et al.* (unreported, January 3, 2007, doc. No. 99-CV-174519) 2007 CanLII 34, (ON. S.C.) 2007. Carswell.

*Meyer v. Gordon* (1981), 17 C.C.L.T. 1 (B.C.S.C.).

*R. v. Anderson* (1985), 35 MVR 128, at p. 133 (Man. CA).

*R. v. Coyne* (1958), 124 C.C.C. 176; 31 C.R. 335 (N.B.C.A.).

*R. v. Sharpe* (1984), 12 C.C.C. (3d) 428; 39 C.R. (3d) 367; 26 MVR 279 (Ont. CA).

*R. v. Sullivan and Lemay* (1986), 31 C.C.C. (3d) 62; 55 C.R. (3d) 48 (B.C. Co. Ct.), appeal dismissed on other grounds (1988), 43 C.C.C. (3d) 65; 65 C.R. (3d) 256; 31 B.C.L.R. (2d) 145 (C.A.).

*Thompson Estate v. Byrne et al.* (1993), 114 NSR (2d) 395, at p. 423 (SCTD).

## Texts and Articles

Canadian Nurses Association (CNA). (2008). *Code of ethics for registered nurses.* Ottawa, ON: Author.

Dunn, D. (2005). Home study program: Substance abuse among nurses—intercession and intervention. *AORN Journal 82*(5), 775–799.

Fischbach, F. T. (1996). *Documenting care: Communication, the nursing process and documentation standards.* Philadelphia, PA: F.A. Davis.

Fleming, J. (1983). *The law of torts* (6th ed.). Sydney, Australia: The Law Book Co.

Linden, A. (1993). *Canadian tort law* (5th ed.). Toronto, ON: Butterworths.

# Chapter 8

## End of Life

### Learning Objectives

The purpose of this chapter is to enable you to understand:

- Some of the legal and ethical issues surrounding death and the process of dying
- The ethical and moral approaches to palliative care
- The value of and challenges associated with advance directives (living wills)
- Why it is important to respect varying cultural perspectives with respect to death and dying
- The special considerations of children and older adults at the end of life
- The legal and ethical implications of withdrawal of treatment
- The difference between euthanasia and assisted suicide
- The legal and ethical challenges surrounding tissue donation and organ transplantation
- The legal definitions of death and challenges with proposed redefinitions

## Introduction

MANY OF THE MOST challenging ethical, legal, and emotional issues in health care today are associated with the end of life. Despite various cultural and religious views of the meaning of death and what happens after it, many people are fearful of death and of the dying process. Death, after all, remains one of life's greatest mysteries.

Nurses play a vital role during this significant transition by providing care and comfort to the patient, support to the family, and ultimately ensuring that the process of dying is dignified and respectful of all involved. Nurses have a significant role in minimizing suffering, ensuring the presence of those the dying person would like to have there, and providing comfort to patients and families when that cannot be possible. For example, if a patient's death is sudden or unexpected, and family members are not able to arrive in time, nurses are able to be present, to provide comfort to the dying person, and to reassure the family that their loved one did not die alone. Though it may not always be possible, ensuring that someone is present at a patient's death should be considered a priority for resource allocation and patient assignments. It is not necessary that it be the patient's nurse, but the nurse can ensure that a volunteer or other member of the team is there with the patient. In a home setting, nurses play a significant role in assisting the family's involvement with care and facilitating the client's wishes to die at home.

The fear of death has led society to find ways to extend life at all costs. Yet, there is a cost when extending life diminishes the quality and dignity that give life meaning. When a person dies in hospital—for example, in a Critical Care Unit—the very technology that extends his or her life may distance caregivers and family members from that person. Ethically and morally, nurses are central to preserving dignity and, through the caring relationship, to supporting not only the patient but also those that person is closest to. In caring for the dying patient, nurses afford that person as much comfort, respect, and freedom from anxiety and pain as possible. Special consideration must be given to the needs of the family or significant others in coping with their impending and subsequent loss (Canadian Nurses Association, 2008, pp. 13–14).

In a multicultural society such as Canada's, patients come from many religious and cultural backgrounds, and view death and dying from varying perspectives. Nurses must be sensitive to these differences and respectful of the values and beliefs of others.

This chapter will examine the complex ethical and legal issues that relate to the end of the life continuum: death and dying.

## Death and Dying

Like so much else in our society, the process of dying has become more complex and, in some circumstances, less humane. In previous decades, and still in some cultures, persons at the end of life died in their own homes, surrounded by their loved ones.

Today, in high-tech environments, patients may be denied the presence of family and friends, especially when death occurs as a result of failed resuscitation attempts. Today's advanced technology even allows parts of human bodies to live on after death through organ donation and transplantation. This is possible because through life-support technology, the body can be kept alive well beyond the point at which the patient's capacity to interact with the world is gone. Consequently, health care professionals have been obliged to explore and redefine the distinction between life and death.

## End-of-Life Issues

### Communication Challenges

Families and patients are confronted with a great deal of unfamiliar information at a time of incredible stress. At this most stressful time, they are expected to make very complex and emotionally laden decisions. They frequently have to struggle to comprehend and retain the information shared with them, and to feel confident with the challenging decisions they are asked to make (Jezewski & Finnell, 1998). A key role for nurses is ensuring effective and respectful communication with patients and families, and creating an environment conducive to sharing information, questioning, clarifying, and listening. An example of the struggles patients and families must face comes in the form of discussions related to end-of-life choices, such as whether cardiopulmonary resuscitation should occur or not.

### Advance Directives (Living Wills)

An advance directive is a person's instruction regarding decisions about care if he or she is ever rendered incompetent. When the person is not able to participate in decision making, advance directives ensure that the patient retains some control of the care he or she receives. Advance directives can take the form of verbal discussion with someone whom the person has identified as a substitute decision maker or be made explicit in writing (Singer, Robertson, & Roy, 1996). There are a number of tools and guidelines available today that serve as a resource for communicating one's wishes in advance.

For most people, it is difficult to envisage all possible scenarios in advance, especially when there is limited understanding of the complexities of future health care decisions relating to the end of life. Advance directives may not be as helpful as initially intended since it is not possible for individuals to anticipate every possibility in advance or their future state of mind and circumstances (Dresser, 1994). One solution is to construct a life-values advance directive, thereby integrating the complexity of acceptable treatment with an expected level of independence, function, and quality of life (Kolarik, Arnold, Fischer, Hanusa, 2002). For example, since one is not able to envisage every future possibility, one can instead express in advance that which is important to him or her. One might value independence, not being a burden on others, being free from pain, or not wanting excessive use of technology when mortality is certain or when the result might be lifelong morbidity. Connection to family may also be an important value that might influence one's decision. For example, would the person want treatment withdrawn immediately if awaiting family coming from out of town?

Advance directives do not have legal sanction in all provinces. However, it is legally recognized in Ontario in the *Substitute Decisions Act*, in Manitoba under the *Health Care Directives Act*, in Nova Scotia under the *Medical Consent Act*, and in Alberta pursuant to the *Personal Directives Act*. Substitute-decision legislation has been passed in British Columbia through the *Adult Guardianship Act* and the *Representation Agreement Act*. The former statute allows the court to appoint a guardian or substitute decision maker. The latter statute allows competent persons over the age of 19 to appoint a person to make substitute decisions for them.

A written advance directive may be created in the form of a living will, a document that enables a patient to specify his or her informed choices well in advance of requiring such care. The living will takes effect only when the patient is incapable of making decisions. People with living wills usually update and revise them on a regular basis. Regardless of whether they are sanctioned by law, living wills are a useful resource for health professionals.

There are usually two components to living wills. An instruction directive allows the person to specify which life-sustaining treatments he or she would not wish in various situations. The proxy directive allows individuals to identify a substitute decision maker should they ever be rendered incompetent.

Individuals who complete a living will are advised to ensure that several appropriate people know the will exists and that copies are distributed, particularly to their doctor, lawyer, and family members. The will should be reviewed and updated regularly to ensure that it continues to reflect its maker's current wishes.

Ideally, individuals who complete a living will consult with physicians, nurses, and perhaps a lawyer or other persons so that they can anticipate the situations that might arise and comprehend the treatments available to them. This helps them to make sound choices and ensures that these are clearly expressed in the living will.

## Ethical Issues Related to Resuscitation

Over the past few decades, advancements in pharmaceuticals and technologies such as defibrillation have made cardiopulmonary resuscitation (CPR) a routine intervention unless the patient or family have refused this in advance and a "no CPR" order is documented in the patient's chart or in some other form of an advance directive (discussed later in this chapter). "No CPR" is frequently used interchangeably with "Do Not Resuscitate" (DNR). DNR, however, is a broader concept that may preclude other interventions, such as ventilation, antibiotic therapy, and so on. A person may agree to aggressive treatment, but may choose not to receive CPR in the case of a cardiac arrest. CPR has proven to be effective in specific cardiac events not related to another terminal condition (Booth, 2006). Such cardiac events may include sudden arrythmias, such as ventricular fibrillation, or sudden asystole, related to cardiac disease. CPR is usually not as effective in circumstances in which a patient's condition is unrelated to a cardiac problem and when the patient's illness is in its final stage (such as emphysema or severe stroke) (Booth, 2006). CPR in these circumstances, however, may influence the quality and dignity of that person's death and the experience of that person's family and friends.

Over the past number of years, various processes and policies have emerged to prevent the inappropriate provision of CPR. These exist in acute-care settings and also in long-term care facilities and nursing homes. Also, mechanisms are now in place to respect the wishes of a person who wants to die at home in the event that emergency services are called. In previous years, when an event, such as the dying patient's experiencing sudden severe respiratory distress, resulted in the family calling emergency services, CPR was initiated even against the wishes of the family. If a dying patient was being transferred home via ambulance, a physician needed to accompany that person in the event of death to avoid CPR and transfer to another hospital's emergency department. Now processes and documentation tools are in place in the community to ensure that the wishes of the patient and family are met, while at the same time the emergency workers can be reassured that they are doing the right thing and are protected in these difficult circumstances.

Recently, however, there has been some reflection on the burden placed on families when they have to make a "no CPR" decision on behalf of an incapable family member (Venneman, Narnor-Harris, Perish, & Hamilton, 2008; Cantor, Braddock, Derse, Murray Edwards, Logue, Nelson, et al., 2003). Recent research suggests that the emotional conflict the family faces may arise from the terminology used when they are asked to make this decision. From their perspective, they are being asked to make a decision not to do something. Some families feel they are making a decision not to prevent death, that they are signing a "death warrant" or "playing God," or that they are making a decision to terminate a loved one's life. The emotions associated with these thoughts would potentially have serious consequences on the family's future bereavement process and on their ability to come to terms with the death by worrying that they played a role in what was, in fact, inevitable (Jezewski & Finnell, 1998).

Emerging are thoughts that the emphasis and discussion about the choice the family is being asked to make should be on whether aggressive therapy should continue or whether the person should be "allowed a natural death." Framing the decision around whether to "allow a natural death" enables a more positive experience in which one is contributing to a dignified and respectful death without the use of inappropriate intervention (Venneman et al., 2008). Knowing that the death was dignified and compassionate may also influence the family's experience and memories of the dying process (Cohen, 2004).

There are other considerations with respect to CPR that include whether this choice or intervention should be offered at all. For example, though a person has the right to refuse any treatment offered, does he or she have the right to demand a particular therapy when it has no likelihood of success? Should the family or patient even be offered the option of CPR when the patient is dying of a terminal illness such as end-stage cancer, extreme cardiac failure, or severe traumatic brain damage? These questions are not straightforward when taking into consideration various cultural views or the family's or patient's reluctance to give up hope (Cantor et al., 2003). Such challenges are best met not through policy but via a fair process based on the shared relationship the nurse and the team have with that patient and family. Each should be explored as a situation arises and through a common understanding of the values and perspectives of all team members, including those of the patient and family. For example, what are the goals behind the family's or patient's wishes? A patient who is near death may want resuscitation if a close friend or family member is soon to arrive from out of town and he or she wants to say goodbye. At the same time, there are challenges within a complex system with limited resources that consistently attempts to meet the needs of all patients (e.g., a critically ill patient may be waiting in the emergency room until a bed is available on the unit).

Nurses are active team members when difficult ethical questions such as these are raised and when decisions around them must be made. These challenges occur in complex sociological, cultural, technological, and legal or political contexts. Decisions are not easy and are made based on probabilities since there are very few absolutes in health care. Every situation is unique and must be decided contextually. Ethical principles, similar cases, professional codes, positions, statements, policies, and procedures can serve as guides, but each case requires a collaborative effort in deciding the most ethical course of action (Hayes, 2004).

## Palliative Care: Ensuring Relief of Suffering

**Palliative care** is introduced once the patient, the family, and the health providers have accepted that a cure is unlikely, death is inevitable, and further treatment would be burdensome. Today, palliative care can be provided in the home, hospice, or institutional settings such as hospitals, nursing homes, and long-term care facilities, and is supported by a palliative care team. The goal of palliative care is to ensure that through emotional and psychological support and effective symptom management, the patient experiences a quality dying process and a dignified death.

Regardless of the environment, nurses can provide superior supportive care to their patients. For example, a dying person may want to recall important life events and ensure an ongoing connection with family by documenting his or her story in a journal or through video, and nurses can facilitate this. Or what may be most important to a dying person is having the opportunity to spend quality time with those he or she loves. Nurses are in an important and significant position to give family and friends the opportunity to be involved in care if they, and the patient, so choose and to aid in this significant transition. Nurses may enable opportunities for the dying person, friends, and family to engage in meaningful conversation and perhaps reach closure on past issues that have remained unresolved. For as long as possible, the nurse should ensure that the patient retains control. For example, the patient should dictate care and decide on the right balance of pain manaagement if he or she is alert and cognitively sound (Hayes, 2004).

## Dying Before Life Begins: The Low-Birth-Weight Neonate

Advances in technology have led to extreme dilemmas with respect to the care of newborn infants with uncertain prognoses. Interventions to support and treat high-risk newborn infants have become more effective, to the extent that it is now possible, in some circumstances, for the child to achieve a normal life. However, these interventions may alternatively result in life with disability or with developmental delays. In some cases, these interventions compromise the quality of the infant's life and prolong the dying process (Committee on Fetus and Newborn (American Academy of Pediatrics), 2007).

When a child is born at 24 to 32 weeks' gestation, parents must make extremely difficult decisions (Paris, Graham, Schreiber, & Goodwin, 2006). They had looked forward to parenthood and the birth of a child but are suddenly faced with extreme dilemmas regarding a person who has not yet lived, whose values they do not yet understand, and whose promise of life is as yet undetermined (McAllister & Dionne, 2006).

Babies born prematurely may simply have arrived early, or in addition they may have conditions such as cardiac or other congenital anomalies. In some cases, multiple challenges are anticipated; in others, they are not. These various scenarios influence the timing and extent to which the health care team can collaborate with the parents to decide on the best course of action. Potential problems may be known in advance or not discovered until the delivery room. Regardless, parents of premature babies need the special support of nurses and the entire interprofessional team.

In these extremely challenging and emotional moments, the health care team and parents have to weigh the benefits and burdens of aggressive intervention for the infant; for example, in circumstances in which:

- Early death is very likely, and survival would be accompanied by high risk of severe morbidity
- Intervention would only prolong dying
- The prognosis is uncertain, and survival may be associated with diminished quality of life
- Significant neurodevelopmental disability is possible
- The infant would suffer significant discomfort (such as pain)
- Survival is likely and the risk of morbidity is low (Janvier & Barrington, 2005)

In most sitations, the infant's future is highly uncertain, making the parents' decisions even more difficult (Meadow, 2006). It is important that the decisions be made collaboratively and that they respect the wishes of the family and ensure that the best interests of the infant are met. These decisions are made in very stressful situations, which is why a collaborative team approach (with the parents as members of the team) to decision making is essential (Baumann-Hölzle, Maffezzoni, & Bucher, 2005).

For the parents and family, continuity of care is extremely important; therefore, whenever possible, one nurse should be designated to provide ongoing support for the family and a core team of nurses should be consistently assigned to caring for the infant. In these strenuous circumstances, the parents need to see strong interprofessional collaboration that can enable effective and meaningful communication (Kowalski, Leef, Mackley, Spear, & Paul, 2005). Parents will view nurses as their primary source of information. Nurses are thereby put in a leadership position to promote parents as active participants in rounds and team meetings.

When the decision is to provide palliative care, nurses must support the parents and family through this very difficult transition. They do this by respecting the special needs of parents whose child's life is about to end before it begins. Nurses may support the family through this emotional transition by:

- Facilitating the opportunity for the parents to hold their child
- Creating memories by taking pictures or videos or making sculptures of the child's hands or feet
- Facilitating breastfeeding, if possible, or ensuring the infant receives the mother's milk (through pumping)
- Enabling the opportunity for the infant to go home
- Ensuring sibling participation
- Influencing organizations to make available family-centred homelike environments that offer privacy and dignity (Ives-Baine, 2007; Epstein, 2007)

Nurses have a responsibility to ensure the comfort of the dying neonate and to provide the parents (and siblings) the opportunity to create memories of the child that can sustain them through their loss. It is important to families that they have memories of the infant as a person. In many settings, rooms are set up to provide a more homelike and peaceful environment where parents can hold and comfort their child and each other.

## The Special Circumstances of the Dying Child

The world of the dying child is highly emotional and challenges nurses with highly complex moral and ethical issues. These include the difficult choices parents and the team must make on behalf of the child who may not be competent or of an age to make these decisions. Moral dilemmas arise when decisions must be made as to whether to maintain life-sustaining therapies when the outcomes may not be clear and the quality of the child's life is compromised. Nurses have expressed concerns of conscience over caring for a critically ill or dying child when they believe the treatments to be overburdensome or when they believe there to be inappropriate use of technology (Solomon, O'Donnell, Jennings, Guilfoy, Wolf, Nolan, et al., 1993). Rarely do nurses cite examples in which the health care team gave up too soon (Solomon, Sellers, Heller, Dokken, Levetown, Rushton, et al., 2005), which is not surprising since our frame of reference is the belief that children have a long life ahead of them and parents usually expect to die before their child. Society is programmed to care for and protect children, and, therefore, it is to be expected that every attempt is made to prevent them from dying. Having said that, health care teams need to address these moral and emotional challenges to ensure that children die in comfort, free of pain, and with dignity.

There are particular challenges when the team disagrees with the family about continuing care or withdrawing treatment (Canadian Paediatric Society, 2004). Consider the example of the seriously brain-injured child whose injury evolves to brain death. The family may not be ready to accept death and may need some time to adjust to this reality. Yet the team may think continuing to care for the patient is a burden on both the child and the system.

Nurses often develop long-term relationships and emotional bonds with patients and their families when caring for children with, for example, cancer or cystic fibrosis, or with those who receive transplants. It is then very emotionally traumatic for them when the child they have grown to know so well and cared for over time nears death. In these circumstances, nurses would not find it helpful to draw on traditional reasoning processes based on theories of justice, for example. However, an ethic of care that focuses on the relationship with the child and family can enable nurses to understand and accept what is right from all perspectives and continue engaging with and supporting the child and family. Though saddened by the loss, nurses are rewarded in knowing that they have provided the most dignified passage for that child.

Issues of consent are challenging for parents who must decide on behalf of their child; even more so when their child is dying or is diagnosed with a terminal illness.

Some of the most challenging circumstances for nurses are those related to life support for neonates and children. There is general agreement that life support may be forgone when children are terminally ill or permanently unconscious, in instances of medical futility, or when the burdens of treatment outweigh the benefits from the child's perspective. Still, these decisions are not easy. They become increasingly challenging when they relate to the withdrawal of treatment already begun versus making an early choice to enable a natural death. Though the family may decide against highly complex technological support for their child, even more difficult are decisions related to the withdrawal of nutrition, particularly given the symbolic nature of nurturing a child through the provision of food and water (Canadian Paediatric Society, 2004).

Nurses recognize the importance of supporting the family by encouraging their involvement in care, in pain and symptom management, and in making the situation as normal as possible for the child, which may be achieved by enabling the child to die at home. If this is not possible, even a hospital room can be arranged to achieve a homelike environment. In all circumstances, it is important that nurses support parents in enacting their parental role with their child.

As discussed, most children are not able to make difficult end-of-life decisions for themselves. They may be too young, too ill, or cognitively impaired. However, there are particular consent challenges regarding treatment decisions when one is dealing with an adolescent. A 13-year-old who is newly diagnosed with cancer may want to refuse treatment because he or she is afraid of the pain and of feeling sick. A 13-year-old with a long history of leukemia who has relapsed on a number of occasions would be in a different pos-ition regarding making a decision not to accept further treatment. Consent by adolescents is discussed further in Chapter 6.

Of particular importance in children's settings is their need to develop emotionally and socially even when they are ill or dying. Consider the story of Layla, a teen who was diag-nosed with osteosarcoma of the tibia at the age of 10.

## Layla's Story

At 13, Layla actively engaged in conversation with the nurses about all the things teens want to talk about. When she was going through chemotherapy, she enjoyed displaying all the stylish wigs she was able to wear and enjoyed her sense of fashion. Layla had been cared for by the same nursing team for almost 3 years before she relapsed and her cancer spread to her lungs.

Layla deteriorated quickly during the relapse and was suffering major respiratory distress. She was very upset that she would not be able to attend her Grade 8 graduation. Layla's pri-mary nurse mobilized the team, organized an ambulance, and, along with one of her physi-cians, escorted Layla and her parents to the graduation.

Layla was able to maintain her stamina, and was wheeled into the graduation hall, where she received a standing ovation from her teachers and fellow classmates. She received her diploma! When Layla returned to the hospital that evening, she died.

In this important transition in Layla's life, her primary nurse understood what mattered to her and her family. To the end, Layla continued to grow and develop as any 13-year-old girl would. She was still a child graduating from Grade 8 and in need of this important rite of pas-sage. In fact, she wasn't ready to go until she reached this milestone. This act of caring ensured that Layla's family, in spite of their grief, would retain the happy memory of their child's experi-ence of achieving her goal of receiving her Grade 8 diploma along with her friends.

This story illustrates the developmental stage of a young adolescent. How might nurses con-sider the phases of development of other clients? What about the infant? The young mother? The husband who has just lost his wife? The older adult who has had so many life experiences? How should these factors be considered in nursing practice?

## Meaningful Lives: Caring for Older Adults

Persons who die late in life may no longer be in a position to care for themselves. It is very sad when those who throughout their lives contributed a great deal to society, their profes-sion, their families, and others become unable to care for themselves because of physical inability, dementia, Alzheimer's disease, or other organic problems. They may feel a loss of dignity and yearn for the respect they received earlier in their lives. Some may be aban-doned by their families; others may worry that they are a burden on their families. People who have been independent their whole life find it difficult to rely on others to accomplish even basic bodily functions.

Nurses are instrumental in ensuring the dignity of those who have lived long enough to experience cognitive or physical deterioration. They can ensure that older adults retain as much control over their lives as possible. They should create an environment of respect and not condone practices or language that is insulting or demeaning. For example, it is inappropriate to infantilize older adults by encouraging the use of adult incontinence products when other nursing interventions, such as regular toileting, can be used to manage incontinence. When these products are required, however, it is disrespectful to use the term "diapers." Nurses must also be sure to refer to patients in respectful ways. A 90-year-old gentleman, for example, may or may not wish to be called by his first name.

Nurses who engage in conversation with older adults about their lives, listen to them, and learn from them are richer for the experience. Older adults need stimulation and socialization, and want to share their stories and to be treated with the respect they have earned throughout their lives.

## Cultural Considerations at the End of Life

An ethical approach to care requires the nurse to understand the particular views and traditions of the patient and family. It is important to build these considerations into the overall initial assessment of the patient and family in order to understand their values. The nurse's attention to such needs can improve the quality of the dying process and constructively influence the bereavement that follows. A general familiarity with the fundamental concepts of various traditions allows nurses to provide competent, compassionate, and respectful care as patients from differing backgrounds approach the end of life (Ross, 2001). By undertaking cultural assessments of patients and families, nurses gain a basic understanding of the values and practices important to them and hence can play a crucial role in supporting the patient and family at the end of life. When nurses do their best to facilitate traditional practices, the family experiences the true meaning of care and respect, and nurses feel valued when the best possible outcomes are achieved.

To understand the importance of cultural assessments, consider a few examples of various perpectives on the end of life. The following illustrations demonstrate why it is not possible to understand the beliefs and rituals of all cultures and why it is therefore important to ask the patient and family what is most significant to them.

### Islamic Views on End of Life

In Islam, death is not viewed as final but, rather, as a transition from this world to eternity. Just as the fetus develops in the womb, Muslims believe that the soul undergoes growth and change in the grave in preparation for the Day of Resurrection (Chittick, 1992; Kramer, 1988). As the Muslim approaches death, he or she must be placed in the supine position, facing Mecca (the spiritual centre of the Muslim faith, located in Saudi Arabia). The room must be perfumed, and anyone unclean must leave it. (This would include women who are menstruating.) Excerpts from the Quran are read by the dying person or a close friend or family member, and the basic tenet of Islam—"There is no God but Allah and Muhammad is his prophet"—is recited (Chittick, 1992; Kramer, 1988), thus making the connection from birth to death, as this statement is the first read to the newborn. Traditionally, families prepare the body for burial almost immediately, and, when possible, the dead are buried on the day they die. Ideally, family members are present at the time of death, both to mourn and to prepare the body (Ross, 2001).

## Buddhist Views on End of Life

Buddhists also have unique rituals associated with death. Undertaking these rituals might be challenging in the institutional setting; however, the following scenario is a compelling illustration of the incredible role nurses can play in supporting a family through the death of a loved one. In this situation, a newborn child with a serious congenital condition was dying, and his nurses supported the parents and grandmother through this emotional time.

# Case Scenario

## HONOURING BELIEFS

When David was 26 days old, he was diagnosed with a fatal congenital condition. When his parents learned of his diagnosis, they were devastated. Earlier, they had given birth to a daughter with the same condition, who died shortly after. How had they had the misfortune to give birth to two children with the same condition? Why them? What had they done in previous lives to warrant such a tragedy? The notion of karma in the Buddhist tradition is the belief that one's actions in past lives have consequences in future lives. The parents understood their child would die soon and, in discussions with the team, agreed that palliative care was in their infant's best interests.

David's parents were not religious. However, his grandmother, who had just arrived from northern China and did not speak a word of English, had strong Buddhist beliefs. David's parents had told her prior to her leaving China that things did not look good for her grandson; however, this gentle woman came to assist her grandson through this very significant transition. When she got to David's hospital room, she began to chant, and continued to chant in spite of her fatigue after such a long journey. The nurses discovered that Buddhists believe that chanting helps to connect the living with the higher being. She was chanting to encourage the higher being to lead her grandson's spirit to a happier place. Although she had not slept for more than two days, she continued her chanting, sometimes falling asleep while doing so. She also wrote messages in Chinese on small cards, which were placed on her grandson's chest. These were also intended to help him get to the next place. The

continued on following page >>

nurses were careful to put the cards back in place whenever they provided care to David that required moving them.

The nurses soon discovered that David's grandmother's belief was that more voices chanting would strengthen the request of calling for the coming of the higher being. They began to chant with her. They further discovered that when David died, it was important for the chanting to continue for an additional 16 hours since it would take this long for the boy's spirit to leave his body. This would ensure the connection with the higher being. Though clearly not the norm that the deceased remain in the acute-care setting that long, the nurses made this possible and transferred David and his family to a private, more peaceful setting. In doing so, they made a significant difference to the family.

At the same time, the nurses learned a great deal. They gained insight into the importance of faith to some families and how faith and tradition give people strength and the ability to survive adversity such as the death of a child. The experience reinforced that language barriers can be overcome by presence and by sharing in rituals, whether understood or not. It also validated that by asking and listening, "we learn much more about the specifics of a family's cultural interpretation than when we assume we know, based on what is written in the books, profiles and guides" (Ives-Baine, 2007).

**Issues**

1. What have you learned from this story?
2. How do you gain insight into the cultural values and beliefs of your patients or clients and their families?
3. The nurses were able to make a difference in this situation. What are the barriers we need to overcome to ensure all families in these circumstances have a meaningful experience?

With the increasing diversity of society, a single policy for the care of the dying and of the patient after death is not sustainable. Nurses can access literature and locate experts to ensure optimal care to dying patients and their families. A meaningful death goes a long way in supporting the family's grieving process and in providing comfort. By facilitating and engaging in traditional practices, nurses can help achieve the right outcomes for the dying (Ross, 2001).

## Choosing Death

The issue of withdrawal of treatment began to gain prominence in the mid-1970s with the case of Karen Ann Quinlan in the United States (*Re Quinlan*, 1975, 1976), followed by Nancy B. in Quebec (*Nancy B. v. Hôtel-Dieu de Québec et al.*, 1992), and Sue Rodriguez in British Columbia (*Rodriguez v. British Columbia*, 1993). Public debate regarding Robert Latimer in Saskatchewan (*R. v. Latimer*, 1997, 2001) has renewed and re-energized controversy over the ethical and legal justifications for and against euthanasia, withdrawal of treatment, and physician–assisted suicide.

## Withdrawal of Treatment

In withdrawal of treatment, nothing active is done to end the patient's life; rather, all life-sustaining treatment is withdrawn, and death is allowed to occur through natural processes. Indeed, it is this approach, previously labelled "passive euthanasia," that the Quebec Superior Court allowed in the Nancy B. decision, discussed in Chapter 4.

A recent case from Western Canada illustrates well the issues relating to withdrawal of treatment and the ethical conflicts that arise for health care professionals. An 84-year-old man was placed on life support after he became unable to speak, breathe, or eat on his own. He had had a portion of his brain removed after a fall a number of years earlier. The treating physicians determined that his chances of recovery were extremely remote, and they recommended to his family that life support be withdrawn. The man was an Orthodox Jew, and his family fought the decision to end life support, arguing that to do so would result in the commission of a sin since their religious beliefs required that all life must be preserved to a natural conclusion. Ending life support, they argued, would hasten the man's death and would, in fact, constitute an assault. Accordingly, the man's family commenced an action against the hospital for an injunction requiring that life support (a ventilator and feeding tube) be continued. The court granted a temporary injunction preventing termination of life support and ordered the matter to proceed to a trial. The physicians relied on Manitoba College of Physicians and Surgeons guidelines for such situations, which stipulated that if the patient was unable to communicate, the physicians would consult with the patient's family to determine what course of action should be taken, but that the ultimate decision on withdrawing treatment would rest with the physicians. They and the hospital maintained the view that given the man's terminal condition and the extremely poor prognosis, keeping him on life support would needlessly prolong his suffering and would be a waste of limited medical resources while other patients were in serious need of those same resources.

The man ultimately died, but not before a number of physicians at the hospital withdrew their services rather than continue to perform what they deemed to be unethical continued treatment ("Orthodox Jew to remain on life support, trial next," 2008; *Golubchuk v. Salvation Army Grace General Hospital et al.*, 2008).

## Euthanasia (Including Assisted Suicide)

A special committee of the Senate of Canada was established in February 1994 "to examine and report on the legal, social and ethical issues relating to euthanasia and assisted suicide" (Government of Canada, 1995). The intention of this study was to assist members of Parliament in preparing for the legislative debate on these issues, and to seek opinions regarding them. The committee presented to the Senate a number of recommendations related to palliative care, pain control, sedation practices, withholding and withdrawal of life-sustaining treatment, advance directives, assisted suicide, and euthanasia.

**Euthanasia**, or "painless death," is defined as an act that brings about the immediate death of a terminally ill patient. Commonly referred to as "mercy killing," it is seen as a means to end the suffering and pain of patients who otherwise would experience a difficult, undignified death. It is viewed as an act of compassion, as its intention is to do a good by relieving pain and suffering. Today's heightened awareness of euthanasia arises partly from advances in health care technology and partly from the growing number of patients with terminal conditions, in which the quality and dignity of the dying process are a concern.

There is an important distinction between euthanasia (or assisted suicide) and withdrawal of treatment. In euthanasia, active steps (e.g., the administration of a drug that is intended to cause death, such as a bolus of potassium chloride) are taken to end the life of a patient who requests this. Such a request might arise in the case of irreversible injury or terminal illness, when the patient deems his or her quality of life unacceptable. This may be due to a complete loss of mobility and the inability to perform even the most basic tasks of everyday life (as in the case of patients with amyotrophic lateral sclerosis [ALS]); the extreme confusion and incapacity to communicate that is typical of Alzheimer's disease; or severe and unendurable pain that requires heavy medication, rendering the patient too sedated and disoriented to take an active part in life.

In the United States, pathologist Dr. Jack Kevorkian publicly admitted assisting the deaths of a number of patients using the "suicide machine" that he designed and built; he was convicted of first-degree murder in Michigan following a broadcast of a videotaped assisted suicide on a well-known U.S. current affairs program. He served 8 years of a 10- to 25-year sentence and was paroled in June 2007. Here in Canada, the federal government has promised a full legislative debate and public hearings on the issue, but these have yet to take place.

Euthanasia under certain conditions has been legalized in the Netherlands. A law passed in 2002 states that physicians who perform euthanasia are no longer criminally responsible, provided they have followed the procedures prescribed in the statute. (See the *Termination of Life on Request and Assisted Suicide (Review Procedures) Act* (the Netherlands).) To be exempt from criminal sanctions, a physician must exercise due care and report the death promptly to the municipal coroner. Physicans who adhere to these two requirements will be exempted from prosecution. It is important to note that persons performing acts of euthanasia that do not conform to this Act may still be prosecuted since this statute does not decriminalize all acts of euthanasia. The due care requirements provide, among other things, that the patient's request to die be voluntary and well-considered, that his or her condition be terminal, that there be no hope of recovery, and that he or she be suffering unbearable pain. Furthermore, a second physician must be consulted, and the euthanasia or assisted suicide must be performed with due medical care.

In assisted suicide, the patient is mentally competent to decide to end his or her life because of its deteriorating quality yet is too debilitated by illness to act on this decision without the assistance of another (e.g., a physician, nurse, family member, or friend).

The following case scenario highlights some of the legal and ethical challenges associated with these issues.

# Case Scenario

## A CRY FOR HELP?

Joan, a 40-year-old mother of two teenage children, was diagnosed 2 years ago with ovarian cancer. She has always been independent and active, a devoted mother who ran a corporate law practice and participated in civic organizations.

Early in her illness, Joan was treated with chemotherapy, radiotherapy, and surgery. For a time, the cancer seemed to be in remission. However, after a year, it metastasized to her liver and lower intestines. Since then, Joan has been in and out of the hospital receiving various treatments. Over the past 2 months, her health has deteriorated to the point that she is in constant and intense pain, especially in her bones. During her last admission to hospital, the team decided that nothing they could do would slow the growth of the tumour. After discussions with the team and her family, Joan decided to enter a home palliative care program that provides her with home care services, a pain control protocol, and a home care nurse. As well, Joan's husband, Bob, has taken a leave of absence from work to remain at home with his wife.

For the past few weeks, Joan's condition has remained unchanged, although the pain is becoming difficult to control, and she suffers frequent bouts of nausea and constipation (side effects of the medication). She has become despondent and distressed by her loss of dignity and the effect her illness is having on her family.

One day, Joan exclaims to the home care nurse: "I've had enough! I can't stand the pain; I've become a burden on my husband and children. Please help me end it!"

## Issues

1. What can the home care nurse do in this situation (a) legally and (b) ethically?
2. What alternatives are available to the nurse?

## Discussion

Sometimes, patients, families, and caregivers are asked to choose between extending a painful, undignified life and death. Even when the best palliative care is available, not all pain and suffering can be relieved. When death is preferred, the means toward achieving it may place caregivers and family under great moral stress—for example, in the case of withholding food and fluids at a patient's request. These situations become even more difficult when the patient is no longer competent and has left no advance directive and a substitute decision maker must make the decision. Hence, it is not surprising that questions around advance directives, withdrawal of treatment, euthanasia, and assisted suicide have surfaced in recent years.

continued on following page >>

Many ethical principles, often conflicting ones, ground decisions about these issues. On the one hand, we have the principle of autonomy, or respect for the rights of individuals to make decisions that affect their lives. But the law places limits on that autonomy and draws the line when it comes to individuals' determining how and when their lives will end. In such cases, the principle of autonomy conflicts with the principle of the sanctity of life, which for many is an absolute principle—that is, it cannot be overridden in any circumstances.

Nurses may experience extreme emotional and moral distress when dealing with challenges related to death and dying. Whether in the institutional or the home setting, they are often in closer contact with the patient and family than any other health care professional. Consequently, they empathize with the physical, emotional, and spiritual experience of the patient and family. Conflict occurs when the patient's wishes, the nurse's loyalty to the patient, and the principle of beneficence (e.g., concern over providing good and avoiding harm when pain control and symptom relief fail) clash with the principle of sanctity of life and the law. These situations, more than any others, represent true dilemmas that nurses face in their practice and provide a poignant reminder that what is legal may not, for some, be what is right.

Joan's situation is an example of one that challenges the ethical and professional integrity of the nurse and the nature of the nurse–patient relationship. Nurses are encouraged to empathize—that is, to enter into the patient's way of seeing and being—so that they can feel what the patient feels and can understand the situation from the patient's perspective. A nurse working closely with a patient such as this might understand the patient's pain and be sensitive to her request. Regardless of their ethical values and beliefs, most nurses would feel frustrated by their limited ability to reduce the patient's physical and emotional pain, and would want to respect and support his or her wishes.

Nurses have a duty to care for the physical, emotional, and psychological needs of the patients and families entrusted to them. The CNA's *Code of Ethics for Registered Nurses* expresses the following responsibilities:

> In all practice settings, nurses work to relieve pain and suffering, including appropriate and effective symptom and pain management, to allow persons to live with dignity. . . .
>
> When a person receiving care is terminally ill or dying, nurses foster comfort, alleviate suffering, advocate for adequate relief of discomfort and pain and support a dignified and peaceful death. This includes support for the family during and following the death, and care of the person's body after death. (Canadian Nurses Association, 2008, p. 12)

Within the context of the caring relationship, the nurse in this scenario cannot assume that Joan has thought through all the issues and choices available to her and has made a reasoned decision to end her life. Joan's nurse has a responsibility to explore with her the reasons behind this request. Has it arisen out of fear and uncertainty about the future and how her death will occur? Has her pain become unbearable? She believes she is a burden to her husband and

continued on following page >>

family. Is she angry about her illness and its inevitable outcome? Is she frustrated with the grow-ing lack of control she has over her life? Finally, does she believe she has little or no dignity left?

Knowing the reasons behind Joan's request, the nurse may be able to intervene to assist in making her remaining life, and her dying, more tolerable. Although Joan is already receiving palliative care, perhaps her symptoms can be managed more effectively; for example, she may require alternative approaches to pain management.

Patients dying of cancer can tolerate extremely high levels of pain medication. The ethical and caring nurse ensures that such patients receive appropriate pain management while attempt-ing to minimize the related complications of drowsiness, confusion, constipation, and diarrhea. Patients should be given choices regarding the level of pain control they receive. Some may elect to experience some pain in order to remain lucid and to continue communicating with others. For other patients, the pain may be so severe that they want it controlled even if it means falling into a semi- or unconscious state. Nurses may be concerned that high levels of pain medication may bring about or hasten the patient's death. The ethical concept of **double effect** helps to resolve this dilemma. The notion of double effect justifies the provision of appropriate pain relief in that the good intention is to eliminate pain, and a subsequent effect of that good intention may or may not result in hastening the person's death. From an ethical perspective, the nurse's primary obligation is to respect the patient's wishes and to provide a good by minimizing the pain, which may or may not hasten death. The obligation to provide palliative care and adequate pain control is also supported in law (Law Reform Commission of Canada, 1980).

Joan's nurse may assist her in taking control over her remaining time. There are ways that her family and caregivers can give her back some control. Perhaps she needs more opportunity to talk about her feelings and the meaning this experience has for her. Joan's husband and fam-ily may have similar needs; the nurse could help them talk about these matters with Joan.

There may be many other nursing interventions that might help Joan. Occasionally, there is nothing else nurses can do to relieve a patient's physical and emotional suffering. It is in these situations that we face one of the most challenging ethical and legal dilemmas in health care today.

## Legal Perspectives

### EUTHANASIA

As mentioned earlier, advances in health care technology and the growing number of patients with terminal conditions have played a large part in bringing euthanasia to the fore. In recent years, we have also seen more cases dealing with "mercy killing" brought before the courts.

A case in point is the story involving Saskatchewan farmer Robert Latimer's conviction for the second-degree murder of his severely disabled daughter (*R. v. Latimer*, 1997, 2001). Convicted after a second trial ordered by the Supreme Court of Canada, Latimer was sen-tenced to time served plus 2 years in jail, notwithstanding the fact that the minimum sen-tence for second-degree murder is imprisonment for life without possibility of parole for at least 10 years. The sentencing judge held that to sentence Mr. Latimer to the minimum term specified in the *Criminal Code* would have constituted cruel and unusual punishment under the circumstances and violated his constitutional right to be free from such punishment. The Court granted Mr. Latimer an extremely rare (and equally controversial) constitutional dispensation from the legally mandated sentence for this offence. In so doing, the judge recognized the agonizing choices and decisions that Mr. Latimer made in the face of his daughter's suffering. Some argue that the Latimer decision signalled a turning point in the law's attitude toward euthanasia. Mr. Latimer's sentence, however, was subsequently overturned on appeal by the Crown to the Saskatchewan Court of Appeal, which substituted the minimum 10-year sentence mandated by the *Criminal Code*. As mentioned in Chapter 4, Mr. Latimer's subsequent appeal to the Supreme Court of Canada in 2001 was dismissed. The Supreme Court of Canada ruled that Mr. Latimer could not invoke the defence of necessity because he did not lack a legal alternative, there was no imminent peril, and the harm he had inflicted was out of all proportion to the harm he sought to avoid. His application for parole was recently granted on appeal from the National Parole Board. A number of special interest groups participated in the Latimer proceedings, including groups advocating for the disabled. These groups were particularly concerned that Mr. Latimer might succeed on grounds of appeal relating to the defence of necessity or the jury properly deciding that he should be judged on the basis of what they thought was "right" according to their own consciences rather than following "black letter law," among other concerns. They were essentially concerned that the human rights and constitutional rights of disabled persons would be gravely and adversely affected were Mr. Latimer to succeed on any of the grounds (*R. v. Latimer*, (1995), 128 Sask. R. 195 (C.A.)). These groups were permitted to participate as intervenors in Mr. Latimer's appeal.

On the subsequent appeal to the Supreme Court of Canada in 2001, other interest groups also intervened, including the Canadian Civil Liberties Association, the Canadian AIDS Society, and the Disabled Women's Network of Canada, as well as a number of religious groups representing various Christian denominations. The religious groups sought to argue that allowing the defence of necessity in this case would legalize euthanasia, a concept to which they were opposed on religious grounds. Women's groups argued that the decision might undermine the autonomy of disabled women.

Similarly, the situation involving Dr. Nancy Morrison in Nova Scotia in 1996 focused attention on the divergent views of the legal system and the public at large on the issue of euthanasia. Dr. Morrison enjoyed a groundswell of public support for her cause after she was charged with the murder of a terminally ill cancer patient. Charges against Dr. Morrison were dropped at a preliminary hearing owing to insufficient evidence that she had done anything to hasten the patient's death. The Crown has since stated it would not appeal a recent ruling dismissing its application to reinstate the charges. Subsequently, Dr. Morrison accepted a reprimand from her provincial College of Physicians and Surgeons.

The attention given to patients' rights and respect for patient autonomy has provoked questions regarding the right to die and the right of patients to choose the time and means of their death.

Some who argue against euthanasia base their reasoning on the principle of sanctity of life and the traditional rules and laws prohibiting the taking of life except in situations of self-defence or war. (Strong advocates of this principle would argue that even in these circumstances, it is unacceptable to kill.) Others are concerned about the potential for abuse if euthanasia were permitted. It would be difficult to limit the act to situations in which patients are terminally ill and actively dying; conceivably, it might extend to the chronically ill, the infirm, the aged, and the demented. This is the "**slippery slope**" argument.

Those who support euthanasia believe that not all life is worth living. They believe that when someone is dying and it is no longer possible to eliminate their physical, emotional, and psychological pain, then euthanasia should be permitted at the request, and with the consent, of the competent patient. Supporters believe that sanctity of life is not an absolute principle and can be overridden out of respect both for patient autonomy and for the dignity of human life. They believe that, since death will occur anyway, euthanasia only makes that process more compassionate and dignified. If rules were in place to control euthanasia, as they are in the Netherlands, they argue, then the potential for abuse would be lessened.

ASSISTED SUICIDE

Suicide is defined as the act of taking one's own life. In assisted suicide, the person lacks the means and physical ability to complete the act and requires the assistance of someone else. For example, an accomplice might provide the person with a lethal dose of medication or help him or her to ingest it. This issue has arisen in cases in which patients with a chronic disease have desired the means to control the time of their death before falling into a state in which such action is no longer possible. An example is the patient with amyotrophic lateral sclerosis (ALS) who wishes to live as long as possible yet not end up in a state of total paralysis, dependent on artificial ventilation. Such persons would require assistance to commit suicide, since generalized weakness would limit their ability to do so on their own.

The arguments for and against assisted suicide are similar to those of euthanasia. However, those who support assisted suicide also argue that by not providing assistance, we set limits on disabled people's autonomy by denying them the opportunity to perform an act that able-bodied persons are capable of.

## The Current Law in Canada

The case of *Rodriguez v. British Columbia* (1993) received much public attention. Sue Rodriguez was diagnosed with ALS, a progressive disease of the nervous system that eventually results in complete paralysis and loss of the ability to speak, swallow, or breathe without a respirator. The patient afflicted with ALS gradually loses control of all bodily functions. Finally, even the heart succumbs to paralysis, and the person dies. Throughout the course of the disease, the patient's mind remains clear. The ability to reason is unaffected by the deterioration of the nervous system, although the disease can take a heavy emotional toll on the patient, family, and friends. The disease is accompanied by painful muscle spasms, though these can be controlled to some degree with medication.

Mrs. Rodriguez was married and the mother of a young son. At the time of her Supreme Court hearing, she had been given a life expectancy of between 2 and 14 months without the assistance of a respirator (*Rodriguez v. British Columbia* (1993), per Lamer J. (dissenting), pp. 530–531 (S.C.R.)). Her concern throughout was that, while she wished to live as long as possible, she did not wish to live through the last and most debilitating stages of ALS and die as a result of asphyxiation. Fearing complete loss of control over her bodily functions, and hence the ability to end her own life when she wished to do so, she brought an application before the Supreme Court of British Columbia for an order declaring section 241(b) of the *Criminal Code* unconstitutional.

Section 241(b) makes it an offence, punishable by up to 14 years' imprisonment on conviction, for anyone to counsel, aid, or abet another to commit suicide, whether or not the suicide is successful. Mrs. Rodriguez sought a declaration on the grounds that the effect of that section was to deprive her of several of her rights under the *Canadian Charter of Rights and Freedoms*, namely, life, liberty, security of person (*Charter of Rights and Freedoms*, 1982, s. 7), equality before the law (*Charter of Rights and Freedoms*, 1982, s. 15(1)), and freedom from cruel or unusual treatment (*Charter of Rights and Freedoms*, 1982, s. 12). She argued that the effect of the law was to deprive her of control over her body and her life. Further, she argued that section 241(b) prevented her from obtaining the assistance of another person in ending her life when she could no longer do so on her own and that this subjected her to cruel and unusual treatment at the hands of the state. Finally, she argued that since suicide was no longer a criminal offence in Canada (the provision in the *Criminal Code of Canada* making it an offence to commit or attempt to commit suicide was repealed in 1972; see *Criminal Law Amendment Act*, 1972, s. 16), she was being discriminated against and treated unequally by the law solely by reason of her physical disability because she was effectively being prevented from doing that which able-bodied people could do legally.

Mrs. Rodriguez's application was dismissed by the Supreme Court of British Columbia and again by the B.C. Court of Appeal. A final appeal to the Supreme Court of Canada was heard on May 20, 1993, and the Court rendered its decision in September of that year.

The Court delivered a five-to-four decision against Mrs. Rodriguez's application. The closeness of the vote illustrates the difficulty of the issues and the lack of consensus in the courts. The majority of the judges felt that while the effect of section 241(b) was to impinge on Mrs. Rodriguez's right to life, liberty, and security of person, such intrusion was not contrary to the principles of fundamental justice. The majority also felt that her right to equal treatment was violated but that this was permitted as being a "reasonable limit which [was] demonstrably justified in a free and democratic society" (*Charter of Rights and Freedoms*, 1982, s. 1). The minority judges opined that both her right to life, liberty, and security of person, and her right to equality before the law had been infringed, and that the infringement by the state through section 241(b) could not be justified in any way under the Charter. Thus, they felt that the section could not stand as valid under the Constitution and that, therefore, Mrs. Rodriguez should be free to seek assistance in committing suicide when she wished it.

Mr. Justice Sopinka, writing the decision for the majority, undertook a historical review of the ethical and legal principles behind the legislative prohibitions against both suicide and assisted suicide. The chief ethical principle that he identified was the state's and society's concern for the sanctity and value of human life and human dignity (*Rodriguez v. British Columbia*, 1993, p. 592), as well as society's role in protecting those who are vulnerable and who could be coerced or encouraged, in a moment of weakness, to commit suicide. The purpose of section 241(b) was to protect such members of society. In recent times, the concept of protecting human life at all costs has become tempered with limitations premised on personal independence and dignity and with quality-of-life considerations (*Rodriguez v. British Columbia*, 1993, pp. 595–596). Further, common law has recognized the right of an individual to withdraw or withhold consent to medical treatment, even if the absence of such treatment would likely result in death. Mr. Justice Sopinka's decision relied on the decision of the Supreme Court of Canada in *Ciarlariello v. Schacter* (1993), the decision of the Quebec Superior Court in the case of *Nancy B. v. Hôtel-Dieu de Québec* (1992), and the decision of the Ontario Court of Appeal in *Malette v. Shulman* (1990).

The majority judgement suggests that the law recognizes a form of *passive euthanasia*— for example, inadvertently hastening a terminally ill patient's death by administering larger and larger doses of pain medication with the intent to control pain. Another example might be withdrawing (with the patient's consent) all treatment and artificial means to prolong life once such treatment has become therapeutically useless. The distinction between passive and active euthanasia is thus seen as a basis for upholding the law's continued prohibition against assisted suicide.

In response, the majority judgement of the Supreme Court notes that the law has always had great aversion to the participation of one person in the death of another, but passive euthanasia is considered acceptable because artificial means to prolong life are withdrawn on the patient's request and death ensues as a natural consequence. While some have criticized the distinction between passive and active euthanasia as artificial (since both take place with the full knowledge that death will ensue) (*Rodriguez v. British Columbia*, 1993, p. 606, citing a *Harvard Law Review* note: Physician-assisted suicide and the right to die with assistance, (1992) 105 *Harv. L. Rev.* 2021, pp. 2030–2031), in the case of passive euthanasia, the exact time of death cannot be known, and death does not result directly from the actions of another. Critics of the active/passive distinction and proponents of euthanasia also note that the outcome in either situation is ethically the same but that in a case in which treatment is merely withdrawn, death can come more slowly and may be more painful.

Another legal concern that justifies maintaining the blanket prohibition on assisted suicide, in the majority's opinion, is that of preventing abuse, together with the difficulties in formulating guidelines and conditions under which assisted suicide would be legally permissible. Mr. Justice Sopinka cited a working paper of the Law Reform Commission of Canada (Law Reform Commission of Canada, 1983) that points out examples of mass suicides, or of one person taking advantage of the depressed state of another to encourage him or her to commit suicide for the other's financial gain, as reasons justifying the continued prohibition. Further, he reviewed the record in the Netherlands, which has the most liberal guidelines on euthanasia and physician-assisted suicide, and noted evidence (without stating his source) of a disturbing rise in cases of voluntary active euthanasia, which is not permitted by those guidelines (*Rodriguez v. British Columbia*, 1993, p. 603). Thus, the "slippery slope" argument, in the opinion of the majority, justifies a complete prohibition on physician-assisted suicide. To Mr. Justice Sopinka, to hold otherwise would "send a signal that there are circumstances in which the state approves of suicide" (*Rodriguez v. British Columbia*, 1993, p. 608).

The minority justices wrote equally compelling dissenting opinions. The Chief Justice, Mr. Justice Lamer, opined that section 241(b) of the *Criminal Code* infringed on the rights of disabled persons such as Sue Rodriguez because it effectively deprives them of choosing suicide, an option available to able-bodied persons (*Rodriguez v. British Columbia*, 1993, per Lamer J. (dissenting), p. 544). Thus, they were not being treated equally before the law as guaranteed under the Charter. Lamer also relied on the fact that it is a fundamental aspect of personal autonomy in common law that citizens have the right to make free and informed decisions about their bodies and to consent (or withhold consent) to specific medical treatment, even when to do so would likely result in death.

The next consideration was whether such violation was "a reasonable limit, demonstrably justified in a free and democratic society" within the meaning of section 1 of the Charter. Here, Mr. Justice Lamer undertook an interesting review of the values and objectives of the prohibition against assisted suicide. He pointed out that the repeal of the attempted-suicide prohibition by Parliament in 1972 (*Rodriguez v. British Columbia*, 1993, per Lamer J. (dissenting), pp. 530–531) reflected its belief that self-determination was now a paramount factor in the regulation of suicide. Thus, if no outside interference with an individual's decision could be shown, then that person's attempting suicide would no longer be a criminal offence (*Rodriguez v. British Columbia*, 1993, per Lamer J. (dissenting), p. 559).

With respect to the "slippery slope" argument, His Lordship felt that despite the concern that decriminalizing assisted suicide would leave the physically disabled vulnerable and open to manipulation by others, this still would not justify depriving a disadvantaged group (i.e., the disabled) of equality before the law, specifically, the right to determine the circumstances in which they end their life. In Mrs. Rodriguez's case, there was no evidence of such vulnerability and plenty of evidence of her free consent (*Rodriguez v. British Columbia*, 1993, pp. 566–567). He thus concluded that the limit placed by section 241(b) of the *Criminal Code* upon Sue Rodriguez's right to equality was not reasonable and could not be justified under the Charter.

Hence, the section was constitutionally invalid. However, he was inclined to suspend the declaration of unconstitutionality for one year, until such time as Parliament could address the issue and either enact legislation that would deal with assisted suicide in cases such as Sue Rodriguez's or simply enact no constitutional legislation to replace section 241(b). This effectively meant that, while the law was unconstitutional, it would nevertheless remain in effect for one year so that the "floodgates" would not be opened, thus negating the objective of protecting the vulnerable from the influence and coercion of others in consenting to assisted suicide.

In the meantime, he would have granted Mrs. Rodriguez an exemption to compliance with section 241(b), provided that:

1. She had applied to a superior court for authorization
2. She had been certified by her attending physician and a psychiatrist to be competent, had made her decision freely and voluntarily, and at least one physician would be with her when she committed assisted suicide
3. The physicians also certify that (a) she is or will become physically incapable of committing suicide unaided and (b) they have informed her of her continuing right to change her mind about terminating her life
4. Notice and access be given to the regional coroner at the time
5. She be examined daily by the physicians
6. The act actually causing her death be her act alone, unaided by anyone else (*Rodriguez v. British Columbia*, 1993, p. 579)

The exemption was to expire 31 days after the date of the physicians' certificate in (1) above. The conditions were described as having been designed with Mrs. Rodriguez's circumstances in mind. However, Mr. Justice Lamer advanced them as guidelines to future applicants in similar circumstances.

The approach taken by two of the dissenting justices (Madam Justice McLachlin, who wrote the dissent, and Madam Justice L'Heureux-Dubé, who concurred in that dissent) is also interesting. Madam Justice McLachlin felt that security of person entails personal autonomy, which protects the dignity and privacy of individuals with respect to decisions surrounding their own bodies (*Rodriguez v. British Columbia*, 1993, per McLachlin J. (dissenting), L'Heureux-Dubé (concurring), p. 618).

Part of that autonomy involves the right of the person to decide what is best for him or her. There was thus no rational basis upon which to deny Mrs. Rodriguez a right that was freely available to others who were more able-bodied than she.

## Application to Joan's Case Scenario

The nurse in Joan's situation clearly is not entitled to assist her to commit suicide, given the Supreme Court's pronouncement on this issue. Section 241(b) is constitutional and prevents the nurse from actively assisting Joan to end her life. It is legal, however, for the nurse to assist in pain control and to make Joan as comfortable as possible. If the nurse proceeded in helping Joan commit suicide, she would run the risk of being found out and criminally charged. The sentence recently handed out to Robert Latimer by a sympathetic Saskatchewan judge, and currently under appeal, cannot realistically afford comfort and encouragement to the nurse.

The following case scenario focuses on a more common dilemma faced by health care professionals.

# Case Scenario

## WHO SPEAKS ON MY BEHALF?

A 70-year-old patient in the Critical Care Unit, Mr. C., has end-stage cardiac disease. He is intubated and dependent on medication to sustain adequate blood pressure. Though his case is seemingly futile, the medical team plans to continue aggressive therapy. One of the patient's sons would like treatment to be withdrawn. The patient's wife and daughter disagree. Mr. C. is unable to speak for himself and made no decisions respecting care in advance, while competent. The treatment plan and the rules of the unit mean visiting is kept to a maximum of 10 minutes per hour.

### Issues

1. In the absence of direction from the patient, how should the health care team make its decision?
2. Who has the right to make the decision in this situation?
3. Would an advance directive have helped? How?
4. What are the responsibilities of Mr. C.'s nurse?

### Discussion

Situations like the one described in this scenario often give rise to conflict among family members, and this is stressful for all involved. The health care team may feel torn between its primary focus—the best interests of the patient—and the competing interests of the family. Decisions regarding withdrawal of treatment are more difficult when the patient is incompetent and unable to participate. Unfortunately, this is often the case in Intensive Care Units. The nurse may experience moral distress when the wishes of the patient are not known and when the decision of the most appropriate next of kin or substitute decision maker conflicts with what the nurse believes is in the patient's best interest. This distress is alleviated if the nurse is confident that decisions regarding care are based on the previously expressed wishes or values of the patient.

### Legal Perspectives

In this case scenario, the facts that the treatment being administered is futile and that the patient seems near death raise an interesting legal point with respect to withdrawal of treatment. The Quebec Superior Court's decision in *Nancy B. v. Hôtel-Dieu de Québec* (1992) dealt with the legality of a lucid patient's request not to be subjected to further medical treatment when that person deems such treatment no longer appropriate. (The details of this case are reviewed

continued on following page >>

in Chapter 4.) This ruling was made in the context of Quebec's *Civil Code*, which places ultimate responsibility for treatment decisions with the patient. Thus, consent-to-treatment issues (as discussed in Chapter 6) may be inseparable from the issue of withdrawal of treatment.

In point of fact, withdrawal of treatment in Mr. C.'s circumstances is supported by common law. For example, in the United States, the Superior Court of New Jersey ultimately supported the concept of withdrawal of treatment in the case of Karen Ann Quinlan, who, following the ingestion of a combination of sleep aid medication and alcohol, was in a permanent vegetative state for more than 25 years. The problem is that common law has historically been hesitant to recognize the right of a spouse or next of kin to make treatment decisions on behalf of an incapable person. In Manitoba, this situation has been remedied in the *Health Care Directives Act* (C.C.S.M. c. H27); in Nova Scotia (to an extent), in the *Medical Consent Act* (R.S.N.S. 1989, c. 279); in British Columbia, in the recently enacted *Adult Guardianship Act* (R.S.B.C. 1996, c. 6, Part 2 of which was not yet in force at the time of writing); in Alberta, in the *Personal Directives Act* (R.S.A. 2000, c. P-6); and in Ontario, in the *Substitute Decisions Act*, 1992 (1992), which enables another person to make decisions on behalf of those who cannot make them for themselves.

At present, in provinces without specific legislation on this subject, the practice is to accept treatment decisions made by an incapable person's spouse or, if there is no spouse, that person's closest living relative, who may make the decision on the basis of what the patient would have wished. This means that the proxy (the person making the decision for the incapable patient) must make every effort to determine what the patient's wishes would have been (Canadian Encyclopedic Digest (Ont. 3d.), Title 72, s. 177, citing an unpublished article).

In the case scenario, the conflict between the son on the one hand and the wife and daughter on the other suggests that the matter may have to be resolved in court through guardianship proceedings (as discussed in Chapter 6). The guardian(s) would be authorized to make treatment decisions respecting the patient. This is a sad, costly, and needless development. Outside of guardianship proceedings, it is fairly certain that the law would not interfere with the decision to withdraw treatment in such a case since treatment is demonstrably futile. However, as we have said above, it draws the line at acts that would constitute assisted suicide.

In the majority of cases, the resolution should not end up in court. It is the health care team's responsibility to meet with the family to present the alternatives and to explore their feelings and views. It is important that the family be fully informed of all the medical facts relevant to the patient's situation. It is also helpful to share with them a framework that might assist them to reach consensus on the best course of action.

Through discussion, the family might remember occasions when Mr. C. expressed thoughts on what he would want in such a situation as this—for example, a comment made about a similar case on television or in the newspapers. Or they might talk about Mr. C.'s lifelong values in order to get some sense of his likely decision, were he capable. With the support of the health care team, clear communication, and time, most situations like this can be resolved.

continued on following page >>

Advance directives are always helpful in cases of incompetence. In future, it is likely that these will play a greater role in treatment decisions, especially since legislative reform in such provinces as Ontario, P.E.I., Newfoundland and Labrador, Saskatchewan, and Yukon already encourages them.

## Organ Donation

The field of transplantation has grown tremendously in recent years. The long-term survival rates for lung, heart, kidney, and liver transplant patients have improved remarkably. Patients who would have died otherwise may live much longer and with good quality of life.

In Canada, organ donation is generally viewed as morally justified when treatment alternatives to transplantation are not readily available and respect for the autonomy of donors and their families is maintained through appropriate legislation and guidelines.

Ironically, recent successes of transplant programs have contributed to the problem of limited availability of organs. The technology has evolved to the extent that more organ disease can be treated with organ replacement; surgical transplant procedures have advanced; and rejection is less of an issue than it was in the past. The supply of donor organs has not kept pace with the growing need. Furthermore, advances in the neurosciences, compliance with seat-belt legislation, and a reduction in drinking and driving have reduced the numbers of deaths that would offer a potential for organ donation. Recent approaches have therefore focused on translating potential donors to actual donors. Strategies explored to maximize the number of donors have included changes to the legislation regarding the consent process, donor incentives, education, and hospital-based policy and resources. For more information, the reader is invited to refer to the following provincial Web sites related to organ donation:

- Yukon Organ Donation Program: http://www.hss.gov.yk.ca/programs/insured_hearing/organdonation
- Trillium Gift of Life Network: http://www.giftoflife.on.ca
- BC Transplant: http://www.transplant.bc.ca

### Promotion of Organ Donation

Low donor rates in relation to the growing number of patients who need organ transplants have raised questions about whether alternative systems for organ donation should be considered. Following is a brief overview of some possible approaches.

### Recorded Consideration

The recorded consideration approach attempts to deal with the issue of health care professionals not asking family members about organ donation (Youngner et al., 1985). It requires that health care staff routinely consider and document the appropriateness of a dying or brain-dead patient for organ donation. If the patient's organs are appropriate, then the family is to be approached. If the organs are not appropriate, or if the family refuses consent, then staff are required to document this in the patient's chart. (This is required by law, for example, in Prince Edward Island's *Human Tissue Donation Act*.)

## Required Request

With this system, all patients are asked about their position on organ donation when admitted to hospital or when they use the health care system in any way. Concerns have been raised about whether such questions are unduly stressful for patients, who hope to have their health care needs met in the hospital and thus may not wish to entertain the possibility of imminent organ donation (Youngner et al., 1985).

## Presumed Consent

This approach is commonly referred to as "opting out." The assumption is that the dying or brain-dead patient would have chosen to donate his or her organs, unless he or she expressed otherwise beforehand. Those who favour this method reason that it would make approaching the family easier and would result in more organs being made available. They argue that autonomy is respected since individuals still have the right to refuse. Those who disagree with this approach say that consent, particularly of the bereaved, cannot be presumed and that it undermines the notion of altruism. It has been noted that in countries where presumed consent is the law (e.g., France, Belgium, Singapore), organ donor rates improved for a while and then levelled off. This phenomenon was apparently related to the continuing reluctance of health care professionals to approach families (Youngner et al., 1985).

## Market Strategies

Some suggest that organ donor rates would improve if there were a financial incentive involved, ranging from a lump-sum payment to coverage of the deceased's funeral expenses. Again, concerns arise that this approach would not only undermine the notion of altruism but might also take advantage of those compromised by poverty. As well, it would introduce a coercive element into the process of consent (Youngner et al., 1985). At present, buying or selling human tissue or organs is prohibited by law in every Canadian province and territory. Penalties for breach of this prohibition vary from province to province, but they include steep fines and several months' imprisonment.

## Education

Educating the public and health care professionals has been encouraged. Further knowledge and better communication would ensure that the notion of brain death is understood, that individuals are aware of the donation options available to them, and that health care professionals understand and accept their role in the organ donation process. It is not adequate to educate only health care professionals working in hospitals. A significant role exists for nurses practising in the community to represent the interests of health care in general and to educate their clients about specific issues such as organ donation (Youngner et al., 1985).

## Ethical Issues Associated With Organ Donation

The ethical issues associated with organ donation include the determination of death, consent, donor management, and recipient responses. The organ donation process, if not managed properly, can be highly stressful for nurses, the interprofessional team, and, most important, the families of donors.

Nurses caring for a donor patient may experience moral distress during the donation process if the challenging transition from trying to save the life of a patient to managing that patient's organs for the benefit of others is not effectively managed. The nurse's focus shifts from the recovery of the patient to advocating for his or her wishes and ensuring the well-being of the recipient in need of the transplant. A strong relationship between the nurse and the patients (both the donor and recipient), together with ethical management of the process by all members of the team, can make this an enriching experience for all involved.

The following case scenario illustrates some of the ethical and legal challenges of organ donation.

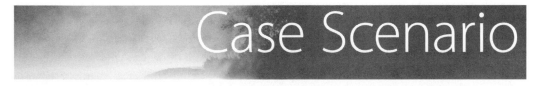

## A GIFT OR AN OBLIGATION?

Mr. R., a patient who has ingested a large quantity of barbiturates, is admitted to an Intensive Care Unit (ICU). The drugs have damaged his brain to such a degree that he has been declared brain-dead. He remains on a ventilator and is presently hemodynamically stable. In the same hospital, another patient, Mr. S., is dying as a result of a rejection episode following a heart transplant. Mr. S. has less than 24 hours to live unless another suitable heart is found for retransplantation.

Mr. R. is judged by the ICU team to be a suitable donor for the urgently required heart. Further, a signed organ donor card was found in his wallet. As is the practice in most hospitals, and despite the existence of this card, the ICU team approaches Mr. R.'s parents and requests that they consent to donating their son's organs. The parents categorically refuse consent. They are not informed about Mr. S. for fear that this would constitute coercion. Mr. S. dies the next day.

### Issues
1. What is the legal status of a signed organ donor card?
2. Is the consent of the donor's family required?

continued on following page >>

3. Could health professionals be more aggressive in encouraging the donor's family to give consent? Should family be told about the recipient in need?
4. Might further legislation in the area of consent help? How?

## Discussion

Canada's current approach to organ donation is a voluntary system of expressed consent. This is based on the principle of beneficence, doing good and avoiding harm. Because society does not oblige us to help others or to be altruistic, the system is based on the notion of voluntarism and encourages organ donation through such mechanisms as a driver's licence, health care card, or organ donor card, on which individuals can state which organs they are willing to donate upon death. Supporters of this system argue that procurement built on voluntarism promotes socially desirable virtues such as altruism while protecting the rights of persons who might refuse to donate (Task Force on Presumed Consent, 1994).

Certain problems have arisen in regard to this approach:

- For reasons such as superstition, individuals may choose not to sign a donor card, even when they support the concept.
- The donor card is not always available to health professionals at the time of a patient's death.
- Regardless of whether a donor card is signed, families are approached, and, in practice, their decision takes precedence.
- Health professionals are still reluctant to approach families or to initiate a complex and time-consuming donation process (Task Force on Presumed Consent, 1994).

The last point raises some ethical issues with respect to the role of the health care team (especially nurses) as participants in organ donation. Some health care professionals cite the grieving process of the family as the reason for not approaching them with regard to organ donation. Others claim that the cultural or religious perspectives of some patients preclude organ donation. The problem is that when health care professionals decide not to raise the issue with the family or fail to look for a signed organ donor card, then they are in fact making the decision for the patient not to donate, and this is disrespectful of the individual's autonomy.

Furthermore, we cannot make assumptions about the views of various cultural and religious groups. In fact, most world religions (including Christianity, Judaism, and Hinduism) support organ donation and transplantation. The Japanese Shinto religion and some sects of Tibetan Buddhism prohibit (or discourage) organ transplantation because of beliefs about the dead, taboos against injuring the body after death, and the extensive purifying rights required after death occurs (Task Force on Presumed Consent, 1994). In Korea, for example, many express aversion to organ donation, believing that the deceased person would be humiliated through the organ procurement process. Many Koreans have a strong belief in Confucianism, in which the body must be intact for burial (Kim, 1998). Lack of knowledge and understanding of the concept and meaning of brain death is also a factor (Kim, Elliott, & Hyde, 2004).

Nurses may experience emotional exhaustion in caring for organ donors and their families (Borozny, 1988; Hibbert, 1995). They may approach the care of the patient with mixed emotions

continued on following page >>

and a sense of contradictions. Research suggests that health professionals' attitudes, knowledge, and willingness to approach a family influence the bereaved family's decision-making process (Bidigare, 1991).

However, nurses are in the best position to raise the issue of organ donation with patients' families. The nurse caring for the patient has the most opportunity to interact with the family throughout this difficult process. Nurses often develop a supportive relationship with patients' family members as they prepare them for the inevitable, and most have the communication skills to raise the issue of organ donation sensitively. Given the fact that families often forget about organ donation in the midst of crisis, it is important that nurses ensure that the issue is raised.

Regardless of the decision, the nurse has represented the interests and wishes of the patient and his or her family. Taking part in this process also eases the nurse's own transition from caring for the patient to maintaining that patient's organs for the benefit of future recipients. The relationship continues, as the nurse ensures that the patient's wish to give to others is fulfilled.

The declaration of brain death remains a controversial process that continues to create emotional tension for health care professionals. It is difficult to accept that a patient is dead when the chest continues to rise and fall and skin colour and body temperature seem normal. Some health facilities use particular rituals to acknowledge the occurrence of a death. For example, some settings observe a moment of silence to respect the deceased and to acknowledge the emotions of family and staff. This observance can also ease the transition to the next phase of the donation process. Such rituals are an issue particularly for nurses in the Operating Room, who may be left alone with the patient after removal of the organs (Youngner, Allen, Bartlett, Cascorbi, Hau, Jackson, et al., 1985). Hospitals should be sensitive to and support the needs of staff left in such a situation.

## Legal Definition of Death

Removal of organ tissues from deceased donors is bound up with the legal and medical determination of death. Few jurisdictions in Canada or the United States provide a legislative definition of the moment of death. Historically, physicians have concurred that a person is dead when all vital signs (heartbeat, pulse, respiration) have ceased. In religious terms, death is seen as the moment when the soul leaves the body, generally at the time when the person's heart ceases to beat. Until well into the twentieth century, the courts recognized that a person was legally dead when the "vital functions [have] ceased to operate. The heart [has] always been regarded as a vital organ" in this determination (*R. v. Kitching and Adams*, 1976, p. 711, per O'Sullivan J.).

In the last half century, sophisticated medical technology has allowed physicians to sustain the lives of seriously ill patients who, in the past, would not have survived their situations. A patient who can no longer breathe on his or her own or whose heart function has ceased can now be kept alive with the aid of respirators and other devices to sustain blood circulation. As well, advances in transplant technology have made possible the transplantation of viable organs from deceased donors into the bodies of living persons. We have also learned much more about the human brain and its role not only in controlling vital bodily systems but also as the source of personality, intelligence, emotion, and a host of other human characteristics.

It has become apparent that the traditional medical criteria for determining the fact of death have become inadequate. The question now is: Can a person whose brain function has completely and irreversibly ceased but whose other bodily functions remain active still be considered a living human being?

In 1975, Manitoba became the first province to enact a legal definition of the moment of death. The Manitoba *Vital Statistics Act* provides that, for all civil purposes (i.e., not for the purpose of criminal law), "the death of a person takes place at the time at which irreversible cessation of all that person's brain function occurs" (*Vital Statistics Act*, s. 2). This definition conforms to the accepted definition of death within the modern medical community. In arriving at a new medical definition of death, a committee of the Harvard Medical School suggested that brain death is established with the cessation of all brain function, both cerebral and brain stem, and that the cessation of such brain function must be irreversible.

With respect to human tissue donation, the laws of most of the provinces require that the death of a prospective donor be determined in the way stated above. (See Alberta: *Human Tissue Gift Act*, R.S.A. 2000, c. H-15; British Columbia: *Human Tissue Gift Act*, R.S.B.C. 1996, c. 211; Manitoba: *Human Tissue Gift Act*, C.C.S.M. c. H180; New Brunswick: *Human Tissue Gift Act*, S.N.B. 2004, c. H-12.5; Newfoundland and Labrador: *Human Tissue Act*, R.S.N.L. 1990, c. H-15; Northwest Territories and Nunavut: *Human Tissue Act*, R.S.N.W.T. 1988, c. H-6; Nova Scotia: *Human Tissue Gift Act*, R.S.N.S. 1989, c. 215; Ontario: *Trillium Gift of Life Network Act*, R.S.O. 1990, c. H.20; Prince Edward Island: *Human Tissue Donation Act*, R.S.P.E.I. 1988, c. H-12.1; Quebec: *Civil Code*, arts. 19, 23–25, 42–45; Saskatchewan: *Human Tissue Gift Act*, R.S.S. 1978, c. H-15; Yukon: *Human Tissue Gift Act*, R.S.Y. 2002, c. 117).

Manitoba's legislation provides specifically that death must be determined according to the definition set out in the *Vital Statistics Act*, with bodily circulation still intact as necessary for the purposes of a successful tissue transplant, and that such determination must be made by at least two physicians (*Human Tissue Gift Act* (Manitoba), s. 8(1)).

Further ethical and legal problems arise with respect to the removal of tissue and organs from the bodies of anencephalic neonates. Brain-stem anencephaly is demonstrated by the absence of the cerebrum, although the mid-brain cerebellum and brain stem are present and functioning. In such a newborn, there is enough lower brain function that the neonate can breathe and maintain a heartbeat for some time. It may be difficult to establish that all brain function has indeed ceased. Furthermore, because an infant's brain cells are resistant to damage, caution must be exercised in applying brain-death criteria to children under 5 years of age. Specific criteria do exist for children under 5, but not for infants under 2 weeks of age (Capron, 1987).

Eventually, an anencephalic child will stop breathing. Yet, he or she can be kept on a respirator to ensure that the organs are kept healthy and viable for transplantation. Since anencephalics are not conscious and have no mental capacity, such a child would never be able to live a meaningful life. He or she is doomed to live in a vegetative state for the rest of his or her brief life, a few days at most.

The question that arises in this situation is whether such a child should be considered legally dead so that his or her organs may be removed for transplant to save another child's life. Clearly, an anencephalic is alive even by modern medical criteria, since the lower brain is still functioning and is able to sustain breathing and circulation, to a degree. The definition of death based on irreversible cessation of all brain function is of no help in this situation. Consequently, physicians and ethicists alike have recently argued for a revised definition of death that would address such a situation.

Some ethicists have argued that anencephalic donors ought to be deemed dead while respiration and circulation are maintained to keep the organs viable. Others opt for a special category of "brain absent" persons, which would include anencephalics. This definition would permit removal of organs for transplant while the infant's "body" is not yet dead. It is argued that this is a more utilitarian solution that preserves the donor child's humanity, spares it from further physical pain, saves the lives of recipients, prevents deterioration of the organs, and allows the parents the dignity and comfort of knowing that their child's condition and brief life were not in vain.

This definition allows for the maintenance of the dead donor paradigm—that organ procurement cannot cause death. Recently, however, a well-known bioethicist has argued for the abandonment of the dead donor rule (Koppelman, 2003). Elysa Koppelman suggests that individuals may be able to specify ahead of time to have their organs donated if cognitive function fails, even if the technical definition of death is not achieved. This, she argues, could apply to persons who have suffered serious irreparable brain injury or to persons in persistent vegetative states. Others argue against abandoning the dead donor rule and for redefining death to include persons with serious irreversible brain damage who have no functioning cerebral cortex (Veatch, 2003; Hester, 2003; Crowley-Matoka & Arnold, 2004; Campbell, 2004; Steinberg, 2003; Menikoff, 2002; Dudzinski, 2003; Trachtman, 2003; Truog & Robinson, 2003; Truog, 2000). Others argue for a debate on what constitutes death in circumstances such as these, but not to have the need for organ donation as the impetus for this; rather, they propose a debate on the meaning of life itself and when it may not be worth sustaining (Koenig, 2003).

## Redefining Death

Some health care professionals have responded to the shortage of organs by suggesting that the definition of death be extended to include cortical death, as in the case of the anencephalic donor. This definition would include patients in a persistent vegetative state, who have no cortical activity although the brain stem is intact. Such persons can maintain their vital functions, and their body can live for years with appropriate nursing care. However, everything that makes them a person—their ability to communicate, to relate to others, to remember—is gone. These patients may live for years or may have treatment withdrawn and be allowed to die.

Those who seek to redefine death argue that we are losing a potential pool of organ donors who may have previously expressed, while competent, the wish to donate organs at the time of death. Those who argue against this redefinition suggest that we cannot redefine death whenever it is convenient to do so. Further, they argue that these questions should be raised not in the context of organ donation but out of a duty and responsibility to the patient in the persistent vegetative state (Keatings, 1990). To do otherwise would be to treat individuals, as Kant would say, as means and not as ends in and of themselves.

Redefining death to include cortical death would present procedural problems. Would this redefinition apply universally or only in cases in which organ donation is viable? In any case, when would biological life be deemed to end? Would this happen immediately after cortical death is declared? Or would it end when convenient—for example, when a transplant recipient is in need (Keatings, 1990)?

## Non-heart-beating Organ Donation

Recently, a new approach to the notion of **non-heart-beating organ donation (NHBOD)** has been reintroduced. In the early days of transplantation, before *brain death* was defined, organs were retrieved from "cadavers" after cardiac death. This approach was abandoned because of the challenges of using nonperfused organs, those deprived of oxygen for a period of time. As the demand for donation grows and rejection technology improves, this approach is being reintroduced (Ethics Committee, ACCCM, 2001).

The death of the NHBOD patient is determined by "traditional" or "cardiopulmonary" criteria: (1) unresponsiveness, (2) apnea, and (3) absent circulation. The "dead donor rule," a recent security convention, states that it is unethical to cause death by procuring organs, which is why the notion of "brain death" was introduced. To ensure death has occurred with NHBOD, there must be a full five-minute observation period after an onset of circulatory arrest, apnea, and unresponsiveness.

Clearly, this approach to organ procurement requires a great deal of psychosocial support for patients and their families.

There are two situations in which NHBOD may occur. Organ donation may follow a death that occurs after a planned withdrawal of life-sustaining therapy. For example, the patient, family, or both, refusing life-sustaining therapy, have opted to withdraw life support and have requested organ donation after death. Other situations may arise when an unexpected cardiac arrest occurs and resuscitation is not successful (Bell, 2006).

## Challenges for Care

The potential donor has the right to comfort, care, and symptom (e.g., pain) management. Knowing death is about to occur, he or she may experience anxiety. Continuity of caregivers is, therefore, extremely important for the patient and family if the patient is transitioned to another setting. He or she has a right to family presence and supports from team members such as social workers and bereavement counsellors. Family members in particular need to understand and be prepared for what the experience may be like. They will need ongoing support, and most provinces have resources in place to provide this.

If we agree that it is legally and ethically justifiable to withhold or withdraw life-sustaining treatment in infants, children, and adolescents when the burdens of those treatments outweigh the benefits, then donation in these situations would be justified using the same criteria, as long as the other special considerations regarding children are followed. Therefore, parental consent, or consent of a competent adolescent, would be required.

The following standards apply to all potential donors:

- Informed consent to withdraw treatment and informed consent to donate must be given.
- Organ procurement must not cause death.
- Death will be determined using appropriate standards.
- End-of-life supportive care must continue to be provided to the patient, and special consideration of the family must be made (Ethics Committee, ACCCM, 2001).

While aggressive treatment and care is being provided, nurses focus on doing what is best for their patient. There may be ambivalence as the patient begins to die or as treatment is withdrawn and the patient proceeds toward death and organ donation. Some may view this as treating the organs, not the person, and see the person merely as a means to an end in organ donation. However, the care relationship the nurse has with the patient must be maintained even as the focus shifts to ensuring that the patient's wish to be an organ donor is realized (Day, 2001; Rassin, Lowenthal, & Silner, 2005).

A challenge unique to NHBOD is that the patient who wishes to become a donor may, unlike a brain-dead donor, be conscious and aware of what is happening. Consider the following scenario.

## Brad's Story

Brad Hoffman, at 28 years of age, became a ventilator-dependent quadriplegic after a serious motor vehicle accident. Against the desires of his family and concerns of the health care team, Brad decided that he did not want to live in this state and asked that life support be withdrawn. Moreover, he volunteered to be an organ donor. This case had numerous ethical and emotional challenges. Was Brad competent to make the decision to withdraw life support? Was he in a depressed state, and was this influencing his decision? Did he have enough time to appreciate that he could still sustain a good quality of life? Was his motivation to be a donor clearly separate from his wish to withdraw treatment? After much consultation with his family, the health care team, and an ethics consultant, his life support was withdrawn and organs donated. The team involved in his care had intense emotional issues about this case. But should it be more difficult or easier when a person's consent is clear and when that person is able to choose the nature of his or her death and have family present through that process? If the team had misgivings, what would that mean? Are there problematic moral issues that are not readily evident (Spike, 2000)?

What are your thoughts on this real-life situation? As a health care professional, what would your position be? What would the role of the nurse be in supporting Brad and his family? If you were in Brad's situation, what do you think you would do? What are your thoughts on the amount of time Brad should have to reflect on his decision in this situation?

## Human Tissue Legislation Across Canada

All provinces and territories have enacted legislation dealing with organ donation before and after the death of the donor (see discussion above). This legislation is remarkably uniform across Canada. The various statutes basically provide a mechanism for obtaining the consent of the donor (or others, if the donor is unable to consent) to the removal of tissue from the donor's body for transplant into the body of another, for medical education, or for purposes of scientific research.

There are two primary situations contemplated by the statutes:

1. The donor is living and has consented to the removal of nonregenerative tissue from his or her body for therapeutic use, such as a transplant to another person's body. This is legally referred to as an inter vivos gift of tissue, from the Latin meaning "among the living"; that is, the donor gives the tissue during his or her lifetime.
2. The donor (or another, if the donor has expressed no wishes on the matter) has directed that specified body parts be removed from his or her body for transplant into another living person after the donor's death. This is legally known as a postmortem gift of tissue.

Legislation in all provinces and territories except Manitoba and Quebec specifically excludes such regenerative tissue as bone, blood or its constituents, skin, or other tissue that is regenerated naturally by the human body. In each of these provinces and territories, an adult who is mentally competent and makes a free and informed decision may legally donate such regenerative tissue under common law. For example, a person donating bone marrow in one of these provinces or territories need only be of the age of majority and mentally competent to orally consent to giving such tissue. (In practice, however, most health facilities require a signed consent for the mutual protection of all parties concerned.)

In contrast, the law in Manitoba excludes only blood or its constituents (*Human Tissue Gift Act*, (Manitoba), s. 1, "tissue" (c)). Thus, its *Human Tissue Gift Act* does not apply to a blood donation. Rather, common law requires merely that the donor be an adult, be mentally competent, and be able to make a free and informed decision. On the other hand, a bone marrow donation, or a donation of skin for a skin graft, would have to comply with the requirements of the Act.

Similarly, the *Civil Code of Quebec* allows any person in Quebec of the age of majority who is mentally capable to consent to the removal of tissue from his or her body while living (*Civil Code of Quebec*, art. 19, para. 1). Since the *Civil Code* does not define "tissue," one can presume that it includes any tissue from the donor's body, including blood and other such regenerative tissue, as well as kidneys.

CONSENT TO TRANSPLANT DURING DONOR'S LIFE

In the case of an inter vivos gift—for example, a donor consenting to give a kidney for transplant into the body of a sibling—the consent is valid if it is in writing and is signed by the donor. Although the statutes are silent on this point, the consent can be revoked (cancelled) at any time thereafter, either in writing or orally.

In all provinces and territories except Ontario, Prince Edward Island, and Quebec, only a person who has reached the age of majority may legally consent to an inter vivos gift of tissue. Ontario and Prince Edward Island allow persons below the age of majority but who are at least 16 years old to give consent without the approval of a parent or guardian (*Trillium Gift of Life Network Act* (Ontario), s. 3(1); *Human Tissue Donation Act* (Prince Edward Island), s. 6(1)).

In Quebec, a minor (a person who has not yet reached the age of majority) may consent to an inter vivos donation of regenerative tissue only with consent of a parent or tutor (in Quebec, the equivalent of a child's legal guardian) and with permission of the court, provided that the procedure does not result in serious risk to the health of the minor (*Civil Code of Quebec*, art. 19, para. 2). The New Brunswick (s. 1) and Northwest Territories (ss. 1(1), (2)) statutes are silent on inter vivos transfers. However, common law would likely permit such transfers if the donor were an adult, mentally competent, and making a free and fully informed decision.

Apart from being of the requisite age, a person in Alberta, British Columbia, Newfoundland and Labrador, Nova Scotia, Ontario, Saskatchewan, or Yukon must be mentally competent to consent and must make a free and informed decision (*Personal Directives Act* (Alberta), s. 3(1); *Human Tissue Gift Act* (British Columbia), s. 3(1); *Human Tissue Act* (Newfoundland and Labrador), s. 4(1); *Human Tissue Gift Act* (Nova Scotia), s. 4(1); *Trillium Gift of Life Network Act* (Ontario), s. 3(1); *Human Tissue Gift Act* (Saskatchewan), s. 4(1); *Human Tissue Gift Act* (Yukon), s. 3(1)). A "free and informed decision" (as discussed in Chapter 6) follows the common law requirements for fully informed consent to medical treatment set out by the Supreme Court of Canada in *Reibl v. Hughes* (1980). The physician must inform the donor of all potential and material risks inherent in the procedure that would be reasonably likely to affect the donor's decision.

For their consent to be valid, Prince Edward Islanders must specifically be able to understand the consequences and nature of transplanting tissue from their body during their lifetime (*Human Tissue Donation Act* (Prince Edward Island), s. 6(1)). If there is any doubt on this point, a physician must determine through an independent assessment whether the transplant should be carried out (*Human Tissue Donation Act* (Prince Edward Island), ss. 6(2) and (8)).

MENTALLY INCOMPETENT INTER VIVOS DONORS AND MINORS

Situations in which the prospective donor is a minor, is mentally incompetent, or is otherwise unable to make an informed decision because of not understanding the nature and consequences of the procedure pose a special problem. Such a situation might arise, for example, if the health risk to the donor, a minor, is minimal and therefore perfectly acceptable and the tissue is urgently required to save the life of that person's sibling.

As mentioned above, the Prince Edward Island statute provides for an independent assessment in a situation in which the donor appears not to understand the nature and consequences of the transplant and yet consents to it. The assessors must consider whether:

- The transplant is the treatment of choice
- The donor has been coerced or induced to give consent

- Removal of the tissue will create a substantial health or other risk to the donor
- The Act and its regulations have been complied with (*Human Tissue Donation Act* (Prince Edward Island), s, 8(6)

This requirement for assessment also applies in the case of a donor under 16, even if he or she understands the nature and consequences of the transplant (*Human Tissue Donation Act* (Prince Edward Island), ss. 7(1) and (4)). In Prince Edward Island, in the case of a minor under 16, parental consent, too, is required for an inter vivos gift of regenerative tissue (e.g., bone marrow). An additional requirement for inter vivos donors under 16 in P.E.I. is that all other members of the donor's family must be eliminated as potential donors for medical or other reasons. The assessors must give written reasons for their decision and must indicate in their assessment that the transplant should be carried out.

The P.E.I. statute further provides that a person may appeal the decision to the Supreme Court of Prince Edward Island within three days (*Human Tissue Donation Act* (Prince Edward Island), s. 9(1)). The Court may confirm, vary, or quash (cancel) the assessors' decision, or return the matter to the assessors for further action. Pending the decision of the appeal, the transplant cannot proceed.

Manitoba's *Human Tissue Gift Act* and Ontario's *Trillium Gift of Life Network Act* permit persons under 18 but at least 16 to consent to the donation of tissue while living. However, a physician who is not and never has been associated with the proposed recipient must certify in writing that he or she believes such person is capable of understanding and does understand the nature and effect of the transplant. Further, in Manitoba, a parent must consent and the donor must be a member of the recipient's immediate family (*Human Tissue Gift Act* (Manitoba), supra footnote 108, ss. 10(1), (2)). The physician who makes the certificate cannot participate in the transplant operation. This provision addresses concerns over potential conflicts of interest.

In Manitoba, persons under 16 may donate tissue while living only if these conditions are met:

- The proposed recipient is a member of the donor's immediate family.
- Only regenerative tissue will be given.
- The recipient would likely die without the tissue.
- The life and health risks to the donor are minimal.
- The donor consents to the transplant.
- The donor's parent or legal guardian consents.
- The transplant is recommended by a physician who is not and never has been involved in any way with the recipient and will not be involved in the transplant.
- Court approval is obtained.

The term *immediate family* specifically includes the donor's mother, father, or stepfather or stepmother, brother, sister, stepbrother or stepsister, or half-brother or half-sister (*Human*

*Tissue Gift Act* (Manitoba), ss. 10(4), 11(3)). This applies in the case of both a donor under 16 and a donor between 16 and 18.

Alberta, British Columbia, Newfoundland, Nova Scotia, Ontario, Saskatchewan, and Yukon do not require an assessment procedure in the case of a minor or mentally incompetent inter vivos donor. Ontario's *Health Care Consent Act* (1996, s. 6, para. 3), for instance, specifically states that its provisions do not affect the law with respect to, among other matters, the removal of regenerative or nonregenerative tissue for implantation in another person's body.

The human tissue donation statutes of most of these provinces are virtually identical. However, they do provide that if the donor giving consent is a minor, is mentally incompetent to consent, or is unable to give a free and informed decision, the consent is still legally valid if the person acting on that consent (presumably, the physician who will perform the transplant) has no reason to believe that the donor is a minor, is mentally incompetent, or is unable to make a free and informed decision. There is thus a requirement of good faith on the part of the person performing the transplant and a duty upon him or her to ensure that a prospective donor is indeed a mentally competent adult who is giving a free and informed consent.

In most cases, this provision does not pose a problem. Most physicians and nurses are competent to assess the general mental capabilities of their patients. A careful review with the patient of all material risks inherent in the transplant, within the criteria stated in *Reibl v. Hughes*, would likely address the problem of a free and informed consent. The case of the minor poses a slightly different problem when that person appears much older than he or she actually is. The level of maturity disclosed in the conversation between the health care professional and the minor cannot be considered conclusive. The statute protects health care professionals acting in good faith in such a situation.

Apart from this, such prospective donors would require some sort of court authorization according to common law. This has been the traditional route in jurisdictions lacking procedures such as those required in Prince Edward Island or explicit provisions for court authorization such as those in Quebec's *Civil Code*. A court reviewing such a case would likely consider factors such as those mentioned in the P.E.I. Act and, further, would consider the impact of the procedure on the donor.

In the case of a minor, some courts have relied on the "competent minor" rule. This rule holds that a person under the age of majority may be sufficiently mature to comprehend fully the nature and consequences of the transplant. Since in these cases, the donor is not receiving a direct health benefit from the transplant, in some American states, the courts have considered that the infant donor still derives an emotional benefit from the survival of his or her sibling. The family is thus relieved from the potential stress of the death of one of its members and can provide full emotional support to the donor. Further, especially in cases in which the infant donor is old enough to have expressed even a rudimentary wish to help the sibling (though not fully comprehending the nature and consequences of the transplant), that child is spared the emotional guilt that may develop later in life from not having had an opportunity to save the sibling's life (Sneiderman, Irvine, & Osborne, 1989).

Interestingly, Prince Edward Island's *Human Tissue Donation Act* deals expressly with the question of regenerative tissue donation by an infant sibling (*Human Tissue Donation Act* (Prince Edward Island), section 7(2)). It provides that, with the consent of the infant donor's parents, and the approval of the independent assessors, bone marrow may be removed from such a child during the child's life for implantation into the child's biological sibling. Of course, the assessors will have eliminated all other eligible family members for medical or other reasons.

POSTMORTEM DONATIONS

Consent to donation of tissue after the donor's death is somewhat different. The policy behind the law in such cases is to encourage the donation of organs after death since there is always a large pool of recipients who urgently need them. Thus, the requirements for lawful consent are more relaxed and flexible.

In all provinces and territories, a person over the age of majority (over 16 in Ontario and Prince Edward Island) may consent in writing to the removal of any and all tissue for therapeutic, medical educational, or medical research purposes. Except in Quebec, the written document containing the consent may be part of a will or other testamentary instrument (e.g., organ donor card, driver's licence), regardless of whether such will is legally valid.

In Manitoba and Ontario, a person under 18 but at least 16 years of age may consent to such removal, but only with the consent of his or her parent or guardian, unless the parent or guardian is unavailable (e.g., dead, physically or mentally ill, or otherwise absent) (*Human Tissue Gift Act* (Manitoba), ss. 2(1), (2); *Trillium Gift of Life Network Act* (Ontario), s. 3). These provisions permit flexibility and promote the availability of organs. Consent given by a person under 16 is deemed valid if the person who acted on it had no reason to believe that the postmortem donor was in fact under 16. This mirrors the provisions of inter vivos donations in most provinces and imposes a requirement of good faith on the part of physicians acting upon the donor's directive.

In Quebec, a minor 14 years of age or older may authorize the removal of organs or tissue or give his or her body for medical or scientific purposes. A minor under 14 may also do so with the written consent of a parent or guardian (*Civil Code of Quebec*, art. 43).

Most provinces allow consent to be made orally by the donor in the presence of two witnesses during the donor's last illness. Manitoba and Prince Edward Island do not specify whether the consent must be written. The statutes of those two provinces speak of the removal of tissue "as may be specified in the consent," which implies a requirement for written consent. However, in a case in which a clear, unequivocal oral consent is given in the presence of two or more witnesses, it is possible that such consent would be permissible as clear evidence of the donor's last wishes. In all cases, the donor may revoke (cancel) his or her consent at any time prior to death. The law will respect the absolute final wishes of the donor and the right to change his or her mind, even at the last possible moment.

The consent is effective upon the donor's death. The determination of death can be problematic, as discussed above. All statutes across Canada require that, in cases in which organs are to be removed, death must be determined by at least two physicians. Neither may be persons associated with the intended recipient such as might influence the physician's judgement nor may either participate in the transplant. This is to avoid potential conflicts of interest.

As mentioned earlier, a valid consent may not be acted upon if the person acting on it has reason to believe that the donor has not reached the age of consent, is not mentally competent, or is not able to make a free and informed consent. Thus, physicians and nurses involved in the transplant should be alert to any such indications. If there is no reason for such suspicions, the consent will be valid even if it later turns out that the donor was underage, was mentally incompetent, or was otherwise unable to make a free and informed consent.

The consent grants complete authority to remove and use parts named in the consent for any purpose specified, unless the person acting on it has reason to believe that consent was withdrawn by the donor before death. This is consistent with the principle permitting the donor to change his or her mind at any time. The withdrawal can be made either orally to witnesses or in writing, signed by the donor.

POSTMORTEM DONATIONS LACKING THE DECEASED'S CONSENT

What of situations in which the deceased expressed no wishes regarding donation of tissues or organs after death, or was incapable of giving consent? This is different from specifically refusing consent since the law requires that such refusal, however unfortunate for the prospective recipient, be respected. Yet, organs or tissue may be urgently needed to save the life of another. In such cases (i.e., the prospective donor has expressed no wishes, and death is imminent in the opinion of a physician), the law in all jurisdictions allows other specific persons to make the decision regarding the removal of tissue or organs from the deceased's body.

There is a hierarchy of persons who may be approached to make this decision:

1. The spouse of the donor
2. If there is no spouse, any of the donor's children over 18
3. If there are no children, either of the donor's parents (or legal guardian, in some provinces; in Prince Edward Island, the person's guardian ranks above his or her spouse)
4. Any of the donor's siblings
5. The donor's next of kin
6. If none of the above is available, anyone who is in lawful possession of the body

The statutes make clear that the sixth category excludes the coroner, medical examiner, embalmer, and funeral director. It might conceivably include the executor or administrator of the donor's estate, since such person is responsible for the proper and respectful disposal of the deceased's remains, either by burial or cremation.

Sometimes, relatives of the deceased will disagree over permitting the removal of organs or tissue. For example, the wife of a patient whose death is imminent might refuse a physician's request for removal of the man's kidneys, whereas the patient's father may be in favour of such a request. The law in most provinces and territories provides a resolution to such a conflict: No person may act on a consent given on behalf of a dying or deceased donor if such person knows of an objection to it by anyone having the same or closer relationship to the donor than the one who gave the consent. Thus, in our case scenario, Mr. R.'s wife's wishes (if he has a wife) would overrule those of the donor's parents. Similarly, in a case in which the donor's sister gave consent and the donor's brother objected, that objection would void the consent and end the matter unless another relative closer in relationship to the donor consented. Manitoba's legislation does not provide a mechanism for resolving such disputes, but it is likely that a health care professional in that province faced with a similar conflict could resolve it in this manner.

In Quebec, the *Civil Code* permits the deceased's heirs or successors to give or refuse consent (*Civil Code of Quebec*, art. 42). There is no mechanism for conflict resolution in the *Civil Code*. However, a person qualified to give consent to care of the donor (when living) may also consent to the removal of tissues or organs from the deceased's body (*Civil Code of Quebec*, art. 45, para. 1). In Quebec, a physician may proceed with the transplant of an organ or tissues from a deceased if two physicians certify that they were unable to obtain such consent in due time and that the operation was urgently required to save a human life or to significantly improve the quality of a life (*Civil Code of Quebec*, art. 45, para. 2).

Finally, the law, as always, respects the deceased or dying donor's wishes. If a health care professional acting on the consent of a donor's spouse or other relative has reason to believe that the donor would object to the removal, or, in Manitoba, that such removal would be contrary to the donor's religion (*Human Tissue Gift Act*, s, 4(3)(a)), he or she cannot proceed on the basis of the consent. Similarly, if the health care professional in charge of the case believes that the deceased's death occurred in circumstances requiring an inquest by a coroner or medical examiner (i.e., the deceased did not die of natural causes and an inquest into the cause of death is required), that professional cannot proceed on the basis of the consent unless the coroner or medical examiner agrees. This requirement preserves the evidentiary value of a postmortem examination of the body.

## Provincial Strategies to Promote Organ Retrieval

Manitoba and Ontario have made an attempt, in their organ donation legislation, to encourage physicians and other health care professionals to identify potential organ donors. The Manitoba Act requires the last physician who attended the deceased to consider, upon the death of one who has given no direction as to organ donation (or whose direction is invalid because the person was incompetent), whether it is appropriate to request permission of the donor's proxy or other relative to remove tissue or use the body for therapeutic purposes (*Human Tissue Gift Act* (Manitoba), s. 4(1)). The physician must take into account the condition of the body and its tissues, the need of these for therapeutic purposes, and the emotional and physical condition of the deceased's survivors. The Manitoba statute specifically provides for the removal of the pituitary gland and eyes (for corneal transplants). Ontario's Act requires a designated health care facility to notify the Trillium Gift of Life Network (described below) of the death or imminent death of a patient in its care. The Network, established under the Act, is then required to determine whether the health care facility should contact the patient or the patient's substitute concerning consent for tissue donation. It must make that determination in consultation with the facility (*Trillium Gift of Life Network Act*, Parts II.1 and II.2). This is to ensure that in every instance in which viable organs might be retrieved, the patient or patient's substitute decision maker is proactively given an opportunity to consider organ donation. The Trillium Gift of Life Network is an arm's-length, not-for-profit organization whose mandate is:

- To plan, promote, coordinate, and support activities relating to the donation of tissue for transplant and activities relating to education or research in connection with the donation of tissue
- To coordinate and support the work of designated health care facilities in connection with the donation and transplant of tissue
- To manage the procurement, distribution, and delivery of tissue
- To establish and manage waiting lists for the transplant of tissue and to establish and manage a system to fairly allocate tissue that is available
- To make reasonable efforts to ensure that patients and their substitutes have appropriate information and opportunities to consider whether to consent to the donation of tissue
- To provide education to the public and to the health care community about matters relating to the donation and use of tissue and to facilitate the provision of such education by others
- To collect, analyze, and publish information relating to the donation and use of tissue
- To advise the Minister of Health and Long-Term Care on matters relating to the donation of tissue (*Trillium Gift of Life Network Act*, s. 8.8)

The ultimate aim is to enhance the efficient and timely retrieval of organs and tissue to meet the demand.

Prince Edward Island law requires an attending physician or other person to record whether he or she discussed tissue donation with any of those authorized to provide consent on behalf of the patient to removal of organs or tissue. If no such discussion has taken place, the reason that it has not must be recorded (*Human Tissue Donation Act* (Prince Edward Island), s. 4). This is as far as the P.E.I. legislation goes. It does not demand that such consultation take place.

**Application to Mr. R.'s Case Scenario**

The misconceptions and misinformation surrounding organ tissue laws in Canada have regrettably contributed to a low rate of organ retrieval across the country. The case scenario of Mr. R. and Mr. S. raises the issue of whether the ICU team ought to have been more persuasive with Mr. R.'s family. This would have been an appropriate role for the nurses in Mr. R.'s team. With the valid organ donor card, the team could have proceeded despite the parents' wishes. Unfortunately, however, in practice, most hospitals do not contravene the wishes of the deceased's next of kin, even with a valid consent from the deceased, possibly because the attempt to persuade the deceased's family to consent might be deemed coercive. However, if the team approaches the family in a gentle, diplomatic, and sensitive way, the request need not be coercive; in fact, a request made in such a manner might garner earnest support from families. Many more lives could be saved if this situation were expressly addressed in each province's legislation.

## Summary

Nurses today belong to a health care culture that constantly strives to overcome the mysteries of life and death. This chapter has explored many difficult ethical and legal issues that nurses face in day-to-day practice.

The emphasis on the principle of sanctity of life in medicine and health care has driven the development of treatment modalities and technologies that can cure many previously terminal diseases and save lives but that can also simply prolong the process of dying. The fear of dying in isolation, and in pain and suffering, has driven society to seek other options to protect people from this fate.

Nurses play an important role in ensuring that patients' rights and dignity are respected throughout the process of dying. The ultimate goal of nursing is that patients are made comfortable, are kept free of pain and suffering, and remain in control of their lives and the nature of their deaths. For example, they should be able to make decisions about where they die and the people with whom they wish to be at that time. As members of Canadian society, nurses share in the debate about the ethics of assisted suicide, euthanasia, and the like. At the least, in their professional role, they should try to ensure that these measures will not be necessary for their patients and clients. Nurses support the wishes of patients at the end of life by ensuring that their advance directives are respected, influencing a respectful organ donation process when that is the person's wish, and being sensitive to the needs of the dying, from premature neonates to older adults.

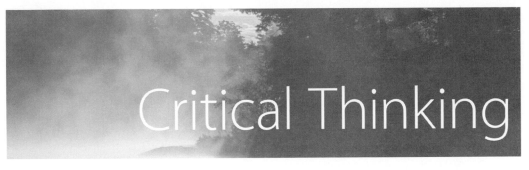

# Critical Thinking

The following scenarios are provided to stimulate reflection, discussion, and analysis. As you review each case, consider the following questions as well as those specific to the case.

1. Have the nurses in these cases violated any ethical or legal standards?
2. If so, what are these standards?
3. Is there risk of any civil or criminal liability?
4. How could these situations have been prevented?

## IN WHOSE BEST INTERESTS?

Ian is a 29-year-old man who sustained a major head injury in a car accident 7 years ago. He is presently in a long-term care facility. Ian cannot communicate in any way, requires total care, and is incontinent of urine and stool. He is likely in a persistent vegetative state, and his prognosis is thought by the team to be hopeless. He has a gastrostomy tube and receives regular feedings.

Ian's parents believe that their son would not wish to be maintained in this way and have requested that the feeding tube be removed. They have made this request several times in past years. However, the hospital's policy does not allow discontinuation of tubes. As tubes are replaced at regular intervals, Ian's family is now asking that their son's tube not be replaced in the event that it accidentally falls out.

### Questions
1. What are your views on this hospital's policy regarding withdrawal of treatment?
2. As a nurse, how would you support this family?
3. Do you agree with the family's plan?
4. In this situation, what would be the legal requirements for organ donation in your home province?
5. What criteria does your hospital use for determining death?

continued on following page >>

## WHOM DO I WANT BESIDE ME?

Saleem is a 74-year-old man who suffered a serious heart attack, causing a small hole in his ventricular septum. His condition is critical; his only option is to be placed on an intra-aortic balloon pump (to assist cardiac output) and to undergo immediate surgery. He agrees to this treatment plan.

Saleem's wife and children remain in the ICU's waiting room during his surgery, which takes about 6 hours. They are relieved when he is wheeled into the ICU; they have been told they will be able to visit within a few minutes of his return. When they inquire about visiting, they are told they will have to wait, as it is the change of shift, and the nurses are giving report. A half hour passes, and they ask again. This time, they are told that the nurses are still organizing Saleem's care; they must wait a bit longer. What is, in fact, happening is that Saleem is still bleeding from the surgery. The nurses are in the process of giving him blood; he is being assessed by the surgeon and a hematologist. An hour and a half later, the family has still not been allowed into his room. After asking again, they are allowed a 5-minute visit.

### Questions

1. What are the nurses' responsibilities to Saleem and his family? Did they meet these responsibilities?
2. What policies in hospitals and intensive care units might restrict nurses from meeting the needs of patients and families?
3. How might nurses and nursing leaders ensure that policies and rules reflect high ethical and professional standards?
4. Can you think of similar situations in your own practice experience?

## CARE AFTER DEATH

Liz has just learned that her only brother, Glen, has been killed in a motor vehicle accident. Though his identity has been confirmed, Liz and her parents wish to see him. They are directed to the hospital's emergency department, where the nurses say little to them beyond indicating that they have called a supervisor.

When the supervisor arrives a quarter of an hour later, she offers condolences and tells them how hard the team worked to save Glen. When Liz expresses her need to see her brother, the family is taken to the hospital morgue. They are distressed to see Glen wrapped in a plastic sheet, his hands bound, and his face covered in blood.

continued on following page >>

## Questions

1. What responsibility did the nurses in the emergency department have to this family? Was the morgue a suitable environment for their viewing the body?
2. Does respect for the person extend beyond life, or do other factors (such as how busy the unit may be) take precedence?
3. How do you think this experience will affect the family's experience of grief?

## THE COST OF COMFORT

Carla, a case manager in the home care setting, is currently coordinating the care of a cancer patient dying at home. Amelia is expected to die within the next few days. Community nurses visit daily, but Amelia's daughters and husband are providing most of her care. Though she receives morphine on a regular basis, she is still in great discomfort. Amelia is emaciated; the skin over her coccyx has broken down, and the cancer has metastasized to her bones. One daughter comments to Carla that during a recent hospital admission, the nurses placed her mother on a special mattress that relieved her discomfort considerably. Carla explains that this mattress is not covered by home care and instead offers special-duty nurses for the next few nights. Since Amelia's death is imminent, Carla is concerned that the family will need their rest. The family refuses the offer of nurses because they want to remain with Amelia and ensure they are with her when she dies. They make arrangements to rent the mattress themselves at their own cost.

## Questions

1. What responsibilities does Carla have to ensure that Amelia's care needs are met?
2. Does it make sense that a more cost-effective and practical intervention (the mattress) be denied? How can nurses change agency policies in order to introduce guidelines that focus on individual needs? (Or should all clients be treated the same way?)

## Discussion Points

1. What are your views on the legalization of euthanasia and assisted suicide? If euthanasia is legalized, what safeguards should be in place? What role should nurses play?
2. What guidelines are in place in your facility to ensure that a person has a peaceful and dignified death? Can these guidelines be improved?
3. Does your facility have any policies or rules that limit family access to patients? Can these rules or policies be supported ethically?
4. Identify the key differences between organ or tissue donation, and transplantation in general, and the new territory of fetal tissue transplantation. Can fetal transplantation be supported by those who oppose abortion?

## References

### Statutes

*Adult Guardianship Act*, R.S.B.C. 1996, c. 6 (British Columbia).

*Charter of Rights and Freedoms*, Part I of the *Constitution Act, 1982*, being Schedule B to the *Canada Act 1982* (U.K.), 1982, c. 11.

*Civil Code of Quebec*, C.c.Q. (Quebec).

*Criminal Code of Canada,* R.S.C. 1985, c. C-46 (Canada).

*Criminal Law Amendment Act*, S.C. 1972, c. 13 (Canada).

*Health Care Consent Act*, 1996, S.O. 1996, c. 2, Schedule A (Ontario).

*Health Care Directives Act*, C.C.S.M., c. H27 (Manitoba).

*Human Tissue Act*, R.S.N.L. 1990, c. H-15 (Newfoundland and Labrador).

*Human Tissue Act*, R.S.N.W.T. 1988, c. H-6 (Northwest Territories and Nunavut).

*Human Tissue Donation Act*, R.S.P.E.I. 1988, c. H-12.1 (Prince Edward Island).

*Human Tissue Gift Act*, C.C.S.M. c. H180 (Manitoba).

*Human Tissue Gift Act*, R.S.A. 2000, c. H-15 (Alberta).

*Human Tissue Gift Act*, R.S.B.C. 1996, c. 211 (British Columbia).

*Human Tissue Gift Act*, S.N.B. 2004, c. H-12.5 (New Brunswick).

*Human Tissue Gift Act*, R.S.N.S. 1989, c. 215 (Nova Scotia).

*Human Tissue Gift Act*, R.S.S. 1978, c. H-15 (Saskatchewan).

*Human Tissue Gift Act*, R.S.Y. 2002, c. 117 (Yukon).

*Medical Consent Act*, R.S.N.S. 1989, c. 279. (Nova Scotia).

*Personal Directives Act*, R.S.A. 2000, c. P-6 (Alberta).

*Representation Agreement Act*, R.S.B.C. 1996, c. 405 (British Columbia).

*Substitute Decisions Act*, 1992, S.O. 1992, c. 30 (Ontario).

*Termination of Life on Request and Assisted Suicide (Review Procedures) Act* (the Netherlands).

*Trillium Gift of Life Network Act*, R.S.O. 1990, c. H.20 (Ontario).

*Vital Statistics Act*, C.C.S.M. c. V60 (Manitoba).

### Case Law

*Ciarlariello v. Schacter*, [1993] 2 S.C.R. 119, aff'g. (1991), 44 OAC 385; 76 DLR (4th) 449; 5 CCLT (2d) 221 (CA), aff'g. (1987), 7 ACWS (3d) 51 (Ont. HCJ).

*Golubchuk v. Salvation Army Grace General Hospital et al.* (2008), MBQB 49 (CanLII).

*Malette v. Shulman* (1990), 72 OR (2d) 417 (CA).

*Nancy B. v. Hôtel-Dieu de Québec et al.*, [1992] RJQ 361; (1992), 86 DLR (4th) 385; (1992) 69 CCC (3d) 450 (SC).

*R. v. Kitching and Adams*, [1976] 6 WWR 697, at p. 711 (Man. CA).

*R. v. Latimer*, [1997] 1 SCR 217; 152 Sask. R. 1 (SCC). Sentence following second trial ordered by Supreme Court of Canada: (1998), 121 CCC. (3d) 326; 172 Sask. R. 161, 185 W.A.C. 161, 22 C.R. (5th) 380, [1999] 6 W.W.R. 118, [1998] S.J. No. 731 (QL); aff'd.

[2001] 1 S.C.R. 3; (2001), 193 D.L.R. (4th) 577; [2001] 6 W.W.R. 409; (2001), 150 C.C.C. (3d) 129; (2001), 39 C.R. (5th) 1; (2001), 80 C.R.R. (2d) 189; (2001), 203 Sask. R. 1.

*Re Quinlan*, 137 NJ Super. 227; 348 A.2d. 801 (Ch. Div. 1975), In *re Quinlan*, 70 NJ 10, 355 A.2d. 647 (SC 1976).

*Reibl v. Hughes*, [1980] 2 SCR 880; (1980) 14 CCLT 1; 114 DLR (3d) 1; 33 NR 361 (SCC).

*Rodriguez v. British Columbia* (Attorney General), [1993] BCWLD 347; (1992), 18 WCB (2d) 279 (SC); aff'd. (1993), 76 BCLR (2d) 145; 22 BCAC 266; 38 WAC 266; 14 CRR (2d) 34; 79 CCC (3d) 1; [1993] 3 WWR 553; aff'd. [1993] 3 SCR 519.

## Texts and Articles

Baumann-Hölzle, R., Maffezzoni, M., & Bucher, H. U. (2005). A framework for ethical decision making in neonatal intensive care. *Acta Paediatrica, 94*(12), 1777–1783.

Bell, M. D. D. (2006, November). Emergency medicine, organ donation and the *Human Tissue Act*. *Emergency Medicine Journal, 23*(11), 824–827.

Bidigare, S. A. (1991). Attitudes and knowledge of nurses regarding organ procurement. *Heart & Lung 20*(1), 20–25.

Booth, M. (2006, January). Ethical issues in resuscitation and intensive care medicine. *Anaesthesia and Intensive Care Medicine, 8*(1), 36–39.

Borozny, M. L. (1988, January). Brain death and critical care nurses. *The Canadian Nurse, 84*(1), 24–27.

Campbell, C. S. (2004, September). Harvesting the living?: Separating "brain death" and organ transplantation. *Kennedy Institute of Ethics Journal, 14*(3), 301–318.

Canadian Encyclopedic Digest (Ont. 3d.), Vol. 14, Title 72, Toronto, ON: Thomson Carswell.

Canadian Nurses Association. (2008). *Code of ethics for registered nurses*. Ottawa, ON: Author.

Canadian Paediatric Society. (2004). Treatment decisions regarding infants, children and adolescents. *Paediatric & Child Health, 9*(2), 99–103.

Cantor, M. D., Braddock III, C. H., Derse, A. R., Murray Edwards, D., Logue, G. L., Nelson, W., et al. (2003). Do-not-resuscitate orders and medical futility. *Archives of Internal Medicine, 163*, 2689–2694.

Capron, A.M. (1987, February). Anencephalic donors: Separate the dead from the dying. *Hastings Center Report, 17*(1), 5–9.

Chittick, W. C. (1992). "Your sight today is piercing": The Muslim understanding of death and afterlife. In H. Obayashi (Ed.), *Death and afterlife: Perspectives of world religions* (pp. 125–139). New York: Greenwood Press.

Cohen, R. W. (2004). A tale of two conversations. *Hastings Center Report, 34*(3), 49.

Committee on Fetus and Newborn (American Academy of Pediatrics). (2007, February). Noninitiation or withdrawal of intensive care for high-risk newborns. *Pediatrics, 119*(2), 401–403.

Crowley-Matoka, M., & Arnold, R. M. (2004, September). The dead donor rule: How much does the public care . . . and how much should we care? *Kennedy Institute of Ethics Journal, 14*(3), 319–332.

Day, L. (2001). How nurses shift from care of a brain injured patient to maintenance of a brain dead organ donor. *American Journal of Critical Care, 19,* 306–403.

Dresser, R. (1994). Advance directives: Implications for policy. *The Hastings Center Report, 24*(6), S2–S5.

Dudzinski, D. M. (2003, Winter). Does the respect for donor rule respect the donor? *The American Journal of Bioethics, 3*(1), 23–24.

Epstein, E. (2007). *Moral obligations of NICU healthcare providers at the end of palliative life.* Unpublished abstract, University of Virginia School of Nursing.

Ethics Committee, American College of Critical Care Medicine, Society of Critical Care Medicine. (2001, September). Recommendations for non-heart-beating organ donation: A position paper by the Ethics committee, American College of Critical Care Medicine, Society of Critical Care Medicine. *Critical Care Medicine, 29*(9), 1826–1831.

Government of Canada. (1995). Of life and death—final report. *Report of the Special Senate Committee on Euthanasia and Assisted Suicide.* Ottawa, ON: Author.

Hayes, C. (2004, January/March). Ethics in end-of-life care. *Journal of Hospice and Palliative Nursing, 6*(1), 36–45.

Hester, D. M. (2003). "Dead donor" versus "respect for donor" rule: Putting the cart before the horse. *The American Journal of Bioethics, 3*(1), 24–26.

Hibbert, M. (1995, September/October). Stressors experienced by nurses while caring for organ donors and their families. *Heart & Lung, 24*(5), 399–407.

Ives-Baine, L. (2007). A lasting and meaningful difference: Bereavement care. The Hospital for Sick Children, *Nursing Matters, 8*(3), 3–6. Retrieved July 21, 2008, from http://www.safekidscanada.ca/CentreforNursing/NursingMatters/2007/special07.pdf

Janvier, A., & Barrington, K. J. (2005). The ethics of neonatal resuscitation at the margins of viability: Informed consent and outcomes. *Journal of Pediatrics, 147,* 579–585.

Jezewski, M. & Finnell, D. (1998). The meaning of DNR status: Oncology nurses' experiences with patients and families. *Cancer Nursing, 21*(3), 212–221.

Keatings, M. (1990). The biology of the persistent vegetative state, legal and ethical implications for transplantation: Viewpoints from nursing. *Transplantation Proceedings, 2*(3), 997–999.

Kim, J. R., Elliott, D., & Hyde, C. (2004, March). Korean health professionals' attitudes and knowledge toward organ donation and transplantation. *International Journal of Nursing Studies, 41*(3), 299–307.

Kim, Y. S. (1998). Organ transplantation: Principles and practice. Seoul, South Korea: Huny-Mon Pub.

Koenig, B. A. (2003, Winter). Dead donors and the "shortage" of human organs: Are we missing the point? *The American Journal of Bioethics, 3*(1), 26–27.

Kolarik, R. C., Arnold, R. M., Fischer, G. S., Hanusa, B. H. (2002). Advance care planning: A comparison of values statements and treatment preferences. *Journal of General Internal Medicine, 17*(8), 618–624.

Koppelman, E. R. (2003). The dead donor rule and the concept of death: Severing the ties that bind them. *The American Journal of Bioethics, 3*(1), 1–9.

Kowalski, W. J., Leef, K. H., Mackley, A., Spear, M. L., & Paul, D. A. (2005). Communicating with parents of premature infants: Who is the informant? *Journal of Perinatology, 26*(1), 44–48.

Kramer, K. P. (1988). *The sacred art of dying: How world religions understand death.* New York: Paulist Press.

Law Reform Commission of Canada. (1980). *Medical treatment and criminal law.* Working paper No. 26. Ottawa, ON: Author.

Law Reform Commission of Canada. (1983). *Euthanasia, aiding suicide and cessation of treatment.* Report No. 20. Ottawa, ON: Author.

McAllister, M., & Dionne, K. (2006, September/October). Partnering with parents: Establishing effective long-term relationships with parents in the NICU. *Neonatal Network: The Journal of Neonatal Nursing, 25*(5), 329–337.

Meadow, W. (2006, June). 500-gram infants—and 800-pound gorillas—in the delivery room. *Pediatrics, 117*(6), 2276.

Menikoff, J. (2002, Summer). The importance of being dead: Non-heart-beating organ donation. *Issues in Law & Medicine 18*(1), 3–20.

"Orthodox Jew to remain on life support, trial next." Retrieved from www.ctv.ca/servlet/articlenews/story/CTVnews/20080213/life_support_080213

Paris, J. J., Graham, N., Schreiber, M. D., & Goodwin, M. (2006). Approaches to end-of-life decision-making in the NICU: Insights from Dostoevsky's *The Grand Inquisitor. Journal of Perinatology, 26*(7), 389–391.

Physician-assisted suicide and the right to die with assistance. (1992). *Harvard Law Review, 105*(Note), 2021.

Rassin, M., Lowenthal, M., & Silner, D. (2005, July/September). Fear, ambivalence, and liminality: Key concepts in refusal to donate an organ after brain death. *JONA's Healthcare Laws, Ethics, and Regulation, 7*(3), 79–85.

Ross, H. M. (2001, April). Islamic tradition at the end of life. *MEDSURG Nursing, 10*(2), 83–87.

Singer, P. A., Robertson, G., Roy, D. J. (1996). Bioethics for clinicians: 6. Advance care planning. *Canadian Medical Association Journal, 155*(12): 1689–1692.

Sneiderman, B., Irvine, J. C., & Osborne, P. H. (1989), *Canadian medical law: An introduction for physicians and other health care professionals* (pp. 220–223). Toronto, ON: Carswell.

Solomon, M. Z., O'Donnell, L., Jennings, B., Guilfoy, V., Wolf, S. M., Nolan, K., et al. (1993, January). Decisions near the end of life: Professional views on life-sustaining treatments. *American Journal of Public Health, 83*(1), 14–23.

Solomon, M. Z., Sellers, D. E., Heller, K. S., Dokken, D. L., Levetown, M., Rushton, C., et al. (2005, October). New and lingering controversies in pediatric end-of-life care. *Pediatrics, 116*(4), 872–883.

Spike, J. (2000, Spring). Controlled NHBD protocol for a fully conscious person: When death is intended as an end in itself and it has its own end. *The Journal of Clinical Ethics, 11*(1), 72–76.

Steinberg, D. (2003, March). Eliminating death. *The American Journal of Bioethics, 3*(1), 17–18.

Task Force on Presumed Consent. (1994). *Organ procurement strategies. A review of ethical issues and challenges* (p. 7). Toronto, ON: Multiple Organ Retrieval & Exchange Program of Ontario.

Trachtman, H. (2003, Winter). Death be not political. *The American Journal of Bioethics, 3*(1), 31–32.

Truog, R. D., & Robinson, W. M. (2003, September). Role of brain death and the dead-donor rule in the ethics of organ transplantation. (Review). *Critical Care Medicine, 31*(5), 2391–2396.

Truog, R. D. (2000, September). Organ transplantation without brain death. *Annals of New York Academy of Sciences, 913*(1), 229–239.

Veatch, R. M. (2003, Winter). The dead donor rule: True by definition. *The American Journal of Bioethics, 3*(1), 10–11.

Venneman, S. S., Narnor-Harris, P., Perish, M., & Hamilton, M. (2008). "Allow natural death" versus "do not resuscitate": Three words that can change a life. *Journal of Medical Ethics, 34*, 2–6.

Youngner, S. J., Allen, M., Bartlett, E. T., Cascorbi, H. F., Hau, T., Jackson, D. L., et al. (1985, August). Psychosocial and ethical implications of organ retrieval. *New England Journal of Medicine, (313)*5, 321–324.

# Chapter 9

## Ethical and Legal Issues Related to Advancing Science and Technologies

### Learning Objectives

The purpose of this chapter is to enable you to understand:

- The extent of advances in genetics and how they might influence existing and future generations
- Recent advances in reproductive science and technology
- The legal, social, and ethical dimensions that arise out of these advances
- The moral issues associated with low-birth-weight neonates
- The unique role of nursing in addressing and supporting clients and patients who are affected by these technologies

## Introduction

EXTRAORDINARY ADVANCES IN TECHNOLOGY have made it possible to influence the very creation of life and to sustain life in the face of overwhelming adversity. In recent decades, there have been significant advancements in the area of reproductive technologies, genetics, and life-sustaining therapies for extremely premature infants.

The introduction of these technologies raises questions as to whether it is:

- Better to be born than never to exist
- The right of every human being to have a child
- Right to control the characteristics and attributes of children yet to be born
- Right to sustain life regardless of the quality of that life
- Right to use technology to predict our future state of health and life expectancy

Existing reproductive and genetic technologies can overcome infertility, eliminate genetic anomalies, manipulate and control the characteristics of potential human beings, predict the risk of future diseases, and ultimately find their cures or identify strategies for their prevention. This power to manipulate the creation and experience of life may ultimately reshape society and redefine future generations.

Nurses who work in settings in which these technologies are used face profound social, psychological, and emotional issues, and are challenged to question their own values and beliefs about life and its potential. Nurses in areas such as neonatal intensive care may struggle with the consequences of these technologies when caring for extremely premature infants. Genetic counsellors, many of whom are nurses, face daily ethical challenges as they support individuals and families in circumstances never experienced by previous generations. In a multicultural society such as Canada's, patients and their families come from many religious and cultural backgrounds, and may view the meaning of life from many varying perspectives. Nurses must be sensitive to these differences and respectful of the values and beliefs of others.

This chapter will examine the complex ethical and legal issues related to technologies such as those in the rapidly advancing areas of genetics, reproductive science, and the care of extremely premature neonates.

## The Emerging World of Genetics

Developments in this field have exploded over the past few decades. The Human Genome Project, launched in 1990, was completed in 2003. The goals of this international project were to:

- Identify all the genes in human DNA
- Determine the sequences of the chemical base pairs that make up this DNA
- Establish databases to store this information

- Improve tools for data analysis of this information
- Transfer appropriate technologies to the private sector
- Address the ethical, legal, and social issues arising from these technologies (U.S. Department of Energy Office of Science, n.d.)

In 1997, scientists in the United Kingdom were able to clone a sheep known as "Dolly" from an adult of her species (Gibson, 1998). To date, a human clone has not been developed, yet it is becoming clear that questions no longer exist as to whether these technologies will advance but rather when and in what ways. However, controversy about the possibility continues. With each development in genetics, more ethical questions are raised with respect to their use.

Today it is possible to:

- Select embryos based on gender
- Diagnose an infant in utero for cardiac anomalies or other congenital conditions
- Screen newborns for conditions and deficiencies including congenital adrenal hyperplasia, congenital hyperthyroidism, sickle-cell disease, and thalassemia (Canadian Organization for Rare Disorders [CORD], 2006)
- Predict whether an individual is a carrier or is predisposed for conditions such as Alzheimer's disease, breast cancer, cystic fibrosis, or Parkinson's disease

## Ethical Issues

People can be screened to determine their susceptibility to conditions, some of which may be prevented and others that may not, raising many questions with respect to whether the screening option imposes a burden or provides a benefit, how privacy rights are affected, and whether this increases the potential for discrimination (Chadwick, 2008).

What if an insurance company imposed mandatory genetic screening and denied benefits to individuals based on their future risk of disease (Chadwick, 2008)? What if employers did the same, and individuals were denied employment or the opportunity to advance in their careers because of future potential illnesses?

With these technologies, how are the vulnerable protected? For example, is it right to screen children for adult-onset disorders that are not preventable? Should such results be revealed to children? To adolescents? How should consent be determined?

There are many questions about the most appropriate use of these technologies. Should people be screened only for conditions that are preventable? Should testing become public policy, or should it be an individual choice? Who should pay for this very expensive technology? Might only those who can afford it have access to this screening, thereby excluding those who cannot afford to pay? How is privacy protected? Do individuals have the right to confidentiality when they are found to be susceptible to a disorder that may also affect their siblings or other members of their family? What if a person refuses to have this information disclosed when others may also be at risk? Do health care professionals have a duty to warn others? What if, through testing, information is revealed that may be of significance to others? Under what circumstances might confidentiality be breached (Shuman, 2008)?

Consider the following case scenarios.

# Case Scenarios

## IS IT OUR BUSINESS?

Richard and Megan are the parents of a newborn baby, Julia, who has been newly diagnosed with cystic fibrosis (CF). They are referred for genetic counselling and DNA testing for common CF mutations.

The initial report from the molecular lab shows that only one CF mutation has been identified in the baby, which has been inherited from Megan. So far, Richard's mutation remains unidentified. They are called and given the results.

Several months later, an updated report is received from the lab indicating that both CF mutations have now been identified in the baby but that Richard is not the carrier of the other mutation. Since he does not carry either mutation, it is clear that he is not the parent of this child.

### Issues

1. Should you reveal the outcome of this testing? To whom?
2. Are there possible future outcomes for the child?
3. Who are your clients in this situation? Can you ensure that all of their rights are respected?

## WHOSE RIGHT TO KNOW?

Marlene is 17 years old and has Down's syndrome. She lives with her family and functions well, but she has the intellectual and emotional levels of a 10-year-old. She works at a local store stocking shelves, where she has met 19-year-old Leonce, who is developmentally challenged. In spite of close monitoring by their employer and Marlene's family, Marlene and Leonce have developed a romantic relationship, and Marlene is pregnant. By the time her condition is noted and confirmed, Marlene is in her second trimester. Marlene is excited about the prospect of being a mother, but her parents are concerned about the baby's health and want genetic testing for the fetus.

### Issues

1. Who has rights in this situation? Who should decide whether testing should be done? Who decides what action should be taken if the fetus's test is positive for Down's syndrome?

continued on following page >>

2. What are the best interests of the parties involved?
3. How would you counsel this family?

## HOW MUCH SHOULD BE KNOWN?

Elena, a 17-year-old woman, is worried about her father, who has been demonstrating changes in personality over the past few years. She has just been told that her father, who is 42, has Huntington's disease. Huntington's disease is a degenerative brain disorder that usually manifests between the ages of 30 and 50. There is no cure. Death usually occurs 15 to 20 years after its onset. The symptoms are behavioural, emotional, and physical. The person displays involuntary movements and a drunken gait. He or she may become depressed and irritable, and may exhibit aggressive outbursts, social withdrawal, and short-term memory loss.

Elena is aware that her grandmother also had this disease but does not know if anyone else in the family had it. Her mother has just told her that there is a genetic test available that could inform her, with 100% accuracy, whether she will develop the symptoms. She thinks her mother wants her to have the test, but she is not sure if she wants to.

**Issues**
1. Do children have a right to privacy and confidentiality, even from their parents?
2. Can parents demand testing?
3. When is a child's dissent determinative?
4. Who has, or should have, a say when genetic information will have implications for other individuals?

Today, information and data that result from genetic testing predict the risk or possibility of conditions that may be incurable. However, other predicted conditions may be curable or prevented. When an individual chooses to seek genetic information, the data he or she receives may also have implications for family members. Should that information be shared? Does the individual who chooses to have the testing done have the right to maintain the confidentiality of that information? Does the health care team doing the testing have a duty to warn others who may be at risk?

There are pros and cons to predictive testing. On the positive side, if a person believes he or she is at risk for a condition, knowing, one way or the other, may lessen the anxieties and uncertainties associated with not knowing. Knowing allows one to prepare for the future; for example, the knowledge that the early onset of an incurable disease is possible may alter how that person leads his or her life. He or she may make lifestyle changes that could prevent or delay the onset of the illness. There might even be treatment interventions that minimize the risk of getting the disease, and others who may also be susceptible may be identified.

On the negative side, individual reactions may vary and be unpredictable. For example, knowing one is possibly destined for a future plagued by serious illness or disability may produce emotional breakdowns, depression, anxiety, and the risk of suicide. Some people may experience guilt, knowing their offspring may also be at risk. Or they may deny themselves having children. They may find themselves treated unfairly with respect to medical treatment, employment opportunities, and insurance coverage (Shuman, 2008).

The ethical issues related to the field of genetics are extremely challenging. There will be more challenges in the future, as genetics has the potential to create profound changes and to open up new possibilities.

## Stem Cell Technologies

### What Are Stem Cells?

The possibilities related to the use of stem cells in the future are astounding. **Stem cells** have characteristics that are different from other cells. They are unspecialized cells that renew themselves for long periods through cell division and can be induced to become cells with special functions when certain biological conditions are met. Scientists are now able to induce stem cells to develop into specific cells, raising the possibility that damaged organs can be repaired. Regeneration through cell renewal has the potential to repair and replace cells and tissues and thereby restore function, whether its loss is related to congenital anomalies, disease, trauma, or aging (Greenwood & Daar, 2008). For example, cardiac cells may be stimulated to regenerate, thereby healing damaged tissues after a myocardial infarction. Cells can also be differentiated to treat diseases such as Alzheimer's, Parkinson's, diabetes, Huntington's chorea, multiple sclerosis, ALS, and acute leukemia, as well as spinal cord injuries and illnesses resulting from radiation accidents (Childress, 1997, p. 302), and, hence, to regenerate the damaged tissues associated with these conditions.

Stem cells obviously exist in the human embryo, which differentiates to become a fetus and then a human being. The 3- to 5-day-old human embryo develops multiple cell types that evolve to become a heart, skin, lungs, and other organs. In the adult, stem cells exist in tissue such as bone marrow, where they differentiate and replicate to produce various red and white blood cells. They also exist in muscle and brain cells, where they generate replacement cells that supplant those damaged through injury and disease (National Institutes of Health, 2008).

Stem cell research has the potential not only to regenerate tissue but to advance pharmacogenetics and "personalized medicine." In the future, it may be possible to predict a person's response to particular treatments and, based on the genetic makeup of that person, identify which medications and therapies are the most appropriate (Shuman, 2008).

## Stem Cell Transplantation

The use of stem cells for the treatment of the conditions discussed above continues to be a controversial area. As the technology evolves, to date, the main source of stem cells is fetal tissue and umbilical cord blood. The controversy over the use of fetal tissue stem cells is recent, even though, historically, fetal thymus and islet cells have been used for research into the treatment of thymus disease and diabetes and in the development of the polio vaccine (Childress, 1997, p. 302). Fetal tissue is highly suited to transplantation because of the lack of differentiation of the cells and, therefore, a reduced risk for rejection. Unlike adult neural cells, which cannot be replaced, fetal neural stem cells grow rapidly (Childress, 1997, p. 302).

The use of fetal tissue for research purposes and for treatment poses a significant ethical dilemma. The controversy around it is fuelled by the fact that the tissue results mainly from elective abortions. Spontaneous miscarriages provide abnormal and unusable tissue and, in most instances, occur outside of the clinical setting. Tissue can be used from ectopic pregnancies and stillbirths, but the numbers are too low to meet the need (Childress, 1997, p. 302).

Outside of the anti-abortion argument, a number of concerns have been raised about the use of fetal tissue, including the potential for the exploitation of pregnant women and the encouragement of abortion or pregnancy for the purpose of donation (Mahowald, 1996). The debate over when life begins, however, remains at the heart of the controversy over fetal transplantation. There are three views on the status of the fetus:

- The fetus is simply tissue.
- The fetus has the potential for human life.
- The fetus is a human being (Childress, 1997, p. 302).

Those who believe the fetus to be simply tissue would have no serious moral concerns with fetal transplantation. They would consider the tissue to be that of the pregnant woman, who may dispose of it in any way she chooses. Those who support the second and third perspectives believe that the fetus has some moral standing given either its potential for life or that life already exists (Childress, 1997, p. 302). On the other hand, it is argued that it is also morally relevant that this potential for life can be fulfilled only through development within women's bodies (Mahowald, 1996).

If one objects to abortion, then it would follow that deriving gain from such a process would be inappropriate. Some with these views, however, might accept the concept of fetal transplantation if they can separate the act of abortion from the use of tissue from dead fetuses (i.e., the decision to abort is separate from the decision to donate). In this case, they would argue that fetal tissue should be afforded the same respect as cadaveric tissue from human donors (Childress, 1997, p. 302).

Guidelines for the use of fetal tissue have been recommended to address the concerns of those who oppose abortion, to reduce the chance that the opportunity for transplantation would influence a woman's choice to abort, and to eliminate the risk of financial incentives.

## Legislative Responses

At present, there is somewhat of a legislative void on the issue of stem cell transplantation. Parliament enacted federal legislation in 2004 (the *Assisted Human Reproduction Act*) dealing with assisted human reproduction. This statute (which is discussed in more detail under

"Gestational Surrogacy") specifically governs and regulates the use of technology in the creation of human life. It does not, however, purport to regulate the use of human reproductive tissue for therapeutic purposes. Nevertheless, this statute does regulate the use of embryos to an extent. Under the Act, an embryo is defined as:

> a human organism during the first 56 days of its development following fertilization or creation, excluding any time during which its development has been suspended, and includes any cell derived from such an organism that is used for the purpose of creating a human being. (*Assisted Human Reproduction Act*, s. 3, "embryo")

The Act defines *fetus* as "a human organism during the period of its development beginning on the fifty-seventh day following fertilization or creation, excluding any time during which its development has been suspended, and ending at birth" (*Assisted Human Reproduction Act*, s. 3, "foetus").

The use of such reproductive tissue for the purpose of creating human life is heavily regulated, and certain activities are prohibited by this statute. It should be noted, however, that parts of this Act were struck down as being unconstitutional by the Quebec Court of Appeal in a recent reference case brought before that court (*Renvoi fait par le gouvernement du Québec en vertu de la Loi sur les renvois à la Cour d'appel*, L.R.Q., ch. R–23). It remains to be seen whether this decision will be appealed further and if the law will remain intact. This decision only applies to Quebec.

Apart from the *Assisted Human Reproduction Act*, the common law of most provinces would likely treat fetal tissue as any other human remains. Human tissue gift legislation governs donations of tissues from living donors but explicitly does not apply to embryos or fetal tissue (see, for example, Ontario's *Trillium Gift of Life Network Act*, s. 1, "tissue," which explicitly "does not include…spermatozoa, an ovum, an embryo, a foetus, …"). In common law, there are no property rights attached to a dead body. A deceased person's executor has a limited right to possession of the body for the purposes of arranging a funeral and burial, but this is clearly not applicable in cases involving fetal tissue. Although proposed amendments to the *Criminal Code of Canada* will regulate embryonic research and surrogacy, they remain silent on the issue of fetal tissue transplantation.

Problems relating to the distinct difference between the use of fetal brain tissue and the use of other organs or tissue for transplantation have also been identified. The brain is deemed a "defining organ of human behaviour and personality," responsible for cognition, the experience of pain and pleasure, consciousness, and sense of self (Mahowald, 1996), which raises the concern that parts of the brain responsible for cognition or self-awareness transplanted into another's brain might alter the recipient's cognition or self-awareness (Mahowald, 1996). These concerns can be eased, however, since the number of fetal brain cells transplanted currently is small, and such tissue is usually removed from the lower parts of the cerebrum not responsible for cognition or self-awareness. Also, through the consent process, the recipient will have been made aware of potential risks as well as benefits (Mahowald, 1996).

Further concerns associated with fetal transplantation relate to consent. Consent for fetal tissue donation is usually provided by the mother and is similar to consents provided in other circumstances, such as organ donation (Childress, 1997, p. 302). Other views suggest that the mother, in choosing abortion, has relinquished the right to make decisions about the tissue or product of the abortion (Childress, 1997). The assumption that parents have the best interests of their child in mind is what affords them the right to make choices on their child's behalf. When a pregnant woman chooses to abort, the validity of her consent is thus in question (Childress, 1997, p. 302; Mahowald, 1996). There are other consent questions related to the role of the biological father.

There are a number of arguments in favour of the use of fetal tissue, particularly related to the potential benefits of treating and curing diseases that reduce lifespan and result in severe morbidity, as well as the associated perceived benefits of reduction in the cost of care, reduction of ongoing physical and psychological suffering, and the ability to save lives. (Childress, 1997, p. 302; Mahowald, 1996)

The field of fetal transplantation is in its early stages. New opportunities for its use will likely emerge, even as the controversy continues.

## Reproductive Technologies

Over the past decade, significant scientific and technological advances have been made in the area of reproductive technologies. In fact, many of these, such as fertility control techniques, labour and childbirth management, and screening procedures to monitor fetal development, have been available for decades (Stanworth, 1987). As there are many divergent perspectives on reproductive technologies, it is important for nurses both to understand a broad spectrum of views and to reflect on their own.

Fertility control includes methods to prevent conception or implantation of embryos, as well as to terminate pregnancy—for example, diaphragms, intrauterine devices, condoms, sterilization, abortion, and contraceptive drugs such as "the pill" (Stanworth, 1987). The reader is encouraged to investigate the many religious and cultural perspectives on these issues.

In recent decades, the management of labour and childbirth moved from the home to the hospital setting. Giving birth, once a family-oriented process in which the mother was assisted by female relatives, friends, or midwives, has evolved into a medical procedure within a hospital environment. Technologies to manage labour and delivery include forceps deliveries, Caesarean sections, induced labour, and fetal heart rate monitoring (Stanworth, 1987). Many hospitals are now attempting to balance ensuring the safety of the unborn child with creating a family-centred, homelike environment and encouraging the use of midwives and labour coaches.

With advancing technology, fetal development can now be monitored from the very early stages of pregnancy. A majority of women now undergo ultrasound at some point during their pregnancy; high-risk and older pregnant women often undergo amniocentesis to identify defects in the fetus early in development, either to facilitate a decision regarding the termination of a pregnancy or to take action to correct problems or to prevent complications (Stanworth, 1987). These procedures also provide parents with the choice to know the gender of their baby in advance.

## Recent Technologies

Once controversial, but now less so, **new reproductive technologies** aim to induce pregnancy by overcoming or bypassing infertility. While many infertile couples have embraced these techniques, the options available raise profound social, legal, ethical, and emotional questions. These technologies have thrust us into previously uncharted territory, related to the creation of life itself.

The need for these technologies stems from the basic human desire—or powerful cultural pressures—to procreate (Stanworth, 1987). Infertile couples or individuals seem prepared to accept the physical, psychological, and emotional risks associated with these interventions for the sake of having a child, regardless of the chances of a successful pregnancy (Robertson, 1995). With an increase in the incidence of sexually transmitted disease (Fluker & Tuffin, 1996), and with today's tendency for couples to marry or have children later in life (after their careers are established), infertility problems have increased. Pelvic inflammatory disease (PID), a consequence of sexually transmitted diseases, often results in blocked fallopian tubes, a major cause of infertility in women.

The birth of the first "test-tube" baby, Louise Brown, in 1978 heralded the beginning of the proliferation of reproductive innovations, including **donor insemination** (DI), **assisted insemination** (AI), in vitro fertilization (IVF), cryopreservation, ovum and embryo donation, and **surrogacy**. Advanced genetic technologies that provide the opportunity for sex selection, embryo research, prenatal diagnosis, and human embryo cloning have also been developed.

There are varying views on whether infertility is a disease (and therefore a medical condition) or whether its influences are primarily social in nature. As discussed in Chapter 2, there are many feminist perspectives on this issue.

### INFERTILITY AS A MEDICAL CONDITION

Infertility is considered by some to be a medical problem related to a dysfunction of the body, specifically, the reproductive system. From this perspective, infertility is an important health issue requiring medical solutions (e.g., infertility treatments) to "fix" the problem. This position is promoted by those who believe that such treatments should be covered under provincial health care insurance plans.

### INFERTILITY AS A SOCIAL CONDITION

Infertile couples seeking assisted reproduction have a strong desire to have a child as genetically closely related to them as possible (Schiedermayer, 1988). Some perceive this desire or need to have biological children as being socially constructed or influenced. The stigma and emotional pain experienced by infertile couples often results from the strong pressure placed on married couples, and most especially women, to bear children (Government of Canada, 1996).

Descriptions of some reproductive technologies follow.

*Therapeutic Donor Insemination*

Therapeutic donor insemination (TDI) is the oldest form of assisted reproduction available. Sperm from a healthy donor is introduced into the fertile woman's uterus. This approach is used when the male partner is infertile or when a single woman, or a lesbian couple, wants a child without association with the biological father. Sperm donors are required to undergo extensive screening for infection and genetic disease.

Donor insemination (DI) technologies raise ethical questions associated with confidentiality, disclosure, screening, and the nature of relationships. Presently, the donor insemination process is confidential. Advocates for this approach suggest that the numbers of donors would decrease if donors' identities were to be revealed to the recipients and their children. Other concerns arise associated with disclosure to the child regarding the nature of the conception and the identity of the biological father, especially if the child experiences medical problems of a hereditary nature. The confidentiality status of this procedure may change as these offspring become adults and assert their right to know the background of their biological parent. Consider a child who develops leukemia and needs a bone marrow transplant. Would breaking rules of confidentiality be justified if the biological father might be a bone marrow donor?

*In Vitro Fertilization*

**In vitro fertilization** (IVF) was developed to overcome various physical conditions associated with infertility that traditional forms of artificial insemination cannot address. These conditions include mechanical obstructions resulting from damaged or absent fallopian tubes, endometriosis, intractable ovulatory problems, unexplained infertility, and some forms of male infertility resulting in low sperm count (Fluker & Tuffin, 1996).

IVF is a process whereby fertilization occurs outside the body and without the need for sexual intercourse. The procedure involves a series of interventions that begin with the use of drugs to hyperstimulate the ovaries to produce excess eggs, followed by the laparoscopic aspiration of these eggs with the guidance of ultrasound. The retrieved eggs are then mixed with the partner's (or donor's) sperm in a Petri dish in the laboratory. After approximately 48 hours, about three of the successfully fertilized eggs (embryos) are transferred into the woman's uterus. The remaining embryos may be cryopreserved (see below) and, if necessary, used at a later date, although this practice raises questions about what to do with any unused frozen embryos (Fluker & Tuffin, 1996). Who owns the embryos? What happens if one of the partners dies? Should the embryos be destroyed, or does the remaining partner have the right to use them? Custody debates over frozen embryos have also arisen in divorce proceedings. There is a recent instance of this in Oregon, where the state's Court of Appeal declared that a divorced wife had the right to dispose of frozen embryos that had been created with her husband's sperm during their marriage (see *Re Dahl and Angle*, 2008). In that case, the agreement between the clinic that provided the storage and retrieval service for the embryos and the husband and wife stipulated that if the spouses could not agree, the wife would have the right to decide on proper disposal.

There is great debate about these challenging questions, but little consensus on their resolution.

### Cryopreservation

The number of embryos transplanted into the uterus is usually limited to three in order to maximize the rate of success and to limit the risk of multiple births. Any additional embryos are usually maintained in liquid nitrogen for future use, if necessary, in a process known as **cryopreservation**. This minimizes the need for further invasive and costly procedures to retrieve eggs. Most programs limit the duration of storage, based on a certain number of years, the onset of a client's menopause, or the breakup of a relationship. However, only about 50% of embryos survive the thawing process (Fluker & Tuffin, 1996). Sperm, too, can be frozen for future use.

### Egg Donation

A variation of IVF, egg donation is used to enable pregnancies in women with normal uteruses but nonfunctioning ovaries. The eggs are donated from healthy, usually younger, donors, who undergo ovarian stimulation, or from women with normal functioning ovaries who are participating in the IVF program. The recipient undergoes the transfer component of the process once the partner's (or donor's) sperm fertilizes the egg (Fluker & Tuffin, 1996). The donor may be known to the recipient or may be part of an anonymous donor program.

### Embryo Donation

Since cryopreservation now enables the freezing of embryos for use in the future, issues arise around what to do with these when they are no longer needed or wanted by the couple. There is apparently a growing inventory of surplus embryos. The options are to destroy them, to use them for research purposes, or to donate them to other couples (Robertson, 1995).

When is there a need for **embryo donation**? This option may be desirable when neither partner is fertile but the woman has sufficient uterine capacity for pregnancy and childbirth. It may also be an option for older, single women who are no longer producing eggs, for lesbian couples for whom sperm donation has not worked, and for couples who cannot afford IVF or egg donation (Robertson, 1995).

A number of ethical issues arise out of the question of whether embryo donation or embryo "adoption" should be an option for couples when both partners are infertile. Should the process be treated similarly to adoption, with similar legal processes, screening, and rules? For example, should recipients undergo the same social and psychological testing to ensure they are fit parents (Robertson, 1995)? Further questions relate to whether the donor couple should be informed about the outcome (positive or negative) of the donation and whether their anonymity should be maintained (Robertson, 1995).

*Gestational Surrogacy*

Surrogate or gestational mothers bear a child for another couple or individual. The gestational mother may be the biological mother (through sperm donation of either the male partner or a donor) or may carry the embryo of the couple, an embryo donated by another couple, or one created from a donor egg and donor sperm. This approach may be considered by infertile couples who have experienced multiple failures with IVF, or by women who have a medical condition that limits pregnancy or an anatomical condition that causes repeated spontaneous abortions, or who have undergone a hysterectomy (Robertson, 1995).

Though surrogacy itself is not a technology, the many possible approaches to it raise complex ethical and emotional issues. These arise in part from the sheer number of parties involved (the infant, the surrogate mother, the infertile couple, society as a whole). Other issues related to surrogacy involve concerns regarding the surrogates' own reproductive future; their producing offspring with whom they will not be involved; the appropriateness of the recipients to raise the child; the process of informed consent; and the possibility of coercion, especially when financial remuneration is a factor (Sherwin, 1992).

The following case scenario highlights only a few of the complex ethical issues associated with reproductive technologies.

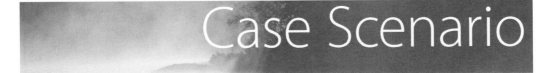

# Case Scenario

## PARENTHOOD—A RIGHT OR A PRIVILEGE?

Marion is a 30-year-old woman with cystic fibrosis who is involved in a lesbian relationship with Sandra, 15 years her senior. They would like to have a child. Sandra has been tested and determined to be infertile. Though Marion is fertile, her medical condition places her at high risk during pregnancy and delivery.

Sandra is a successful lawyer, and Marion inherited some money from her parents. Since the couple can afford the technology, they present themselves at an infertility clinic, where they are interviewed by a nurse and an infertility specialist.

Marion and Sandra ask for IVF. They would like eggs from Marion's ovaries to be retrieved and fertilized by donor semen. Once there is successful fertilization, they would like the embryos transplanted into Sandra's healthy uterus. Since Marion is concerned about passing on the genes for cystic fibrosis, they also request genetic testing on the embryos, and the destruction of any having those characteristics.

continued on following page >>

## Issues

1. Reflecting on your values, what is your response to this situation? Should your response influence your approach to supporting and counselling this couple?
2. What ethical and social questions does this case raise for you?
3. What are the rights of the various parties: the couple, the nurse and physician, the potential donor, and the offspring?
4. How will these emerging technologies influence the future of society?
5. How might various cultures view this scenario and the opportunities this technology offers?
6. What is the nursing role, and what should the nature of the nursing relationship be to this couple?

## Discussion

This case highlights the extent of ethical challenges associated with this new science. On the surface it would appear that only good can result from this couple's request. They would have the privilege of parenthood, and the resulting child or children would have the opportunity of life. Yet, a number of questions have raised debate about this field.

What are the rights of the two women in this case scenario? Is procreation a right or a privilege? Is it a privilege only granted to those who are physically able to procreate? What constitutes "good" parents? Is one parent enough? What are the rights of the potential child? Should criteria be established to screen potential parents? Should this couple's status as lesbians be a factor? What about the fact that one parent, Sandra, is older and that Marion is likely to have a short life expectancy because of her disease? Should the donor have any say relative to potential recipients of his sperm? What should Sandra and Marion tell their child, or children, when asked about the biological father? Should the donor process remain private and anonymous? Is it fair that this technology is available only to affluent people? Should health professionals be using genetic technology to screen out abnormalities such as cystic fibrosis, or further, to manipulate physical characteristics such as sex or hair and eye colour? (People with even minor disabilities are concerned about the negative social attitudes that may emerge as we attempt to create "perfect" humans.) Is it right to destroy "imperfect" embryos? Who would be the legal mother of this child? Who should have custody if the two women separate? What should be done with the surplus embryos? If the couple chose to donate them, should the recipients be told about the potential for genetic abnormalities? If the donated embryos produced an abnormal child, would Marion and the medical team bear any legal liability? Would that child have the right to know about his or her origins and other siblings?

The issues that arise from these technologies are endless, and the answers are not clear. The potential impact on future generations is daunting.

continued on following page >>

## Legislative Perspectives

As mentioned, to deal with the legislative and regulatory void in this rapidly evolving area of biotechnology, Parliament enacted the *Assisted Human Reproduction Act* in 2004 (portions of which have been recently declared unconstitutional by the Quebec Court of Appeal and may not be enforceable in that province). This federal statute recognizes and declares that:

(a) the health and well-being of children born through the application of assisted human reproductive technologies must be given priority in all decisions respecting their use;

(b) the benefits of assisted human reproductive technologies and related research for individuals, for families and for society in general can be most effectively secured by taking appropriate measures for the protection and promotion of human health, safety, dignity and rights in the use of these technologies and in related research;

(c) while all persons are affected by these technologies, women more than men are directly and significantly affected by their application and the health and well-being of women must be protected in the application of these technologies;

(d) the principle of free and informed consent must be promoted and applied as a fundamental condition of the use of human reproductive technologies;

(e) persons who seek to undergo assisted reproduction procedures must not be discriminated against, including on the basis of their sexual orientation or marital status;

(f) trade in the reproductive capabilities of women and men and the exploitation of children, women and men for commercial ends raise health and ethical concerns that justify their prohibition; and

(g) human individuality and diversity, and the integrity of the human genome, must be preserved and protected. (*Assisted Human Reproduction Act*, 2004, s. 2)

The Act makes it illegal to clone a human being or to create any life form that is a hybrid of a human and another animal species. It also bans, among other things, the use of assisted reproductive technologies for the purpose of sex selection or the transplanting of human genetic material or an embryo that was previously transplanted into a nonhuman life form.

The Act also bans the payment of money to any woman for a surrogacy arrangement or to arrange for the services of a surrogate mother. It is also illegal to counsel a woman under the age of 21 to become a surrogate mother or to perform a procedure on such a person for the purposes of assisting her to become a surrogate mother (*Assisted Human Reproduction Act*, 2004, s. 6). The Act also makes it illegal to purchase embryos, sperm, or ova, or to advertise sale of such items (*Assisted Human Reproduction Act*, 2004, s. 7). The Act licenses controlled activities aimed at creating a human embryo. The Act may be exempted from application in provinces in which the federal government is satisfied that an equivalent provincial statute is in force.

## Special Considerations Regarding Fertility Preservation in Patients With Cancer

The situation of people with cancer deserves discussion, as the treatment of cancer poses a serious threat to fertility. Male fertility can be affected by:

- The disease itself
- Anatomic problems related to the disease or to treatment interventions, for example, surgery.
- Primary or secondary hormonal insufficiency
- Damage to or depletion of the germinal stem cells

Female fertility can be affected by:
- Treatment that causes a reduction in the primordial follicles
- Hormonal imbalance
- Interference in the functioning of the ovaries, fallopian tubes, uterus, or cervix
- The early onset of menopause

Evidence suggests that cancer survivors have identified an increased risk of emotional distress related to infertility. Though adoption is a consideration for those who become infertile, most people would prefer to have biological offspring when possible. Therefore, to prevent infertility, young women with cancer, in particular, sometimes choose a less toxic regimen of chemotherapy even though the chance of a recurrence may be higher.

Finding ways to restore fertility in men, women, and children with cancer is a factor in helping patients cope emotionally with their cancer diagnosis and treatment (European Society of Human Reproduction and Embryology [ESHRE] Task Force on Ethics and Law, 2004; Poirot, Martelli, Genestie, Golmard, Valteau-Couanet, Helardot, et al., 2007). In the meantime, sperm cryopreservation is an option available to most men. The biggest challenges, however, relate to finding methods to preserve fertility in women and pre-pubescent males and females.

### SPECIAL CONSIDERATIONS FOR CHILDREN WITH CANCER

Today, the majority of children with cancer can be expected to be cured and become long-term survivors (Jemal, Murray, Samuels, Ghafoor, Ward, & Thun, 2003; Goodwin, Oosterhuis, Kiernan, Hudson, & Dahl, 2007). With today's reproductive technologies, parents are in a position to influence the extent to which their children's fertility may be preserved. This is possible through the cryopreservation of sperm or eggs for future use. The following options are available for their consideration; however, they are not without ethical challenges.

*Sperm Cryopreservation*

Sperm cryopreservation in adolescent boys and young men is an option since sperm production occurs at the age of 13 or 14. However, there are significant implications for the adolescent, as this option of sperm collection requires masturbation. Depending on their developmental stage, some young men may be reluctant to proceed because of a lack of understanding of the purpose or because of emotional reactions such as embarrassment. Further, there may be issues associated with the young man's understanding of all the issues, which may affect a valid informed consent. Parental consent with the child's consent or assent may be necessary in these circumstances. Though postpubertal males are capable of ejaculation, the issue itself is highly sensitive. Therefore, the health provider's approach to these children needs to be supportive and sensitive of their stage of development. If ejaculation is not possible, then sperm extraction or aspiration via testicular biopsy may be an option, as is the case with prepubescent boys. These options, however, raise other challenges with respect to the child's understanding of the issues and whether they have truly and freely consented to the intervention (Bahadur, 2004; Robertson, 2005).

*Oophorectomy and Ovarian Cryopreservation*
Oophorectomy and ovarian cryopreservation can be offered for premenarcheal girls in advance of cancer treatment that might induce ovarian failure (Weintraub, Gross, Kadari, Ravitsky, Safran, Laufer, et al., 2007). There are two approaches to this option. Slices of the ovarian cortex may be grafted into tissue in the forearm, where the eggs would continue to mature. Ovarian tissue must be retrieved prior to treatment and grafted after treatment is completed. Later, in vitro fertilization is necessary to ensure conception. Alternatively, the tissue may be grafted to the remaining ovary or into the adjacent peritoneum, and pregnancy may occur spontaneously.

However, these options raise many challenging and complex questions around consent regarding future unknowns. When the eggs in the graft mature, what if the child dies before these eggs can be used? What are the options for donation? If donation takes place and is effective, what of the welfare of resulting offspring (Lee, Schover, Partridge, Patrizio, Wallace, Hagerty, et al., 2006)?

*Challenges Regarding Consent*
Considerations related to future fertility are highly stressful for the child and the parents. At a time when they are dealing with the trauma of a cancer diagnosis, they must also deal with the challenge of deciding what is in their child's best interest regarding his or her future ability to procreate. In this context, "best interest" includes both the present circumstance of minimizing risk and the child's future interest in procreation. There are some risks with fertility-preservation procedures, though minimal, so the parent must balance these with the possible future wishes of their child. For all procedures, the parent's consent is required, but, depending on the age and level of maturity of the child, his or her consent may also be necessary. Obtaining the child's agreement to such procedures may be challenging since young children may not be comfortable with or totally understand the discussions around them. However, although these circumstances may be difficult for a child, dealing with infertility once he or she has matured can be traumatic (Grundy, Larcher, Gosden, Hewitt, Leiper, Spoudeas, et al., 2001).

There are two phases to the consent process in these circumstances. By electing for the child to undergo fertility-preservation treatments, the parents are making a decision to ensure that their child's rights are held in trust so that in the second phase of the consent process he or she can exercise the right to have children or not (Grundy et al., 2001). In obtaining consent, there would need to be clarification of the risks associated with the procedure itself and details regarding future potential risks and benefits. An important consideration is the actual risk of sterilization associated with the cancer treatment.

## Regulating New Reproductive and Genetic Technologies: Setting Boundaries, Enhancing Health

A royal commission on new reproductive technologies was initiated in 1989 to examine the social, medical, legal, ethical, economic, and research implications of these new technologies (Government of Canada, 1996). The mandate of the royal commission, which issued its final report in November 1993, was to recommend policies and safeguards, and to direct special attention to the implications for women's reproductive health and well-being and the prevention of infertility (Government of Canada, 1996). The royal commission made 293 recommendations that focused on the prevention of infertility, the management of assisted reproduction, sex selection for nonmedical reasons, prenatal diagnosis techniques and gene therapy, judicial interventions in pregnancy and birth, and the use of fetal tissue (Government of Canada, 1996).

In response to the report, the federal government established a moratorium on the use of specific practices, established an advisory committee, and proposed a legislative framework intended to "protect the health and safety of Canadians, ensure the appropriate treatment of human reproductive materials and . . . protect the dignity and security of all persons, especially women and children" (Government of Canada, 1996). The strategy was to manage reproductive and genetic technologies through a plan that would prohibit unacceptable technologies and develop a legislated regulatory process to manage technologies deemed acceptable.

The moratorium in July 1995 focused on nine problematic areas. It was proposed that the following practices be prohibited:

- Sex selection for nonmedical purposes
- Buying and selling of eggs, sperm, and embryos
- Germ-line genetic alterations
- **Ectogenesis** (maintaining an embryo in an artificial womb)
- Cloning of human embryos
- Creation of animal–human hybrids
- Retrieval of sperm or eggs from cadavers or fetuses for fertilization and implantation, or research involving the maturation of sperm or eggs outside the body
- Commercial preconception or surrogacy arrangements

In the proposed legislative framework, additional practices were added (Government of Canada, 1996):

- Transfer of embryos between humans and other species
- Use of human sperm, eggs, or embryos for assisted reproduction or research without the informed consent of the donors
- Research on human embryos 14 days or more after conception
- Creation of embryos for research
- Offering to provide or to pay for prohibited services

Eventually, limited legislation regulating the use of embryos, fetal tissue, and human reproductive material (i.e., genetic material, sperm, and ova) was enacted in the form of the *Assisted Human Reproduction Act* (discussed in more detail earlier in this chapter), but apart from this, there has been no further legislative activity in this area. Nevertheless, under the *Assisted Human Reproduction Act*, all of the activities listed above are prohibited, and the use of human reproductive tissue and material is now regulated and licensed under the Act (subject, of course, to the recent declaration of unconstitutionality of much of this statute by the Quebec Court of Appeal—see the discussion above).

## Ethical Perspectives

FEMINIST VIEWS

Reproductive technologies are primarily practised on women's bodies and have implications for women's reproductive autonomy; thus, they are of strong interest to feminist thinkers. Feminists argue that the focus of the related ethical discussions has been too narrow, avoiding the broader social implications of these technologies' introduction (Sherwin, 1992). According to Susan Sherwin, a Canadian feminist, these practices must be evaluated "within the broader scheme of oppressive social structures" (Sherwin, 1992). She argues the need to explore the possibility that new approaches to reproduction will bring about "profound cultural change" and that their social, political, and economic effects also need to be evaluated (Sherwin, 1992). The lower social and economic status of many women may make them susceptible to the risks associated with reproductive technologies (especially the high risk of failure and the unknown long-term effects of the drugs used to hyperstimulate the ovaries). There is also a need to evaluate those social influences that contribute to the expectations placed on people, especially women, to procreate. Although the intention of these technologies is to give couples or individuals the right to reproductive choice, some feminists are concerned that, in practice, the actual control will belong to others, specifically the male-dominated medical profession (Sherwin, 1992; Overall, 1987).

Additional concerns arise from the potential to commercialize and, therefore, commodify women's reproduction. This possibility was underlined by the placement of an advertisement in a University of Toronto newspaper a number of years ago, seeking a white female, between the ages of 23 and 32, who was willing to donate her eggs for money. This ad was published in spite of the moratorium established by the royal commission. In fact, the going rate for egg donors in the United States in 1995 was about US$2400 (McIlroy, 1996).

### IMPLICATIONS FOR OFFSPRING

A number of known and unknown risks exist for the children who are produced through reproductive technologies. Thirty percent of IVF deliveries are multiple births; thus, these babies are at high risk for low birth weight or problems during delivery (Government of Canada, 1996). Further, little is known about the long-term effects on the resulting children of the drugs used throughout the procedure.

Legal uncertainties regarding family relationships may result in the future, since, in some situations, the legal parenthood of the child may be unclear or challenged. Inheritance, custody, access, and support issues may be raised in future years.

Some parents choose to keep their use of donor insemination secret from family members, friends, and the child, who is usually presented as their biological offspring. This practice has been encouraged in the past by many infertility programs. This conspiracy of silence means that many children born as a result of assisted reproduction do not even know the circumstances of their birth (Sherwin, 1992; Schiedermayer, 1988).

With regard to sperm donors, the present practice is to maintain the anonymity of the donor. Thus, if children conceived in this manner were made aware of the circumstances of their birth, they would not (as is the case with adoption) be able to find or contact their biological fathers. Anonymity is usually a factor in a male's decision to donate semen. There might be many legal and emotional difficulties for future donors if this practice were to change (Government of Canada, 1996).

### CONSENT

As we saw in Chapter 6, informed consent requires that the client, in this case, the recipient and donor, be fully informed of all material risks, uncertainties, and benefits and that the process be free from coercion. The last is especially important when surrogates or donors are friends or relatives, who may be subjected to personal pressures to participate. Factors influencing consent in the area of reproductive technologies include the emotional nature of the process and the psychological effects on both recipients and donors.

### FINANCIAL INCENTIVES

A major concern, for feminist thinkers in particular, is the potential exploitation of poor and middle-class women as breeders for the upper class (Zipper & Sevenhuijsen, 1987). Feminists note that, while women now can make their own reproductive choices, they are still forced to make these decisions under social conditions that remain controlled by men and that stress the importance of female fertility.

Presently, there is no payment to egg donors, although typically they are not required to bear the costs of the procedure. Ironically, men have long been paid for semen donation—a far less invasive procedure. Defenders of this practice claim that payment only covers expenses and that without such payment, the rate of donation would decrease.

Many current reproductive technologies are expensive and are not covered by the Canadian health care system. Thus, their availability is limited to those who are able to pay, creating inequity of access. Further, concerns may arise in the area of embryo donation when the decision to donate may be influenced by the prohibitive costs associated with cryopreservation.

PSYCHOLOGICAL IMPACT

What must be remembered is that reproductive technologies are new, evolving, and imperfect. Success rates are low, leaving potential parents at risk for feelings of extreme loss and grief. Nurses must help their clients deal with the pain associated with grief and mourning, as well as the psychological effects arising from the technological processes themselves.

These processes place a great burden on the relationships of the people involved. The drugs used to stimulate ovum production can cause emotional lability. The regimentation of the process, and the coldness of the environment for procreation, is at the opposite extreme of the normally private and intimate experience. Fear of failure adds further strain. Nurses must consider all these factors in the care that they provide. They need to understand the issues and be prepared to support and guide their clients through a difficult, emotionally charged process.

With the introduction of each new technology in this field, more possibilities, as well as more ethical questions, emerge. As we discuss the explosion of reproductive and genetic technologies, it is worth reflecting on the following statement by Dr. Bernard Dickens, a legal ethicist from the University of Toronto:

One may recall ... the words perceptively written in 1966 about artificial insemination, which were proven true ... and have significance in other reproductive means ... : "Any change in custom or practice in this emotionally charged area has always elicited a response from established custom and law of horrified negation at first; then negation without horror; then slow and gradual curiosity, study, evaluation, and finally a very slow but steady acceptance." (Dickens, 1987)

## The Low-Birth-Weight Neonate: Ethical Implications

Over the past 20 years, survival of extremely premature and low-birth-weight infants has improved significantly due to technological and therapeutic advances. Up until now, a relative marker for viability has been 26 weeks of gestation, though there is debate with respect to the "unknown" zone between 22 and 25 weeks of gestation. The futures of these infants are uncertain, and outcomes are difficult to predict. Some preterm infants have other complications, such as congenital heart disease, or genetic anomalies, which may contribute further to their morbidity and mortality. Some parents are aware of such problems in advance, since these conditions can be diagnosed in utero; others are not. Some may also be aware that their infant may be born prematurely. These circumstances further complicate the difficult choices that parents and the health care team must make in the best interests of these infants. For extremely preterm infants (<26 weeks of gestation), it is unclear whether resuscitation or comfort care is the best option (see the section in Chapter 8 regarding end-of-life care for neonates) (Hellmann, 2008).

Providing intensive care for neonates with high risk of severe impairment and the possibility of prolonged dying is a frequent ethical challenge, since their outcomes are difficult to predict. Time spent in the Neonatal Intensive Care Unit (NICU) also increases the risk of serious life-threatening complications related to long-term ventilation, invasive procedures, and exposure to infectious agents. The following summarizes some of the significant challenges such neonates may face.

NECROTIZING ENTEROCOLITIS (NEC)

NEC is an inflammatory bowel disease that affects 1 to 5% of neonates, and has a mortality of between 10 and 50%, depending on the gestational age of the infant. Neonates born at <36 weeks have the greatest incidence of NEC and the highest rates of mortality. Even those who survive have a great number of long-term sequelae.

The extent of bowel disease is a predictor of mortality, and morbidities include strictures, malabsorption, malnutrition, short gut syndrome, and liver failure as a complication of total parental nutrition, which is required with many of these infants. These complications, inflammation of the bowel, and necrosis also cause extreme pain. If the pain is not well managed at the onset, the children may be at high risk of future chronic pain (Pillai-Riddell, Stevens, McKeever, Gibbins, Asztalos, Katz, et al., 2008). Over the long term, these children may also have neurodevelopmental delays (Gibbins, Maddalena, Moulsdale, Garrard, Mohamed, Nichols, et al., 2006).

NEONATAL BOWEL OBSTRUCTION

Neonatal bowel obstruction may result as a consequence of congenital anomalies of the gastrointestinal tract, such as atresia or stenosis, or from acquired conditions, such as meconium plug syndrome, which is more common in premature infants, and paralytic ileus. Intestinal obstruction can lead to major problems, such as fluid and electrolyte imbalance, shock, sepsis, and renal failure (De Silva, Young, & Wales, 2006). These are potentially life-threatening complications that add to the complexities of care for preterm infants.

MORBIDITY AND MORTALITY

Over the past 20 years, the mortality rates in NICU have decreased due to advancements in technology. At the same time, morbidity and the incidence of long-term problems have risen (Levene, 2004). Hence, it is very challenging to determine the premature neonate's best interests, now and into the future. Though new drugs and therapies are available to treat the above complications and save the lives of smaller and sicker babies, they may face significant problems later in life.

The largest study to date of the long-term consequences of premature birth compared the long-term outcomes for infants born at fewer than 33 weeks' gestation with those born at term. The retrospective study reviewed 1.1 million single births in Norway from 1967 through 1988. The investigators followed all of these children until 2002 and a subset through to 2004. Most of the premature infants had good health and normal reproduction rates, though they were at a higher risk of infertility. They were also at greater risk for lung problems, disability, mental challenges, and delays in school. As expected, premature infants were more likely to die during their first year, but this risk of death did not subside as they aged. They showed a doubled risk of death from the ages of 1 through 5, with birth defects and cancer playing a strong role in causation. Prematurity was linked to lower levels of education, and women who had been premature had a higher risk of giving birth to a premature baby. However, since 1988, when the last of these children was born, there have been even greater advances in the care of such infants, and those born at an even lower gestational age are surviving, so it continues to be a challenge to predict survival and when—and if—problems will exist later in life (Swamy, Østbye, & Skjaerven, 2008).

## Challenging Decisions

In an environment in which existing and evolving technologies are available to support and sustain life, who should be deciding what is in the best interests of the infant? This is an extremely complex issue, as the choices made will also influence the future of the parents and existing or potential siblings. A child with complex challenges and disabilities will have a strong impact on the whole family into the future. At the same time, there is the potential of the life worth saving.

Decision making is always challenging when outcomes are uncertain and when the comfort and quality of life of someone is at stake, even more so in these emotionally charged circumstances. Parents who were anticipating with excitement the birth of a healthy child face an unexpected reality. Instead of basking in the joy of having given birth, they are asked to choose between possibly prolonging the dying of their infant and taking the chance that aggressive interventions will help their infant survive though future outcomes for him or her are uncertain (McAllister & Dionne, 2006).

A study undertaken by Orfali and Gordon (2004) compared a system that emphasized parental authority (in the United States) with a system in which the physicians make the decisions (France). Interestingly, the mothers in France were much more satisfied with the process and outcomes than those in the United States. The factors that influenced their higher levels of satisfaction indicated the importance of strong doctor–patient relationships, continuity of care, the presentation of information with little ambiguity, the emotional empathy of the health care team, and the mothers' belief that what was being done was best for their babies. In the United States, mothers indicated that a lot of information was provided to them but that the uncertainty of outcomes was always emphasized and that little support was given to assist them in decision making. Also shown was that the French mothers coped better with the death of their infants and almost never expressed feelings of dissatisfaction or guilt. This study suggests that a model that focuses entirely on principles—in this case, autonomy—does not respond to the needs of parents in this context. The conclusions of this study reinforced the importance of alternative approaches to ethical challenges that build on relationships of trust and care.

Parental choice must be respected, as parents have the moral and legal authority to ensure the best interests of their infant. However, the health care team should engage in a collaborative process with the parents and, through this, reach mutual agreement on the best course of action for the infant. In these extremely difficult circumstances, the parents are at their most vulnerable, and the serious illness of their infant may diminish their capacity to reason or enact their autonomy (Cassell, 2005). A team approach that ensures that all perspectives are shared, in which there is active listening and shared decision making, results in less guilt and doubt, and the belief that, in most circumstances, the right decision

# Case Scenario

## CONFLICT IN VALUES

Gillian, a registered nurse, works on a busy gynecology unit. One evening, two of her patients experience abortions. Sue, a 24-year-old single woman, has had a saline abortion, as she and her boyfriend decided late (at 16 weeks) that they did not wish to proceed with the pregnancy. The process was painful, and Sue found it disturbing to see the fetus. Afterward, she was tearful and unable to sleep.

Gillian's other patient, Linn, has spontaneously aborted at 24 weeks. She has just returned from having a D & C. Linn and her husband were part of the in vitro fertilization program at the hospital. This was her third pregnancy; she aborted each time. As there are no embryos left, she and her husband will have to begin the process again, and her obstetrician does not recommend this. Linn is also very upset and cannot sleep.

Gillian's time is limited. Now, she wonders which patient needs her most.

### Issues
1. What would you do in Gillian's situation? What principles would guide your actions?
2. Should both these patients be on the same unit? Should both have been assigned to Gillian?
3. What responsibilities do nursing leaders have to ensure that hospital environments and structures minimize ethical conflicts for nursing staff?

was made (McHaffie, Laing, Parker, & McMillan, 2001). From the beginning, these parents need a great deal of support from the health care team and, most especially, the nurses caring for their child.

In the NICU, parents are exposed to multiple health care professionals, whose approaches may vary, and technology that distances them from their infant. In fact, it may be weeks before it is safe for them to hold and comfort their infant. Breastfeeding is not an option, though pumping is encouraged since breast milk is important to the development of the infant. Infants can be in the NICU for weeks or months, so the continuity of relationships, processes, and information is vital to supporting the parents and other family members through this challenging experience. Nurses are essential to ensuring that a climate of caring and trust is established in order to ensure the well-being of the infant and to guide the mother and father in assuming their parenting roles, in spite of the many challenges they face (McAllister & Dionne, 2006).

## Summary

In this chapter, some of the complex technologies in health care today were described and the associated ethical challenges explored. These technologies have the ability to influence not only the creation of life but the nature of future persons and the potential to eliminate illness and disease.

There have been significant advancements in the areas of reproductive technologies, genetics, and life-sustaining therapies for extremely premature infants.

In a multicultural society such as Canada's, patients and their families come from many religious and cultural backgrounds, and may view the meaning of life from varying perspectives. Nurses must be sensitive to these differences and respectful of the values and beliefs of others.

Nurses must be aware of new technologies since they may influence practice and policy in many settings; for example, the field of reproductive sciences is no longer limited to clinical arenas that focus on reproduction. Nurses in, for example, oncology settings may now be exposed to these interventions and will be in a position to support their clients through the fertility process.

Genetics has the potential to influence practice in many settings, not only in the clinical arena but also in the community, and it is sure to have an impact on future policy development.

Premature neonates now have a greater chance of survival, but those who survive may have lifelong needs within the health care system.

New technologies have the potential to reshape society and redefine the nature of future generations.

# Critical Thinking

The following case scenarios are intended to facilitate further reflection, discussion, and analysis.

## I AM AFRAID: YES, I WANT TO HAVE BABIES WHEN I GROW UP

Lara is 9 years old and has just been diagnosed with leukemia. Indications are that she will likely be cured. However, the chemotherapy will definitely make her infertile.

The team offers her parents the opportunity to have Lara's ovarian tissue cryopreserved to ensure that her eggs develop in the future and hence to enable in vitro fertilization. Her parents are split over whether this should be done. Her mother, knowing that her daughter often talks about having babies, thinks this should be done. Her father disagrees, believing their daughter is going through enough.

They agree to discuss the options with Lara. Lara agrees she wants to have children when she grows up but cries when the procedure is described to her. She does not understand what a lot of this means but says she is afraid and does not want the surgery.

### Questions
1. What are the competing ethical issues in the scenario?
2. How can the parents decide what is in Lara's best interests?
3. How would you as the nurse support Lara and her parents through this highly emotional process so that they can make the best choice for their child?
4. If Lara was your child, what might you do?

## THE PERFECT CHILD

Xavier and Adelina tried for some time to conceive before they took the route of IVF. They were successful in the first attempt and have five healthy embryos. They have asked the health care team to test the embryos for positive traits and characteristics they might have inherited from the family. They would like a male embryo to be implanted first and a female frozen for later

continued on following page >>

use. Red hair is a recessive gene in the family, and, if possible, they would like a girl with red hair. They ask whether it is possible to predict the intelligence of their future children, as they would like to take that into consideration.

### Questions

1. Do you think these choices should be made available to these parents?
2. Do you think reproductive technologies have the possibility of influencing future generations?

## A LITTLE MORE TIME

Olivia is pregnant with her first child. Things have been going very well with her pregnancy, and she and her husband, Larry, are looking forward to meeting their baby. Olivia is 24 weeks into her pregnancy when she suddenly experiences severe abdominal pain. Larry rushes her to the hospital, where she is found to be in active labour and is rushed to Labour and Delivery. The health care team attempts to slow her labour, but they are not successful. Meanwhile, they do an emergency ultrasound to evaluate the baby's condition. They find that the baby has significant cardiac problems that, if not addressed immediately after birth, will result in death soon after. It is possible for the nearest pediatric centre that performs cardiac surgery to send a team to the hospital to resuscitate the baby and transport it immediately to the pediatric facility. For this option to be successful, Olivia will have to undergo a Caesarean section. The potential outcomes for the baby are not known.

Olivia and Larry are presented with another option. The baby can be delivered vaginally and receive palliative care.

One hour has passed since Olivia started to have abdominal pain. She and Larry have to make an immediate decision.

### Questions

1. What are the ethical issues associated with this scenario?
2. How can the health care team support the parents?
3. Who should be involved in the decision?
4. How might this decision be made? What are the factors to consider?

### Discussion Points

1. What are the major challenges related to genetics? Have you been exposed to genetic challenges in your practice?
2. Should society pay for all genetic screening? Should society pay for some? What kind?
3. Identify the key arguments in favour of new reproductive technologies. In your opinion, are these arguments valid? What are the opposing arguments?

4. How can exploitation of women be prevented as new reproductive technologies emerge? What concerns in this regard have been expressed by feminist thinkers?

5. How far should society go in regard to using technologies for the extremely premature infant? What potential technologies can you see coming in the future? Should scientists be working on the development of an artificial womb? What would be the implications of that?

## References

### Case Law

*Re Dahl and Angle*, Doc. DR04090713 A133697, Oct. 8, 2008.

*Renvoi fait par le gouvernement du Québec en vertu de la Loi sur les renvois à la Cour d'appel, L.R.Q., ch. R-23, relativement à la constitutionnalité des articles 8 à 19, 40 à 53, 60, 61 et 68 de la Loi sur la procréation assistée*, L.C. 2004, ch. 2 (Dans l'affaire du), 2008 QCCA 1167 (CanLII) (Quebec).

### Statutes

*Assisted Human Reproduction Act*, S.C. 2004, c. 2 (Canada).

*Trillium Gift of Life Network Act*, R.S.O. 1990, c. H.20 (Ontario).

### Texts and Articles

Bahadur, G. (2004). Ethics of testicular stem cell medicine. *Human Reproduction, 19*(12), 2702–2710.

Canadian Organization for Rare Disorders. (2006). Newborn screening in Canada status report. Toronto, ON: Author.

Cassell, E. J. (2005). Consent or obedience? Power and authority in medicine. *The New England Journal of Medicine, 352*(4), 328–330.

Chadwick, R. (2008). Genetic testing and screening. In P. A. Singer & A. M. Viens (Eds.), *The Cambridge textbook of bioethics*. Cambridge, England: Cambridge University Press.

Childress, J. F. (1997). *Practical reasoning in bioethics*. Bloomington, IN: Indiana University Press.

De Silva, N. T., Young, J. A., & Wales, P. W. (2006, September/October). Understanding neonatal bowel obstruction: Building knowledge to advance practice. *Neonatal Network: The Journal of Neonatal Nursing, 25*(5), 303–318.

Dickens, B. M. (1987). Artificial reproduction, infertility treatment and artificial conception. In G. Sharpe (Ed.), *The law and medicine in Canada* (2nd ed., p. 642). Toronto, ON: Butterworths.

European Society of Human Reproduction and Embryology Task Force on Ethics and Law. (2004, February). Ethical considerations for the cryopreservation of gametes and reproductive tissues for self use. *Human Reproduction, 19*(2), 460–462.

Fluker, M. R., & Tuffin, G. J. (1996). Assisted reproductive technologies: A primer for Canadian physicians. *Journal of the Society of Obstetrics and Gynecology Canada, 18*, 451–465.

Gibbins, S., Maddalena, P., Moulsdale, W., Garrard, F., Mohamed, T. J., Nichols, A., et al. (2006). Pain assessment and pharmacologic management for infants with NEC: A retrospective chart audit. *Neonatal Network: The Journal of Neonatal Nursing, 25*(5), 339–345.

Gibson, J. P. (1998, February/March). Cloning Daisy: The genetic future? *Info Holstein Newsletter.* Guelph, ON: University of Guelph.

Goodwin, T., Oosterhuis, E. B. Kiernan, M., Hudson, M. M., & Dahl, G. V. (2007). Attitudes and practices of pediatric oncology providers regarding fertility issues. *Pediatric Blood & Cancer, 48*(1), 80–85.

Government of Canada. (1996). *New reproductive and genetic technologies: Setting boundaries, enhancing health.* Ottawa, ON: Author.

Greenwood, H. L., & Daar, A. S. (2008). Regenerative medicine. In P. A. Singer, & A. M. Viens (Eds.), *The Cambridge textbook of bioethics* (p. 153). Cambridge, England: Cambridge University Press.

Grundy, R., Larcher, V., Gosden, R. G., Hewitt, M., Leiper, A., Spoudeas, H. A., et al. (2001). Fertility preservation for children treated for cancer (2): Ethics of consent for gamete storage and experimentation. *Archives of Disease in Childhood, 84*(4), 360–362.

Hellmann, J. (2008). *Autonomy and conflict in the neonatal intensive care unit.* Unpublished manuscript.

Jemal, A., Murray, T., Samuels, A., Ghafoor, A., Ward, E., & Thun, M. J. (2003). Cancer statistics. *CA: A Cancer Journal for Clinicians, 53,* 5–26.

Lee, S. J., Schover, L. R., Partridge, A. H., Patrizio, P., Wallace, W. H., Hagerty, K., et al. (2006). American Society of Clinical Oncology recommendations on fertility preservation in cancer patients. *Journal of Clinical Oncology, 24*(18), 2917–2931.

Levene, M. (2004, February). Is intensive care for very immature babies justified? *Acta Paediatrica, 93,* 149–152.

Mahowald, M. B. (1996). The brain and the I: Neurodevelopment and personal identity. *Journal of Social Philosophy, 27*(3), 49–60.

McAllister, M., & Dionne, K. (2006, September/October). Partnering with parents: Establishing effective long-term relationships with parents in the NICU. *Neonatal Network: The Journal of Neonatal Nursing, 25*(5), 329–337.

McHaffie, H. E., Laing, I. A., Parker, M., & McMillan, J. (2001). Deciding for imperiled newborns: Medical authority or parental autonomy? *Journal of Medical Ethics, 27,* 104–109.

McIlroy, A. (1996, April 8). Ottawa to regulate baby trade. *The Globe and Mail,* p. A1.

National Institutes of Health, U.S. Department of Health and Human Services. (2008). Stem cell basics. In Stem Cell Information. Retrieved January 7, 2009, from http://stemcells.nih.gov/info/basics/defaultpage

Orfali, K., & Gordon, E. J. (2004) Autonomy gone awry: A cross-cultural study of parents' experiences in neonatal intensive care units. *Theoretical Medicine, 25*(4), 329–365.

Overall, C. (1987). *Ethics and human reproduction.* Boston, MA: Allen & Irwin; Oakley, A. (1987). From walking wombs to test-tube babies. In M. Stanworth (Ed.). *Reproductive technologies: Gender, motherhood and medicine* (pp. 5–116). Minneapolis, MN: University of Minnesota Press.

Pillai-Riddell, R., Stevens, B., McKeever, P., Gibbins, S., Asztalos, E., Katz, J., et al. (2008). *Conceptualizing chronic pain in hospitalized infants: Health professional perspectives.* Manuscript submitted for publication.

Poirot, C. J., Martelli, H., Genestie, C., Golmard, J. L., Valteau-Couanet, D., Helardot, P., et al. (2007, July). Feasibility of ovarian tissue cryopreservation for prepubertal females with cancer. *Pediatric Blood & Cancer, 49*(1), 74–78.

Robertson, J. A. (1995, November). Ethical and legal issues in human embryo donation. *Fertility and Sterility, 64,* 885–894.

Robertson, J. A. (2005). Cancer and fertility: Ethical and legal challenges. *Journal of the National Cancer Institute Monographs, 34,* 104–106.

Schiedermayer, D. L. (1988, Fall). Babies made the American way: Ethics and interests of surrogate motherhood. *The Pharos of Alpha Omega Alpha-Honor Medical Society, 51*(4), 2–7.

Sherwin, S. (1992). *No longer patient: Feminist ethics and health care.* Philadelphia, PA: Temple University Press.

Shuman, C. (2008, April). Genetic counselling—Translating genetic information for patients and their families. Symposium conducted at the Canadian Medical Hall of Fame/Pfizer Canada Discovery Day in Health Sciences, University of Toronto, Toronto, ON.

Stanworth, M. (1987). Reproductive technologies and the deconstruction of motherhood. In M. Stanworth (Ed.), *Reproductive technologies: Gender, motherhood and medicine* (pp. 11–35). Minneapolis, MN: University of Minnesota Press.

Swamy, G. K., Østbye, T., and Skjaerven, R. (2008). Association of preterm birth with long-term survival, reproduction, and next-generation preterm birth. *Journal of the American Medical Association, 299*(12), 1429–1436.

U.S. Department of Energy Office of Science. (n.d.). Human Genome Project Information. Retrieved January 6, 2009, from http://www.ornl.gov/hgmis

Weintraub, M., Gross, E., Kadari, A., Ravitsky, V., Safran, A., Laufer, N., et al. (2007). Should ovarian cryopreservation be offered to girls with cancer? *Pediatric Blood & Cancer, 48*(1), 4–9.

Zipper, J., & Sevenhuijsen, S. (1987). Surrogacy and feminist notions of motherhood. In M. Stanworth (Ed.), *Reproductive technologies: Gender, motherhood and medicine* (pp. 118–138). Minneapolis, MN: University of Minnesota Press.

# Chapter 10

## Patient Rights

### Learning Objectives

The purpose of this chapter is to enable you to understand:

- The rights and responsibilities of patients and the obligations of health care professionals
- A person's right to confidentiality and the conditions under which disclosure is permitted
- A patient's right to information, respect, and discharge from a health care facility
- A patient's right to safety within the health care environment

## Introduction

INDIVIDUALS USING CANADA'S HEALTH care systems have the right to respect, privacy, and confidentiality; to be told the truth; and to give or refuse informed consent. Also, as explained in Chapter 6, persons have the rights to refuse treatment (or to request that it be withdrawn) and to die with dignity. When an individual has a right, then others have an obligation to ensure that right is protected.

Nurses are obliged to ensure that patients' rights are respected and upheld. As they fulfill their responsibilities as caregivers, nurses advocate on behalf of their patients and clients, especially those who are unable to speak for themselves. These obligations are clearly expressed throughout the CNA's *Code of Ethics for Registered Nurses*:

Nurses question and intervene to address unsafe, non-compassionate, unethical or incompetent practice or conditions that interfere with their ability to provide safe, compassionate, competent and ethical care to those to whom they are providing care, and they support those who do the same." (Canadian Nurses Association [CNA], 2008, p. 9)

Many agencies and health care organizations demonstrate their commitment and respect for patient rights through the publication of a bill of rights or through their mission statement. Others adopt the values of a professional code such as the *Code of Ethics for Registered Nurses*.

In this chapter the relationship between rights and obligations is clarified and illustrations are provided to demonstrate the important rights of patients and clients within the health care system.

## What Is a Right?

A **right** is a claim or privilege to which one is justly entitled, either legally or morally. Legal rights make explicit an individual's claim to such entitlement. For example, one explicit right under the *Canadian Charter of Rights and Freedoms* is the freedom of an individual to think, say, write, or otherwise act in accordance with his or her beliefs (*Charter of Rights and Freedoms*, 1982). This suggests another aspect of rights—that is, autonomy, or the right to act on one's own, free of interference or control by the state or others. However, this right is not absolute. Laws also regulate the behaviour of citizens, and this somewhat limits the freedom of each citizen to do as he or she pleases.

A right carries a corresponding **obligation**. For example, in the context of health care, if someone has the right to access care, then another person (or, more often, the state) has the corresponding obligation to provide that care. Otherwise, the right becomes meaningless.

The rights of patients are made explicit and clear through standards contained in professional codes of ethics. These impose an obligation on health care professionals to provide a minimum standard of safe and competent care to patients.

Legal rights are enforced by individuals through court action—that is, through the coercive power of the state to compel individuals to act or refrain from acting in particular ways. Chapter 4 describes the basic legal and political rights and freedoms held by Canadians under the *Charter of Rights and Freedoms* and in various statutes of Parliament and the provincial legislatures.

Moral rights include the right to be treated with respect for one's autonomy. In a health care context, patients have the moral right to be informed not only of the risks of treatment (for purposes of granting or refusing informed consent) but they also have the right to more general information as to what the facility and its caregivers can and cannot do. This would include information about the condition of a patient's health, the treatment resources and alternatives available, the role of the facility's health care professionals, the proposed treatment plan, and the plan of care after discharge. Of course, this also includes the patient's right to refuse or otherwise control the information he or she receives.

These rights are not all necessarily formally recognized in law, but they are acknowledged as societal norms of the Canadian culture. They are based on the ethical principles of autonomy, beneficence, and nonmaleficence (as discussed in Chapter 2). That is, the patient has the ultimate right to make any and all decisions respecting treatment. These rights are enforced, not necessarily through the courts but through the maintenance of practice standards and the ethical values and rules practised by health care professionals every day. If necessary, however, these rights could be enforced through court action in civil negligence or criminal proceedings, should their breach bring harm to the patient.

## What Are the Responsibilities of the Patient or Client?

Not all rights are absolute, and they come with responsibilities. Patients or clients have responsibilities to themselves, the professionals caring for them, the health care organization, and the system, which include treating others with respect, respecting the privacy of other patients or clients, and disclosing information appropriate for safe care.

When patients do not agree, for example, with the treatment provided or the medication prescribed, they should disclose their concerns to their health care professionals so that a more appropriate plan can be put in place. It is not respectful, and it may be unsafe, to decide not to follow a treatment plan without communicating this to the team. At the same time, health care profesionals must listen to their patients' concerns about treatment plans and work with them to resolve their concerns.

Patients also have a responsibility to meet certain standards, which may include:

- Calling ahead if an appointment needs to be cancelled so that another patient may be scheduled
- Arriving on time, having followed instructions related to a treatment or procedure, such as a bowel prep for a colonoscopy and abstaining from food and fluids prior to anesthesia

- Respecting the needs of other patients (for example, maintaining a peaceful and quiet environment and managing visitors appropriately)

Some organizations post patients' responsibilities, along with a patient bill of rights (Dana-Farber Cancer Institute, n.d.; Canadian Pain Coalition, 2008; Settlement.Org, 2008). In academic environments, students' role in providing care as part of their learning experience should be posted.

## What Are Obligations?

We have noted that moral and legal rights carry corresponding obligations for others. An **obligation** is anything that a person must do or refrain from doing in order to permit the full exercise of the rights of another. For example, in order for a patient to exercise the right to make an informed consent, the health care professional charged with that person's care is obliged to ensure that all relevant information has been provided, that the patient has been told of all relevant material risks and consequences inherent in the procedure, and that the patient's questions and concerns have been answered to the best of the health care professional's ability.

The health care practitioner must also ensure that he or she acts in a professional manner and observes all applicable standards of practice. These include the obligation to be informed and aware of the latest developments in his or her area of practice, to maintain up-to-date knowledge and competency, and to treat patients with respect, dignity, and courtesy.

## Informed Consent

The right to informed consent has been discussed at length in Chapter 6. This is not only a legal but also a moral right based on the ethical principles of autonomy, individual respect, respect for self-determination, and the right of individuals to make decisions about the course of their lives. In order to exercise these rights, patients must be fully informed regarding their health condition, prognosis, and treatment options, together with the consequences and risks. Lack of information, or the giving of incorrect or insufficient information, deprives the patient of the right to make a truly informed decision about the course of treatment. As discussed in previous chapters, the provision of treatment without a fully informed consent can lead to legal liability for negligence—even battery, if no consent was given.

As discussed earlier, the *Code of Ethics for Registered Nurses* makes explicit the rights of patients to control their own care: "Nurses recognize, respect and promote a person's right to be informed and make decisions" (CNA, 2008, p. 11). Nurses have a responsibility to inform patients of the nursing care available to them and to welcome patients as active participants in their own care. The patient also has the right to know the extent of the assessment that the health care agency is performing.

# Case Scenario

## A LEARNER'S RIGHT?

Ming has consented to have vaginal polyps removed. Her gynecologist has explained the procedure in detail. Ming is also aware that while she is under the anesthetic, she will undergo a thorough pelvic exam. However, the gynecologist has not told her specifically that there will be nursing and medical students present during the procedure. This is a teaching hospital, and all patients are expected to be informed, when they are admitted, of the role of students.

Third-year medical students are present during Ming's procedure. To give them experience in conducting pelvic exams, the gynecologist allows three of them to undertake separate examinations. Roger, the circulating nurse, expresses his concerns about this to the gynecologist, who tells Roger that Ming has consented to the examination and that there is nothing wrong with giving the students some experience. How else are they going to learn?

### Issues
1. Who is right?
2. In the circumstances, is Ming's consent to this examination legally and morally valid?
3. Were any of Ming's rights violated?
4. What should Roger do?
5. What is the hospital's responsibility?
6. How may appropriate learning experiences for students be ensured?

### Discussion
Chapter 6 explores the elements and aspects of a truly informed consent. Not only must the consent be informed; it must also be free of undue interference by others. There must be no coercion, inducement, or other pressure placed upon the patient to give the necessary consent, nor should the patient be forced to receive information that he or she does not wish to receive. Any fraud perpetrated on the patient to obtain consent would vitiate (negate) it.

As part of the obligation to provide general information, the health care team should, upon a patient's admission to a health care facility, provide him or her with an orientation to the roles of the caregivers, their functions, the physical layout of the unit, and the unit's routines, procedures, and schedules. This orientation should include information about promoting health and preventing disease. Such information is usually provided by primary care nurses (in a clinical setting) and community nurses (such as those in public health).

continued on following page >>

In the case of teaching hospitals, patients should be made aware of the role of students within the facility and the nature of their relationships within the health care team. However, a general overview of the involvement of students (e.g., interns, residents, student nurses) does not fulfill the additional obligation to provide more explicit information in particular circumstances in which the patient may be at greater risk (such as a medical student's performing a thoracentesis for the first time or a nursing student's establishing his or her first intravenous) or if their privacy will be invaded (such as the students' being present during a vaginal examination). For example, patients should be informed when residents are to play a primary role during an operative procedure. In our case scenario, the gynecologist had an obligation to inform Ming and to seek her consent to allow the students this learning opportunity. Teaching hospitals should ensure that processes are in place to meet this standard.

## Right to Health Information and Teaching

Nurses across the system are expected to facilitate a smooth, safe, effective transition to the community for the patient and family (for example, nursing standards ensure nurses inform clients that home care resources are available and are initiated in a timely way). Further, nurses are required to provide discharged patients with the knowledge and skills to care for themselves (to the extent that they are able) after they are released from the hospital. When the patient is not able to provide self-care, family members or friends may be involved. Client teaching might include information on nutrition, the proper use and maintenance of medical equipment, the proper administration of medication, and the changing of dressings. Clients should also be given a means of seeking further information.

Knowledge of how to gain access to the health care system is invaluable to all clients. Nurses can provide a service by informing clients about the workings of the system, treatment alternatives and facilities, alternatives to traditional Western medical care, and so forth. For discharged or older patients, providing information as to available home care services is essential. Where incompetent patients are concerned, nurses should discuss these matters with the substitute decision maker(s). This is important, as the nurse involved in the day-to-day care of such a patient will be intimately aware of all aspects of his or her treatment and progress—what is and is not effective—and will be able to relate this information to the family, the decision maker, or both. This will also enable the substitute decision maker to make better-informed treatment decisions in the patient's best interests.

One challenge that nurses may face is a patient's request for a diagnosis. In such a situation, the nurse must proceed carefully. In Ontario, for example, under the *Regulated Health Professions Act* (1991, s. 27(2), p. 1), "communicating to the individual or his or her personal representative a diagnosis identifying a disease or disorder as the cause of symptoms . . . in circumstances in which it is reasonably foreseeable that the individual or his or her personal representative will rely on the diagnosis" is a **controlled act**. The nurse would be permitted to make a diagnosis according to the rules and regulations governing the delegation of controlled acts only if authorized to do so under the *Nursing Act* (1991), as the holder of one of the following:

- An extended certificate (which allows the holder to deliver an expanded scope of nursing practice, including prescription of tests and treatments, assessments, diagnoses, and health promotion that holders of the regular class of certificate do not have the ability to do)
- A primary health care specialty certificate
- A pediatrics specialty certificate
- An adult specialty certificate
- An anesthesia specialty certificate

Ontario's *Nursing Act* (1991) includes the communication of a diagnosis among those controlled acts that may lawfully be performed by a primary-care nurse practitioner (*Expanded Nursing Services for Patients Act*, 1997). Other provinces may or may not legally restrict the making of a diagnosis, for example, in their medical professional statutes.

Ethical challenges for nurses arise when physicians refuse to communicate a diagnosis to a patient, for example, to protect the patient from emotional harm. If the nurse is aware of the diagnosis, should he or she inform the patient, regardless of the physician's refusal? In such a case, the nurse, as advocate for the patient, should endeavour to influence the physician, stressing the patient's right to be informed. If this strategy is not effective, the nurse may have to turn to the physician's superiors or higher authorities in the health care facility. In most cases, in answering a patient's question, the nurse need not entail the communication of a diagnosis but simply the confirmation of what the patient sees as self-evident. For example, suppose that a female patient was previously told that she may have breast cancer. Surgery is performed to explore the extent of the tumour and to remove it. The patient, once awake in the Recovery Room, asks the attending nurse whether a tumour was found and if so how much, if any, of her breast was removed. She already feels some pain from the incision and knows that her breast does not feel right. The patient's physician has left for the day without having had a chance to talk to her about the results of the operation. Should the patient be left in suspense while awaiting the physician's return? The nurse, by exercising professional judgement, could properly confirm the patient's suspicions to ease her mind and lessen the emotional stress of not knowing. The nurse should be prudent, exercise judgement, and consider all the alternatives, including paging the physician to return to discuss the situation with the patient.

## Cardiopulmonary Resuscitation

Special challenges are also posed by no-CPR (no cardiopulmonary resuscitation) and DNR (do not resuscitate) directions from a patient, which must be respected as part of the patient's autonomous right to refuse treatment. Consider the following scenario:

# Case Scenario

## A DIGNIFIED DEATH—WHOSE CHOICE?

Geoff, an 18-year-old man, is dying of lymphoma. He has expressed his wish to die at home. All aggressive treatment attempted so far has failed, and for the past few weeks, Geoff has been receiving palliative care at home.

One night, Geoff experiences sudden shortness of breath. His family panics and calls 911. By the time the ambulance team arrives, he has settled, but the attendants insist he be taken to the closest emergency department. Geoff is admitted to a medical unit while the physician on call attempts to locate his primary physician.

Meanwhile, as two of the nurses are settling him into his room, Geoff stops breathing. The nurses, aware of his history, are faced with a dilemma. His family is outside in the waiting room. Since the nurses have not heard from the primary physician, they do not have a no-CPR order. They have two choices: They can call a code and perform CPR, or they can invite Geoff's family into the room and give them some privacy.

### Issues

1. What are Geoff's rights in this situation?
2. How would the policy in your institution (if applicable) guide you in this scenario?
3. What is the role of policy in assisting nurses to make the right decision?
4. What is the right decision in this case, legally and ethically?

### Discussion

A distinction should be made between "no CPR" and "DNR." The latter is a broader concept that includes any treatment given to sustain life (e.g., blood transfusion, artificial ventilation, dialysis, antibiotic therapy). CPR is limited to the technique of compressing the patient's chest without applying artificial ventilation. It is important to document carefully the precise nature of the patient's wishes (or those of the substitute decision maker) in this respect. The order withholding CPR in no way limits the administration of other treatment to which the patient has not withheld consent.

Some caregivers may feel that honouring the patient's wishes regarding resuscitation conflicts with the principles of beneficence and nonmaleficence—that is, to promote the patient's well-being and prevent harm. Certain guidelines have been developed to resolve such conflicts. These guidelines are similar to those followed in other treatment situations and outlined, for example, in Saskatchewan's *Health Care Directives and Substitute Health Care Decision Makers Act* (1997) and Ontario's *Substitute Decisions Act* (1992).

continued on following page >>

In a situation like Geoff's, the patient should first be assessed to determine whether his or her life would likely be prolonged by the intervention of CPR. When possible, the results of the assessment should be disclosed to the patient, and his or her wishes obtained and respected. The course of action to be followed, and any discussions held among caregivers, the patient, and the patient's family with respect to the decision, should be carefully documented in the patient's chart. Further, the reasons for the decision should be documented and communicated directly to the health care team. The no-CPR decision should be reviewed at regular intervals decided upon by the decision maker, either the patient or his or her substitute. It should also be communicated to the health care team of any other unit to which the patient is subsequently transferred.

In cases in which the patient is incompetent, his or her advance directive should be respected, subject to any changes expressed by the patient after making it. Such changes should be documented and made known to the attending physician. If there is no advance directive and no substitute decision maker appointed, the decision to implement or withhold CPR will be made by others on the basis of their knowledge of the patient's values and wishes.

In this case scenario, the information available to the nurses indicates that Geoff and his family had accepted the inevitability of his death. Geoff chose a course of action inconsistent with aggressive medical intervention. Clearly, he had chosen to die in his own environment, close to his family and friends. Policies are meant to guide action. Rigid adherence to "rules" in every circumstance may, in fact, contradict good judgement and conflict with individual choice.

## Right to Confidentiality

In some circumstances, a patient's right to confidentiality may conflict with the health care professional's broader obligations to provide care and to prevent harm.

### Statutory Duty of Disclosure

In many provinces, statute law requires certain patient information and conditions to be disclosed. For example, many public health laws require health care professionals to disclose to their local medical officer of health (usually employed in the municipality by a local board of health or other such authority) the identity of anyone diagnosed with certain communicable or sexually transmitted diseases (such as gonorrhoea and HIV/AIDS, among others). This is especially important with respect to HIV/AIDS. (See Alberta: *Communicable Diseases Regulation*, Alta. Reg. 238/85, sched. 4, "Human Immunodeficiency Virus (HIV) Infections,"; British Columbia: *Health Act Communicable Disease Regulation*, B.C. Reg. 4/83, sched. A; Manitoba: *Diseases and Dead Bodies Regulation*, Man. Reg. 338/88 R, Part II; New Brunswick: N.B. Reg. 86-66, s. 94(1)(s); Newfoundland and Labrador: *Communicable Diseases Act*, R.S.N.L. 1990, c. C-26, sched.; Nova Scotia: *Reporting of Notifiable Diseases and Conditions Regulations*, N.S. Reg. 195/2005, sched. A; Ontario: R.R.O. 1990, Reg. 569, s. 5, as amended; Prince Edward Island: *Notifiable and Communicable Diseases Regulations*,

# Case Scenario

## CONFLICTING OBLIGATIONS

Jim is a 34-year-old man who is well known to the community health centre that he and his family have attended for several years. He is married and has two young children. His wife is eight months pregnant. He is a computer salesman and spends much time away from home travelling to see clients across the country.

A few weeks ago, Jim presented to the clinic complaining of generalized fatigue and lethargy. He had recently lost five kilograms and had noticed some unusual lesions on his inner thighs. As part of the blood screening done at that time, an HIV test was undertaken. It turned out to be positive. Given his clinical picture, it was likely that he had already developed AIDS.

Jim's primary care nurse is present when his physician relays the bad news to him. Clearly distraught, Jim admits that he has had sexual intercourse with a number of women during his business trips and, on several occasions, did not bother to use a condom. Fearful of the effects that this revelation would have on both his family and his business contacts, Jim pleads with his caregivers to keep this information, and his diagnosis, confidential. Given his wife's pregnancy, he feels this knowledge might cause her undue harm. He assures them that he and his wife have not had intercourse since her pregnancy. He refuses any treatment for his AIDS-related symptoms since it would make the diagnosis obvious to everyone. Instead, he asks that his family, including his wife, be told that he has terminal and incurable cancer. Jim's physician (who is also his friend) says that he will respect Jim's wishes for now.

## Issues

1. Did the clinic have the right to test Jim for HIV without his knowledge or consent?
2. Should the health care team keep Jim's diagnosis confidential from his wife?
3. Should the fact that Jim's wife is also the clinic's patient influence their actions and decisions?
4. What about the potential risks to the fetus and infant once born?
5. Does the team have an obligation to follow Jim's instructions and misrepresent his diagnosis to others?
6. If the primary care nurse disagrees with the decision of the physician, what can he or she do?

## Discussion

The patient has the right to know the extent of the assessment that the agency is performing. In some provinces, public health laws require that a health care agency obtain consent for HIV testing.

continued on following page >>

The primary legal rule with respect to any information that the health care practitioner obtains from the patient during the course of their professional relationship is that such information is confidential and may not be disclosed to anyone who has no valid purpose for requesting it. There are exceptions to this rule, both in common law and as provided by statute. But, as discussed in Chapter 5, in many provinces, the improper disclosure of confidential information about a patient constitutes professional misconduct. (See New Brunswick: *Nurses Act*, S.N.B. 1984, c. 71, s. 42(1); Northwest Territories: *Nursing Profession Act*, S.N.W.T. 2003, c. 15, s. 32(2)(d); Ontario: *Professional Misconduct Regulation*, O. Reg. 799/93, s. 1, para. 10; Saskatchewan: *Registered Nurses Act*, 1988, S.S. 1988–89, c. R-12.2, s. 26(2)(h).)

For example, it may be necessary for one health care professional to share with another selected information contained in the patient's medical records for consultative purposes. Or a health care practitioner who has become involved in a patient's treatment may need to know what treatment has been provided thus far, and the progress of the patient's recovery. This is a normal part of obtaining a history, which the patient should expect upon being admitted to a health care facility. No specific consent need be obtained in such a case since it is clearly implied that all persons involved in the patient's treatment have a valid reason for inspecting that patient's records. Nevertheless, the patient always has the right to expect that any information divulged to a nurse or other health care practitioner will remain confidential until and unless another professional has a valid need for it.

In this scenario, the nurse and physician are faced with a challenge to the patient–professional relationship. They should consult with and support Jim, giving him time to digest and understand his situation, and clarify with him why his wife should be involved. If necessary, they should support him in disclosing this information to her. Because there is still the potential for harm to Jim's wife and their unborn child, the team has a moral and professional obligation to inform her of Jim's infection. Certainly, the clinic owes Jim's wife an equal duty of care, since she, too, is a patient. Further, the nurse and physician must tell Jim that, given the high risk of infection with HIV, they have a legal obligation to inform the local medical officer of health of his infection. This is required by law in all provinces and territories.

The nurse should discuss these points carefully with the physician. If he still refuses to manage this situation as required, it would be appropriate for the nurse to appeal to the next level of authority until she is satisfied that action is taken. The nurse should not simply let the matter drop.

P.E.I. Reg. EC 330/85; Saskatchewan: *Disease Control Regulations*, R.R.S. c. P-37.1 Reg. 11, Table II.) Through this disclosure, the potential spread of such diseases can be controlled to some extent. The virulence and seriousness of these illnesses are deemed sufficient to justify the infringement on the patient's right to confidentiality. For example, in the case scenario, it would be unlawful for the physician at the clinic not to divulge the fact that Jim is HIV positive (and may, in fact, have full-blown AIDS) to the local medical officer of health.

Similarly, there may arise instances in which a patient tells a nurse that he or she intends to hurt or kill another person. Such a remark may be a manifestation of a patient's illness; nevertheless, if the patient has a history of violent behaviour through which others have been hurt or killed, or if the patient seems likely to harm him- or herself or others, such a statement should be reported to the authorities in the institution and to the police.

In general, however, the nurse's duty of confidentiality toward the patient is somewhat analogous to a lawyer's duty toward a client. A lawyer is under a continuous duty to ensure that any information that a client discloses during the course of their professional relationship remain confidential. For example, a lawyer may not divulge the fact that his or her client admitted to committing a crime. Such disclosure is unethical and may constitute professional misconduct. The law has not recognized a corresponding privilege of confidentiality among other client–professional relationships such as those with doctors, psychologists, nurses, counsellors, accountants, or clergy. For instance, legally, there is no obligation for a health care professional to aid police in investigations. However, as mentioned above, if a patient poses a threat to others, there is an ethical obligation to report this.

The right to confidentiality may be limited in cases in which there is a legal obligation to divulge the information, such as in a disciplinary hearing of the health care professional, a civil or criminal trial, or a coroner's inquest or other government-authorized inquiry. The right is also limited when the information must legally be disclosed to avoid harm to the patient or to a third party. In practice, however, most courts will not readily violate the client–professional relationship without a strong or compelling reason to do so (*A.G. v. Mulholland*, 1963; *Slavutych v. Baker et al.*, 1976). For example, if required by a court, the health care professional must answer any and all questions put to him or her. Failure to do so would place the practitioner in danger of being found in contempt of court and liable to a heavy fine or possible imprisonment.

A patient's confession of prior illegal activity (e.g., use of illegal drugs) made to a health care professional may not have to be disclosed. But it is possible that at some point a court may compel the practitioner to disclose such a fact. The only professional who would be exempt from disclosing such facts would be a lawyer (yet even a lawyer would have to guard against being an accessory to the client's crime). Although the health care professional is under no obligation to aid police, concealing the whereabouts of a fugitive could be construed as aiding and abetting such a person. This is especially likely in light of the *Criminal Code* offence of being an accessory to a crime after the fact (*Criminal Code of Canada*, 1985, s. 23(1)). One is an accessory when one "knowing that a person has been a party to the offence, receives, comforts or assists that person for the purpose of enabling that person to escape" (*Criminal Code of Canada*, 1985, s. 23(1)). By not divulging the information, with the intent that the patient should avoid detection by the police, the health care practitioner may be subject to criminal charges.

Another instance in which provincial law requires disclosure is in cases of suspected child abuse. Many provinces have set up child abuse registries. The laws that establish these are intended to encourage the reporting of situations in which a child has been sexually or physically abused. Indeed, these laws require child care workers, physicians, nurses, and other health care professionals to report suspected cases of child abuse, either to the police or to the local Children's Aid Society for further action. In most cases, it is an offence punishable by fine or imprisonment for a health care practitioner to fail to report an instance of suspected child abuse encountered in the course of practice.

Chapter 5 discusses the obligation of the health care professional in Ontario and some other provinces to disclose incidents of sexual abuse of patients by other health care practitioners. Indeed, even in provinces that have no such explicit requirement with respect to abuse by health care professionals, such behaviour is a reportable criminal offence and constitutes professional misconduct.

DISCLOSURE OF INFORMATION IN WORKERS' COMPENSATION MATTERS
Some nurses are employed as case managers by various Workers' Compensation Boards across Canada. All information regarding employers and workers gathered by such boards in the course of their investigations remains strictly confidential. Indeed, in British Columbia, the Northwest Territories, Ontario, Manitoba, and Saskatchewan, it is an offence to disclose such information without proper authority. The laws in these jurisdictions include substantial fines for contravention. The remaining provinces also impose sanctions and penalties for improperly divulged information. In some provinces, nurses employed by such boards may be required to take an oath of confidentiality as a condition of employment.

Through their freedom of information and privacy protection acts, Ontario and British Columbia provide a full right of access by a worker to his or her file. Generally, a worker, his or her dependants in the case of death, the worker's personal representative (such as a guardian or attorney for personal care), and the employer may have access to information respecting the worker. In Ontario, access by employers to health information about a worker is restricted to only those details related to the specific injury and its treatment. The worker must be notified by the Board of its intention to divulge health information to his or her employer.

The Boards also generally have the right to a health care professional's health information and records that are relevant to the injury or illness in the claim of a worker. A worker who files a claim for benefits is deemed to consent to the release of such information by the practitioner on request. Delays associated with such release can harm the worker in that payment of benefits is often conditional on the Board's receiving this information.

DISCLOSURE OF CONFIDENTIAL INFORMATION IN COURT TESTIMONY
There will be occasions, such as in a medical malpractice action or an inquest into a death, when the nurse must disclose information in court testimony. Most provincial nursing statutes and regulations permit such disclosure. However, even when lawfully disclosing patient information, the nurse should be prudent. Only those details that are relevant to the issues in the hearing, trial, or inquiry should be disclosed. The nurse should not give

a "blanket" disclosure of all possible information, which may not be relevant to the issues under inquiry. The nurse must use discretion and common sense.

## Ensuring Confidentiality in the Treatment Setting

A nurse may inadvertently disclose confidential information in casual conversations with colleagues, friends, or relatives who have no valid right to such details. Thus, nurses must take care at all times not to divulge confidential patient information when engaged in casual conversation in social settings unconnected to their work and duties.

Likewise, the old saying "the walls have ears" applies to hospitals and other health care facilities. For example, care should be taken when discussing details of a patient's condition in hallways, stairways, and elevators. Even when discussing a case with a colleague, only such disclosure should be made as is absolutely necessary for that person's participation in the patient's care and treatment. This requires great caution and discretion on the part of the nurse.

There are other instances in which confidential information may inadvertently be disclosed. For example, when a patient is being seen by a nurse in an Emergency Room in the presence of other people, the nurse should speak in a low voice in discussing the problem so as to avoid being overheard. The best way to address such a situation is to segregate the patient in a private room or area where privacy can be assured. Often, simply closing a door or drawing a curtain around the patient's bed will suffice.

## The Patient's Right to Privacy and Health Information

At the turn of the twenty-first century, we live in a more open society where concepts and issues that were once taboo (e.g., sex and issues of sexuality, euthanasia, and the right to die with dignity) are publicly addressed. Along with this openness, and with the dizzying pace of technological advances, there has been a concomitant increase in society's expectations with respect to the protection and promotion of personal privacy, especially in matters of personal health and finances. In response, all provinces and territories have passed privacy legislation to protect individuals' rights to control the disclosure of such information. Nurses, in their day-to-day practices, are privy to a great deal of health information about their patients, and, in all cases, they must treat such information as strictly confidential. The information must be used only in connection with the treatment and care of the individual patient to which it pertains and can be disclosed only with the consent of that person or, in cases in which the person is not competent to consent, the consent of a person authorized to make treatment and consent decisions on the patient's behalf.

Most provinces have enacted legislation regulating access to personal health information. See, for example, Alberta's *Freedom of Information and Protection of Privacy Act* (2000); British Columbia's *Personal Information Protection Act* (2003); Manitoba's *Personal Health Information Act*; Newfoundland and Labrador's *Personal Health Information Act* (2008); Ontario's *Personal Health Information Protection Act* (2004); and Saskatchewan's *Health Information Protection Act* (1999).

Ontario's statute is one of the most comprehensive in terms of specific protection of individual health and medical records. The Ontario statute states as its main purpose:

(a)  to establish rules for the collection, use and disclosure of personal health information about individuals that protect the confidentiality of that information and the privacy of individuals with respect to that information, while facilitating the effective provision of health care;

(b)  to provide individuals with a right of access to personal health information about themselves, subject to limited and specific exceptions set out in this Act;

(c)  to provide individuals with a right to require the correction or amendment of personal health information about themselves, subject to limited and specific exceptions set out in this Act;

(d)  to provide for independent review and resolution of complaints with respect to personal health information; and

(e)  to provide effective remedies for contraventions of this Act. (*Personal Health Information Protection Act, 2004*, s. 1)

Such statutes generally make it an offence to disclose any personal health information about an individual without that person's written or implied consent. Ontario's Act, for example, provides that health information means:

identifying information about an individual in oral or recorded form, if the information

(a)  relates to the physical or mental health of the individual, including information that consists of the health history of the individual's family,

(b)  relates to the providing of health care to the individual, including the identification of a person as a provider of health care to the individual,

(c)  is a plan of service ... for the individual,

(d)  relates to payments or eligibility for health care, or eligibility for coverage for health care, in respect of the individual,

(e)  relates to the donation by the individual of any body part or bodily substance of the individual or is derived from the testing or examination of any such body part or bodily substance,

(f)  is the individual's health number, or

(g)  identifies an individual's substitute decision-maker. (*Personal Health Information Protection Act, 2004*, s. 4(1))

Thus, the range of what is considered to be "health information" is broad and should be carefully considered by nurses in possession of any personal information about a person in their care.

Under Ontario's Act, a health information custodian (usually the management of the health care institution) is charged with safeguarding the privacy, accuracy, and confidentiality of personal health information and must have policies and practices in place to accomplish these goals. This means that nurses who practice in such institutions must abide by the institution's policies concerning the compiling, storage, use, retention, sharing, and disclosure of such information.

As stated earlier, the disclosure of health information can only be done legally either with the express or implied consent of the person to whom the information pertains. Express consent must be made by that specific individual, must be an informed consent, and must not be obtained by fraud, deception, or coercion. Implied consent would include situations in which a health care professional involved in the person's care discloses health information about that patient to another professional who is part of the health care team (or "circle of care") treating the patient. For example, there would be implied consent by a patient to a nurse to disclose treatment orders to a physician who is consulted by the patient's treating physician or to other nurses involved in his or her care. Where the disclosure is to be made to a non–health care professional, however, the patient must give express and informed, or "knowledgeable," consent. It cannot be implied. A patient's consent is considered knowledgeable if the patient knows why it is being collected or disclosed, what specific information is being sought, and that he or she may give or withhold consent. Consent can be given conditionally, for example, if information is to be disclosed only in the case of a certain event or circumstances.

As discussed in Chapter 6, those giving consent must be capable of doing so. They must be mentally capable, such that they fully understand what it is they are consenting to. The law recognizes that patients can be capable of such understanding at certain times while not capable at others, or that they can understand certain types of information and not others. In most cases, the law will presume that a person is capable unless the health care professional has a reason to suspect that the person is not in fact capable. Such suspicions can arise when a patient does not appear to be coherent or is confused or behaving irrationally. In such situations, legal proceedings may be taken to determine whether the patient has the necessary capacity and to determine a substitute decision maker if the person is found to be not capable to give consent.

## Computer Records and Confidentiality

Many hospitals and other health facilities now use computerized systems to maintain patient and other records. Consequently, there is wider access to a great deal of information by a potentially greater number of people. Access in most cases is controlled by means of magnetized cards and passwords. It is important for nurses to use their own passwords and not to use others' means of access since, in many cases, the use of the password and card is the nurse's electronic signature. Thus, if a nurse were to share his or her access code with another care provider, any action or documentation undertaken on the system would be attributed to the nurse who "owns" the code.

Many computer systems document the fact that a particular person gained access to a particular patient's record. The date and time of such access will also be noted in the computer record. Hospital nursing staff who use their access cards for improper and unwarranted access to patient files are subject to disciplinary action.

Automated records provide many benefits for patient care and for improving the nurse's efficiency. Some of the positive aspects include greater accuracy and validity of documentation, timeliness of recording, and ready access to important information—across the system—about that patient's episode of care, previous admissions, and treatment.

## Right to Privacy

The right to privacy goes hand in hand with the right to confidentiality; one cannot have one without the other. As we have seen in the context of consent to treatment, this implies a right to be free from control by the state or others in choosing the treatment one wishes to follow.

But the right to privacy with respect to nursing carries with it more practical aspects. For example, when a patient is bathing, and to the extent that it is safe to leave the patient alone, he or she should be ensured complete privacy. This right extends to treatment situations and examinations. Thus, care should be taken when examining a patient to ensure that the room is not fitted with mirrored windows, that unauthorized persons are not permitted into the room, and that pictures not be taken without the patient's permission, even if done for educational purposes.

Similarly, in instances in which the nurse feels that a consultation with clergy or a social worker may benefit the patient, the nurse may request such a consultation on the patient's behalf. However, the patient may refuse such help, in which case his or her privacy must be respected.

# Case Scenario

## WHO ADVOCATES FOR THE PATIENT?

Alain underwent emergency coronary artery bypass surgery 10 days ago, and his condition has remained critical. He has not yet completely regained consciousness. Owing to a lung infection, he remains on a ventilator under heavy sedation. In the past week, he has developed one complication after another—total body sepsis, a life-threatening arrhythmia, hypotension, and some liver failure—for which he has received a number of drugs. Now he is in kidney failure and requires dialysis.

Alain's family members, who have been at the hospital since his ordeal began, have been allowed only short visits once or twice per shift. The nurse and doctor informed them of the kidney failure and then left them alone to discuss whether they should consent to dialysis.

continued on following page >>

Alain's family knows his prognosis is poor. They also know he would not wish his life to be extended in this way. They believe he has suffered enough and decide to refuse the dialysis, knowing he will die. They request a meeting with the health care team to communicate their decision.

While visiting Alain a short while later, his wife notices that he is still receiving drugs to maintain his blood pressure, as well as the antibiotics that so far have not improved his condition. Further, the nurse informs her that because Alain's potassium is elevated, he will be given calcium polystyrene enemas in an attempt to bring it down.

The family is distraught. Together, they gather the courage to tell Alain's nurse that they do not wish to subject him to these enemas, which, if effective in the short term, will only prolong his dying. Further, they insist that the drugs be discontinued and that they be allowed to remain with him in privacy.

Alain's nurse supports the family's position and communicates their wishes to the physician on call. The family is permitted to stay with Alain until he dies peacefully a short time later.

## Issues

1. How did this case evolve to the point where Alain's family needed to advocate on his behalf?
2. How could this situation have been avoided? What process would have resulted in a better outcome for everybody?
3. What rights did Alain and his family have? Were these rights respected?
4. Identify the contradictions in this story.

## Discussion

The right to respect includes the right to be treated courteously, to privacy, and to be addressed by one's preferred name or title, and the corresponding obligation of the nurse to introduce himself or herself by name to the patient. It is important for the nurse to listen carefully, to focus on the patient's perceptions and needs, to respect his or her culture, religion, values, and relationships with friends and family. For example, talking about the patient as if he or she were not present diminishes that person's humanity and is disrespectful, as is administering needless medical treatment that will do nothing to improve the patient's welfare and will cause more pain and suffering. This is especially important when caring for patients who are dying.

The process of dying is a significant one for all involved, including patients, families, and caregivers. It is a time that requires all the nurse's powers of empathy. Providing as dignified a death as possible means being concerned about the patient's pain and symptom control, respecting the patient's privacy, and knowing when he or she wishes to be left alone or with family and friends. It also means being concerned with where the patient wants to die. Some patients may wish to remain in the hospital or be referred to a palliative care facility. Others may prefer to be at home yet may not be aware of the resources available to make this choice possible. Rarely does anyone want to die alone.

continued on following page >>

As much as possible, nurses should keep the patient's family and friends informed of the patient's status so that they will be available when necessary. When the patient's condition deteriorates, the family should be informed promptly. The nurse does not need permission to telephone a family member to let that person know what is happening and that his or her presence may be necessary.

Unfortunately, many patients in hospitals die during the process of cardiopulmonary resuscitation. It is common that, during this procedure, families are removed from the patient's room. This limits the patient's right to have a caring family member or friend present when death is imminent. Caregivers are uncomfortable with the idea of family members witnessing what is often a distressing experience. Nevertheless, the family's presence is the patient's right and the family's choice. When it appears to be their wish, the arrest procedure should be explained in detail to family members who choose to be present. Sometimes, loved ones present at arrests will sit quietly, stroking the patient's face, apparently oblivious to the resuscitation efforts. As part of their role in patient advocacy and leadership, nurses might attempt to change systems and processes within their facility to ensure that this can happen more frequently.

Certain aspects of the right to respect find formal recognition in the law. For example, all patients have the right to equal access to health care resources and facilities without regard to sex, colour, mental or physical disabilities, ethnicity, creed, or religion. These rights are enshrined in provincial and territorial human rights codes.

## Right to Respect

Health professionals have an obligation to treat all clients with respect and dignity. Nurses who fail to involve clients in decisions relevant to them violate nurses' ethical responsibility to those in their care.

## Right to Be Kept Safe

Baker and Norton undertook a study in 2004 to determine the extent of error in Canadian hospitals. According to this study of 20 hospitals in five provinces, one in 13 patients experiences an adverse event. The greatest number of these adverse events occurred in teaching hospitals, where patient care is generally more complex and acute. Furthermore, Baker and Norton insist that of the 185,000 adverse events that occur in Canadian hospitals each year, 70,000 are preventable (Baker, Norton, Flintoft, Blais, Brown, Cox, et al., 2004).

The health care system is made up of humans, and humans are imperfect—they make mistakes. This is why it is so important that highly effective systems are put in place to compensate for human limitations. Many reasons account for human error. In health care, these commonly include communication breakdown, fatigue, workload, the complexity of processes, and reliance on memory over checklists.

Errors in health care are most often the result of system problems rather than of individual acts. Yet, historically, the tendency has been to blame individuals for errors and adverse events (Rankin, 2004). Not surprisingly, health care professionals are instinctively defensive when it comes to being questioned or talking openly about medical errors and disclosure of errors. However, when error is not acknowledged, there is a missed opportunity to learn and to improve patient safety. Across the country, there is a growing focus on changing the systems and processes that contribute to or influence the occurrence of error or adverse events.

## A Culture of Patient Safety

Leadership is one of the most important factors in ensuring a culture of safety and transparency. If safety is important in an organization, then its leaders are discussing it on a regular basis and actively participating in strategies to promote safety (Morath, 2006).

To create a culture that ensures patient safety, these leaders must demonstrate commitment through clearly articulated values and actions. In a culture in which adverse events or mistakes are openly reported and communicated, people are made accountable and are recognized for providing an opportunity for learning and ensuring the mistake does not happen again. Often, a series of events or missteps precedes errors, so, today, there is a greater focus on system issues, rather than on individual blame, and recognition that failed processes may contribute to errors.

## A Patient's and Family's Right to Know: Disclosure of Error

In patient safety literature, **harm** is defined as "an outcome that negatively affects a patient's health and/or quality of life" (Disclosure Working Group, 2008, p. 8). It is an adverse event related to the care or services provided to the patient rather than to the patient's underlying problem or illness. When harm occurs, the ethically responsible action is full disclosure of that harm to the patient or family. **Disclosure** is the process by which health care professionals communicate an adverse event to the patient (Disclosure Working Group, 2008).

As discussed, patients are entitled to information about themselves, so when errors are made and harm results, patients and families have the right to be informed of them. Ethical and professional obligations to be open and honest are consistent with professional codes of ethics and patients' rights. When harm results as a consequence of error, others beyond the patient suffer. The health care professionals involved can experience serious guilt and remorse. For the healing of all concerned, disclosure to the patient and or family is necessary to begin the healing process.

Sadly, sometimes a patient dies as the result of error. Understandably, families hope for some acknowledgement of the error and its role in the death of a family member, especially when the death was unforeseen. Such acknowledgement is important for a family in dealing with their loss and provides them with some assurance that the errors will not be repeated, thereby preventing another family from suffering a similar tragedy. A family wants clear and honest answers as to what happened to their loved one, and hospitals have an ethical and spiritual obligation to sit down with the family and, with compassionate grace, disclose the truth.

The disclosure process needs to be open and transparent. With the patient's or family's consent, the physicians, nurses, and other relevant members of the team involved in the patient's care should be present. The process may not be completed in only a single conversation—several meetings may be necessary to ensure that all of the patient's or family's issues, concerns, and questions are addressed (Disclosure Working Group, 2008, p. 16; Morath, 2006; Keatings, Martin, McCallum, & Lewis, 2006).

The absence of full disclosure of medical errors means the loss of one of the most effective tools for improving systems and patient safety, and inevitably results in repetition of these same errors.

## The Claire Lewis Story

On October 14, 2001, three days after undergoing surgery to remove a craniopharyngioma, 11-year-old Claire Lewis died in the Intensive Care Unit of a Canadian hospital. The circumstances of her sudden death, believed by the ICU staff to be due to postoperative complications, may have been overlooked had it not been for her father, John Lewis, and his certainty that his daughter's death could have been prevented.

When Claire died, the health care team who had cared for her for three days in the ICU believed they had provided the most appropriate care. However, even if the team had believed that serious errors had been made, there was no system in place for reporting a critical event such as this error and alerting the hospital's senior leadership to the concern.

Claire's father, John, was a registered nurse working at the hospital where his daughter died and had been at her bedside for most of the three days following her surgery. He was present when she died. Following her death, he reviewed Claire's medical records and arrived at a clear understanding of the errors that had been made and the system failings that had contributed to his daughter's preventable death.

It was almost four months, however, before the hospital's senior leaders became aware of the issues surrounding Claire's death. The silence on the part of the hospital following Claire's death, coupled with a coroner's report that found nothing untoward in her care, infuriated the grieving father. Understandably, the family had hoped for some form of acknowledgement from the hospital in terms of its role in Claire's death. Disclosure of adverse events that lead to morbidity and mortality is important for the families involved as they struggle to deal with their losses.

Immediately following Claire's death, an initial review of her care was conducted. Led by physicians and risk management staff, the review failed to address the critical aspects identified by her father. Furthermore, the hospital's legal advisors edited the report that was sent to the family. Failing to answer many of the family's questions, the report served only to deepen their feelings of distrust and anger.

continued on following page >>

A meeting between the family and hospital about four months after her death resulted in Claire's family feeling an even greater sense of alienation. They were upset about the report; the team who met with them was unprepared for the meeting; and too many people, including a physician whom the family had specifically requested not attend, were in attendance. According to Claire's father, "the meeting was a disaster, as middle management, with wagons in a circle and with a wall of white coats present designed specifically to intimidate two devastated parents, tried to chalk Claire's death up to complications of surgery." Understandably, the family felt offended by the seemingly insincere efforts on the part of the hospital to address their concerns.

Subsequently, a second review identified the errors in Claire's care. However, the debate about what to disclose continued. There were differing perspectives and concerns among the executive team and the legal advisors. Finally, once the question about disclosure made its way to the hospital's senior leaders, the decision was quickly made by them that there would be a full disclosure.

The review of Claire's care in the ICU, the admission of error, and the full disclosure of those errors set the stage for those involved to begin a process that produced 19 recommendations for change to address both system and competence issues.

A letter was sent to the family, along with the conclusions of the second review and a list of recommendations for changes at the hospital. The family, however, was so deeply hurt by the hospital's failure to make this disclosure earlier and the previous failed attempt at dialogue that they refused to meet with hospital leaders. Despite this refusal, the senior leaders persisted in maintaining contact with the family and making offers to meet and engage in open discussion.

It was almost three years after Claire's death that the family was finally able to accept the hospital's invitation to work together to set the stage from which everyone could start to heal and move forward. According to Claire's father, "the hospital's disclosure brought with it unforeseen and unimaginable benefits for the family, the hospital, physicians, and nurses alike." The silence that followed Claire's death had felt like a cover-up to the family and led to the feeling that there had been some intent to harm. "The apology melted this horrific feeling away, slowly opening the door to a meaningful dialogue between the family and the hospital staff" (Keatings et al., 2006, p. 1085).

The bereaved need to create meaning in the seemingly senseless deaths of their loved ones, but when medical errors occur, there are many victims. A number of the staff who had cared for Claire were deeply affected by her death, the review, and the subsequent disclosure process. The disclosure provided staff, as well as the family, the opportunity to "make sense" of Claire's death, to begin to heal and move forward, and to become part of the process of change that would improve patient safety.

### More Than One Victim

Not only did Claire and her family suffer the consequences associated with her death; nurses and physicians were also affected, both personally and professionally. Throughout this sad journey, two of Claire's nurses repeatedly expressed a desire to meet with her family. They wanted the opportunity to apologize for what they may or may not have done that might have contributed to Claire's death and to acknowledge the family's loss and grief. But their legal advisors cautioned against this. When they did meet with the family, it was their decision and taken despite the advice not to do so.

When John, Claire's father, met with the nurses, he was accompanied by his eldest daughter Jessie, who had lacked a clear understanding of what had happened to her sister the day she died. During the meeting, she became aware of the complexity of factors that had led to Claire's death. Both she and John came to understand the pain and heartache experienced by these nurses. The nurses simply said how sorry they were to John and Jessie, who, not feeling the need for further explanation, gave them a hug (Keatings et al., 2006). These professionals, through disclosure and forgiveness, were then able to move on with their professional careers, richer from the experience.

Sources: Hicock, L., & Lewis, J. (2004). *Beware the grieving warrior: A child's preventable death, a father's fight for justice.* Toronto, ON: ECW Press; Keatings, M., Martin, M., McCallum, A., & Lewis, J. (2006). Medical errors: Understanding the parent's perspective. A. Matlow & R. M. Laxer (Eds.), *Pediatric Clinics of North America, 53*(6), 1079–1089.

Health care professionals need to approach the question of full and open disclosure of adverse events with the same commitment and hold it to the same standard of practice applied to any other treatment or decision. When this does not happen, they betray the trust of patients, families, and each other. Health care organizations have to introduce practices and processes to consistently and accurately recognize the occurrence of adverse events. It is essential that such recognition of adverse events be inextricably tied to full and open disclosure. Simply put, it is the right thing to do.

## Right to Be Discharged From a Health Care Facility

### Discharge From Hospital

Can a patient be prevented from being discharged from a hospital? In many cases, a patient who wishes to leave a hospital or other health care facility against medical advice must sign a waiver acknowledging that he or she has been advised that leaving is not recommended at this time. If a competent patient refuses to sign the waiver, the fact that he or she is leaving against medical advice (AMA) should be carefully documented in the chart. Ultimately, there is nothing hospital staff can do to prevent a patient from leaving. A hospital is not a prison.

In cases involving psychiatric patients of unsound mind, the mental health statutes of most provinces may permit such persons to be prevented from leaving if they pose a threat or danger to themselves or to others.

When a patient is discharged, the hospital has an obligation to ensure that he or she arrives home safely. For example, in cases involving same-day surgery, a patient should not be sent home if the sedative has not yet worn off. Such a patient may have to be sent home by taxi or other means, as he or she would not be in a condition to drive. There have been reported cases in which patients still under the effect of sedatives have driven home and have been charged with impaired driving. In many hospitals and health care agencies, patients who have been sedated are required to wait a specified period of time and to be accompanied by another person when they leave the institution.

## Discharge From a Mental Health Facility

Most provinces have legislation governing admission to and discharge from a mental institution. (See Alberta: *Mental Health Act*, R.S.A. 2000, c. M-13; British Columbia: *Mental Health Act*, R.S.B.C. 1996, c. 288; Manitoba: *Mental Health Act*, C.C.S.M. c. M110; New Brunswick: *Mental Health Act*, R.S.N.B. 1973, c. M-10; Newfoundland and Labrador: *Mental Health Act*, R.S.N.L. 1990, c. M-9; Northwest Territories: *Mental Health Act*, R.S.N.W.T. 1988, c. M-10; Nova Scotia: *Hospitals Act*, R.S.N.S. 1989, c. 208; Ontario: *Mental Health Act*, R.S.O. 1990, c. M.7; Quebec: *Protection of persons whose mental state presents a danger to themselves or to others*, R.S.Q. c. P-38.001; Saskatchewan: *Mental Health Services Act*, S.S. 1984–85–86, c. M-13.1; Yukon: *Mental Health Act,* R.S.Y. 2002, c. 150.)

As a rule, if a person's state of mental health is such that he or she poses a threat either to self or to others, such a person may be committed to a mental health facility for treatment upon the order of an examining physician. In most provinces, the determination that such a state of mind exists must be made by a physician (see, for example, *Mental Health Act* (Ontario), s. 15(1)). In Newfoundland, a person may be detained in such a treatment facility only if two physicians certify that the patient is a danger to self or others by reason of a mental disorder (*Mental Health Act* (Newfoundland and Labrador), s. 5(2)).

Generally, there are two categories under which a person suffering a mental disorder is admitted to a mental institution: persons who are not a threat to themselves or others and persons who pose a threat to themselves or others. The former are usually voluntary patients, and they cannot be detained without their consent.

The latter, violent patients who pose a threat to their own or others' safety, generally may be admitted to an institution on an involuntary basis and may be detained without their consent. The matter does not end there, however. There are procedural safeguards in place to provide for a review of the detention of involuntary patients and to ensure they are not arbitrarily detained or detained without proper grounds. If they cease to pose a danger to themselves or others, the law generally requires that they be released when they wish.

The *Mental Health Act* of Yukon articulates the rights of mental patients. As in many provinces, only minimal physical restraints may be used on such patients—that is, only what is reasonable and necessary, considering the person's physical and mental condition (*Mental Health Act* (Yukon), s. 5(1)). Other patient rights in Yukon include the right to receive and make phone calls (*Mental Health Act* (Yukon), s. 40(4)(a)); to have reasonable access to visitors (*Mental Health Act* (Yukon), s. 40(4)(b)); to have access at any time to his or her legal representative, guardian, or other authorized person (*Mental Health Act* (Yukon), s. 40(4)(c)); to send and receive correspondence; to vote; to wear clothing of his or her choice; to security of his or her person; to confidentiality (*Mental Health Act* (Yukon), s. 40(5)(6)(7)); and to be informed (if detained) of the reasons for detention (*Mental Health Act* (Yukon), s. 41). In other jurisdictions, similar rights exist in common law if they are not expressed in statute.

## Summary

This chapter has dealt with the rights and responsibilities of patients and clients within the health care system, and the obligations of health care professionals to ensure that these rights are respected. A health care professional's obligations to respect patients' rights are not always clear; in fact, they may conflict with equal obligations to respect the rights of others. These rights and obligations evolve from the ethical theories and principles described in earlier chapters.

Nurses are obliged to ensure that patient rights are respected and upheld. The pressures of diminishing resources, workload, and other factors in today's health care setting may impose barriers to providing even such basic patient rights as privacy and dignity. Regardless, nurses should always be mindful of their duty and obligation to ensure the rights of patients, while at the same time assuring they themselves are treated with respect. Most important, in today's complex health care environment, health care professionals have a responsibility to ensure the safety of clients and a duty to inform them when mistakes are made. Professional codes of ethics and patient bills of rights help to make certain that patients and clients are informed of their rights and nurses' obligations to protect them.

# Critical Thinking

The following case scenarios offer an opportunity for reflection, discussion, and analysis.

## TO INTERVENE OR NOT?

Margaret, a registered nurse, is visiting her mother, a patient in a long-term care facility. Upon hearing raised voices in the next room, Margaret leaves her mother's bedside to investigate. She witnesses a nurse shouting at a patient that he wasn't doing enough to help her move him. When the nurse leaves the room obviously frustrated, Margaret goes in to see if the patient is all right.

This patient is a 60-year-old man with Guillain-Barré syndrome. Most of his body is paralyzed, but he does have minimal function in his upper body. He tells Margaret that "everything is okay." He does not want her to discuss the event with anyone on the unit. He says, "It's easier this way. I'm totally dependent on the staff here, and the nurse didn't hurt me. She's just overworked."

### Questions
1. Is there a violation of ethical or legal standards?
2. Is there risk of any civil or criminal liability?
3. What are the patient's rights in this situation? Are there conflicting rights here?
4. Does Margaret have any obligation since she is not an employee of this facility?
5. What should Margaret do?

## A CONFIDENCE SHARED

Cynthia is an occupational health nurse in a large manufacturing company. She is managing the case of an employee, Eric, who fractured his wrist when a heavy piece of equipment fell on him. Eric has had problems in the workplace; his manager has often spoken to him about his tendency to become distracted. This is a concern because of the safety risk to Eric and his coworkers.

Now Eric's wrist has healed, and he is functionally able to return to work. However, he confides to Cynthia that he is currently under great personal stress: His wife is dying of cancer, and he is so depressed that he can think about nothing else. Cynthia recognizes that this stress may have contributed to Eric's injury and that, unless addressed, it might cause him further harm.

continued on following page >>

However, Eric asks Cynthia to keep this information confidential. He does not want his manager to know anything about his personal life. He simply wants to return to work.

**Questions**

1. Is there a violation of ethical or legal standards?
2. Is there risk of any civil or criminal liability?
3. Does Eric have the right to ask Cynthia to keep this information confidential?
4. What other rights does Eric have that Cynthia must respect?
5. Does the company, its managers, and other employees have any rights here?
6. What should Cynthia do?

## ACCESS AND DISCLOSURE

Klara is a registered nurse in the emergency department of a local community hospital. One evening, a neighbour, Rohini, presents at Emergency with abdominal pain of unknown origin. Klara is on duty when Rohini is admitted to a surgical unit.

Some days later, another neighbour asks Klara how Rohini is doing. At work, Klara accesses her chart via the hospital's computer system and discovers that Rohini has been diagnosed with advanced liver cancer and, further, that this information has been kept from Rohini. The surgeon caring for Rohini is well known for his paternalistic attitude. Klara recognizes that she must not share this information with anyone. However, she is unsettled to discover that Rohini has been kept ignorant of her diagnosis and prognosis.

**Questions**

1. Is there a violation of ethical or legal standards?
2. Is there risk of any civil or criminal liability?
3. As an employee of the hospital, did Klara have the right to access Rohini's chart?
4. Should the hospital have a policy to ensure privacy with the use of computerized information systems? What should this policy say?
5. In the circumstances, can Klara ensure that Rohini's right to information is respected?

**Discussion Points**

1. Does your work setting or areas in which you have had a clinical placement have a bill of rights for patients or clients? How is this statement communicated? Do you believe it is the nurse's responsibility to ensure that patients know their rights?
2. Can you think of situations in which the rights discussed in this chapter might potentially conflict with the rights of the institution? Of the nurse? Of other patients and families? How do we balance these rights?
3. How do visiting hours in your facility support the rights of patients or clients? What processes are in place to support families of the terminally or seriously ill?
4. What procedures and policies need to be in place to guard against sexual harassment of patients by staff?

## References

### Statutes

*Charter of Rights and Freedoms*, Part I of the *Constitution Act, 1982*, being Schedule B to the Canada Act 1982 (U.K.), 1982, c. 11.

*Communicable Diseases Act*, R.S.N.L. 1990. c. C-26, Schedule (Newfoundand and Labrador).

*Criminal Code of Canada*, R.S.C. 1985, c. C-46 (Canada).

*Expanded Nursing Services for Patients Act, 1997*, S.O. 1997, c. 9 (Ontario).

*Freedom of Information and Protection of Privacy Act*, R.S.A. 2000, c. F-25 (Alberta).

*Health Care Directives and Substitute Health Care Decision Makers Act*, S.S. 1997, c. H-0.0001 (Saskatchewan).

*Health Information Act*, R.S.A. 2000, c. H-5 (Alberta).

*Health Information Protection Act*, S.S. 1999, c. H-0.021 (Saskatchewan).

*Hospitals Act*, R.S.N.S. 1989, c. 208 (Nova Scotia).

*Mental Health Act*, C.C.S.M., c. M110 (Manitoba).

*Mental Health Act*, R.S.B.C. 1996, c. 288 (British Columbia).

*Mental Health Act,* R.S.A. 2000, c. M-13 (Alberta).

*Mental Health Act*, R.S.N.B. 1973, c. M-10 (New Brunswick).

*Mental Health Act*, R.S.N.L. 1990, c. M-9 (Newfoundland and Labrador).

*Mental Health Act*, R.S.N.W.T. 1988, c. M-10 (Northwest Territories).

*Mental Health Act*, R.S.O. 1990, c. M.7 (Ontario).

*Mental Health Act*, R.S.Y. 2002, c. 150 (Yukon).

*Mental Health Services Act*, S.S. 1984–85–86, c. M-13.1 (Saskatchewan).

*Nurses Act*, S.N.B. 1984, c. 71 (New Brunswick).

*Nursing Act, 1991*, S.O. 1991, c. 32 (Ontario).

*Nursing Profession Act*, S.N.W.T. 2003, c. 15 (Northwest Territories).

*Personal Health Information Act*, C.C.S.M., c. P-33.5 (Manitoba).

*Personal Health Information Act*, S.N.L. 2008, c. P-7.01 (Newfoundland and Labrador).

*Personal Health Information Protection Act, 2004*, S.O. 2004, c. 3, Schedule A (Ontario).

*Personal Information Protection Act*, S.B.C., 2003, c. 63 (British Columbia).

*Protection of persons whose mental state presents a danger to themselves or to others, An Act respecting the*, R.S.Q. c. P-38.001 (Quebec).

*Registered Nurses Act, 1988*, S.S. 1988–89, c. R-12.2 (Saskatchewan).

*Regulated Health Professions Act, 1991*, S.O. 1991, c. 18 (Ontario).

*Substitute Decisions Act, 1992*, S.O. 1992, c. 30 (Ontario).

### Regulations

*Communicable Diseases Regulation*, Alta. Reg. 238/85, Schedule 4, "Human Immunodeficiency Virus (HIV) Infections" (Alberta).

*Disease Control Regulations*, R.R.S., c. P-37.1 Reg. 11, Table II (Saskatchewan).

*Diseases and Dead Bodies Regulation*, Man. Reg. 338/88 R, Part II (Manitoba).

*Health Act Communicable Disease Regulation*, B.C. Reg. 4/83, Schedule A (British Columbia).

N.B. Reg. 86-66, s. 94(1)(s) (New Brunswick).

*Notifiable and Communicable Diseases Regulations*, P.E.I. Reg. EC 330/85 (Prince Edward Island).

*Professional Misconduct Regulation*, O. Reg. 799/93 (Ontario).

*Reporting of Notifiable Diseases and Conditions Regulations*, N.S. Reg. 195/2005, Schedule A (Nova Scotia).

R.R.O. 1990, Reg. 569, s. 5 (Ontario).

## Case Law

*A.G. v. Mulholland*, [1963] 2 Q.B. 477.

*Slavutych v. Baker et al.*, [1976] 1 S.C.R. 254.

## Texts and Articles

Baker, G. R., Norton, P. G., Flintoft, V., Blais, R., Brown, A., Cox, J., et al. (2004). The Canadian adverse events study: The incidence of adverse events among hospital patients in Canada. *Canadian Medical Association Journal, 170*(11), 1678–1686.

Canadian Nurses Association. (2008). *Code of ethics for registered nurses*. Ottawa, ON: Author.

Canadian Pain Coalition. *Charter of pain patient's rights and responsibilities*. Retrieved September 26, 2008, from http://rsdcanada.org/parc/english/resources/coalition.htm

Dana-Farber Cancer Institute. (n.d.) *Patient rights and responsibilities*. Retrieved January 6, 2009, from http://www.dana-farber.org/pat/patient/patient

Disclosure Working Group. (2008). *Canadian disclosure guidelines*, 1–34 [pdf]. Canadian Patient Safety Institute. Retrieved January 6, 2009, from http://www.patientsafetyinstitute.ca/disclosure.html

Hicock, L., & Lewis, J. (2004). *Beware the grieving warrior: A child's preventable death, a father's fight for justice*. Toronto, ON: ECW Press.

Keatings, M., Martin, M., McCallum, A., & Lewis, J. (2006). Medical errors: Understanding the parent's perspective. A. Matlow & R. M. Laxer (Eds.). *Pediatric Clinics of North America, 53*(6), 1079–1089.

Morath, J. M. (2006). Patient safety: A view from the top. A. Matlow & R. M. Laxer (Eds.). *Pediatric Clinics of North America, 53*(6), 1053–1065.

Rankin, D. (2004). *Disclosure of harm: Good medical practice* (p. 2). Wellington, NZ: Medical Council of New Zealand. Retrieved September 2008 from http://www.menz.org.nz/portals/1/guidance/disclosure_of_harm

Settlement.Org. (2008). *Information newcomers to Ontario can trust*. Retrieved September 2008 from http://www.settlement.org

# Caregiver Rights

## Learning Objectives

The purpose of this chapter is to enable you to understand:

- The rights of nurses as citizens, professionals, and employees
- When the right to a conscientious objection can be invoked
- The accountabilities of nurses as employees
- The position of the law with respect to discrimination and sexual or physical abuse
- The crucial importance of a healthy work environment
- The nature of workplace violence and how it should be prevented and addressed
- The role of labour relations and collective bargaining in nursing
- Occupational health and safety standards

## Introduction

ALTHOUGH MOST OF THIS book focuses on the rights of patients and clients within the health care system, nurses also have rights. Along with all other Canadian citizens and landed immigrants, under the *Charter of Rights and Freedoms* (1982), nurses have the right to privacy, respect, and freedom of expression—to think, say, write, or otherwise act in accordance with their beliefs. However, these rights are not absolute. For nurses, professional rules and regulations, and ethical responsibilities to patients, may limit individual freedom. For example, when caring for a patient whose values and religious beliefs differ from one's own, it is not professionally or ethically appropriate for the nurse to attempt to influence the patient toward his or her opinions, values, and beliefs.

Nurses are entitled to respect from one another, from other professionals, and from patients and clients. As individuals, they are entitled to freedom from any form of discrimination, harassment (sexual or otherwise), and physical or sexual abuse. As employees, nurses have the right to have their values respected and to function within a work environment in which risks of harm are minimized. This chapter explores some of these rights.

## Conscientious Objection

As employees, nurses are under a contractual obligation to provide competent care to patients and clients. There are times, however, when the duty to provide care may conflict with the nurse's personal values—for example, having to participate in a procedure or provide care that he or she finds objectionable on moral or religious grounds. Must the nurse still provide care in these circumstances?

Most such situations will not be emergencies. In an emergency, the nurse's foremost ethical obligation is to assist patients and to protect them from harm. Refusing to act would go against the ethical principles of beneficence and nonmaleficence and of their professional duties and responsibilities. Therefore, in an emergency, the nurse is bound to assist the patient until alternative care is available. Consider the case scenario on the following page.

## Discrimination Issues in Employment

The case scenario below also raises an employment law issue and illustrates the competing interests of employees' and employers' rights. Legally, the matter involves the application of provincial human rights legislation. This legislation is virtually identical among all provinces and territories and is essentially designed to prohibit discrimination against persons on the basis of race, sex, sexual orientation, creed, religion, physical or mental disability, nationality, or ethnic origin. The thrust of the legislation is that employers are obliged, to the greatest extent possible, to structure work conditions and requirements so as to cause the least possible interference with the religious or cultural views, or physical or mental handicaps, of their employees. For example, employers must accommodate work conditions such that no employee is unduly inconvenienced by reason only of his or her sex, as in the case of providing adequate washroom facilities.

In the case scenario, Marie-France's religious views conflict with her employer's work requirements. If we alter the circumstances and say that she was reassigned to the unit by a supervisor who held her religious views in contempt and merely wanted to harass her by requiring her to work in a setting to which she strongly objected, she would have valid grounds for a complaint before the provincial Human Rights Commission. If her rights have been infringed, Marie-France may be awarded compensation, depending on the laws of her province or territory. She should not be forced to work in a setting to which she objects on moral or religious grounds, subject, of course, to the ethical rules and legal considerations discussed above.

# Case Scenario

## A CONSCIENTIOUS OBJECTION?

Marie-France, a registered nurse of five years' standing, works in the obstetrics department of a secular public hospital in a large urban centre. She is religious and deeply opposed to abortion. Marie-France accepted her position with the understanding that no therapeutic abortions were performed in Obstetrics. In this hospital, abortions are usually performed in the gynecological department; some such procedures involve saline injections. Marie-France would never be asked or required to work on this unit.

Recent cutbacks in funding to the hospital have meant staff reductions and bed closures. Consequently, when beds are tight, an abortion might occasionally be performed in Obstetrics. One afternoon, Marie-France discovers that she has been scheduled to assist in a second-trimester saline abortion that is to take place in Obstetrics later that day. Angry and upset, she accosts her manager: "There's no way I'm going to assist with this! Find another nurse!"

### Issues

1. What are the hospital's ethical and legal obligations to Marie-France and to the patient seeking the abortion?
2. How can the conflict between these interests be resolved?

### Discussion

Whenever possible, employers are obliged to respect the conscientious objections of employees who decline to participate in certain actions on moral or religious grounds. Here, we are not speaking of indulging the employee's prejudices. The employee has the right not to be forced to engage in actions to which he or she objects on ethical grounds. In this case scenario, the

continued on following page >>

treatment in which Marie-France is being asked to participate is not an emergency. If it were, she would be ethically bound to render any and all assistance needed of her—it would take priority over her conscientious objections. For example, if the patient were suffering complications as a result of an abortion, such as internal bleeding following a saline injection, regardless of Marie-France's personal opinion of the patient's actions, it would be her duty to render assistance. While Marie-France can refuse to participate in the abortion, she would be compelled to render emergency life-saving treatment after the fact.

In a different circumstance, a nurse working in a Palliative Care Unit caring for a male patient with AIDS could not ethically refuse to treat him on the grounds that he might be a homosexual or a drug abuser. This would be a clear case of prejudice, which an employer is not obliged to indulge.

Problems relating to conscientious objection are best avoided by informing the prospective nursing employee, prior to employment, of the functions, roles, duties, and responsibilities expected of him or her. The nurse should be advised that, once employment is accepted, he or she will have no option but to provide the care required. Thus, a prospective nursing employee applying for a position in the gynecological department of a secular hospital should be made to understand that the duties may include assisting during abortions. The informed nurse may then decline such employment.

However, if the nature of the nurse's job changes after he or she has begun employment, the agency or hospital is obligated to reassign that nurse to areas in which the objectionable activities are not performed. Yet, since in emergency situations nurses are ethically obliged to provide care, there are no guarantees. They may withdraw from such situations only when to do so does not endanger the patient or when others are available to provide the required care. In very small facilities, it may not be possible to reassign nurses or to guarantee exemption from involvement. In these cases, the nurse may face the difficult choice of seeking employment elsewhere.

The ethical principles that apply in these cases are justice (the patient's right to be treated fairly and equitably), beneficence (the nurse's obligation to do good for the patient), and nonmaleficence (the nurse's duty to do the patient no harm). For example, if a nurse were to withdraw his or her services arbitrarily because of an objection and thereby placed the patient in danger, that nurse would be violating the principle of nonmaleficence and the duty to provide care.

As stated in the Canadian Nurses Association's *Code of Ethics for Registered Nurses*, nurses are not obliged to act on the wishes of a client or patient when those actions pose a serious moral conflict for the nurse. However, the nurse is obliged to ensure that other arrangements are available to a patient or client when the care required conflicts with the nurse's beliefs but is legally acceptable:

> If nursing care is requested that is in conflict with the nurse's moral beliefs and values but in keeping with professional practice, the nurse provides safe, compassionate, competent and ethical care until alternative care arrangements are in place to meet the person's needs or

continued on following page >>

desires. If nurses can anticipate a conflict with their conscience, they have an obligation to notify their employers or, if the nurse is self-employed, persons receiving care in advance so that alternative arrangements can be made. (Canadian Nurses Association [CNA], 2008, p. 15)

In some cases, however, the responsibilities of the nurse may put him or her at risk, and the question of refusal of care may not be related to conscientious objection. Consider the outbreak of severe acute respiratory syndrome (SARS) in Canada, notably in Ontario and British Columbia, in 2003. This highly contagious infection originated in China and spread to Canada through international travel. Many people were infected, including health care providers, and many people died, including the nurses caring for them. This was a true test of the professionalism and dedication of the nursing profession. These professionals were exposed to serious risk, and others will certainly experience other such situations in the future (University of Toronto Joint Centre for Bioethics, 2008). The standards these nurses met are embedded in the *Code of Ethics for Registered Nurses*: "During a natural or human-made disaster, including a communicable disease outbreak, nurses have a duty to provide care using appropriate safety precautions" (CNA, 2008, Appendix D).

It is the responsibility of the system and organizations to put strategies in place to prevent harm to caregivers in these high-risk situations. As a result of the SARS outbreak, and in preparation for future lethal outbreaks or pandemics, many strategies have been implemented.

## The Right of Nurses to Be Protected From Harm and to a Healthy Work Environment

### Right to a Healthy Work Environment

Nursing in Canada has moved beyond legislation to address the fundamental factors that influence nurses' work environment. A key study illustrating the components of a healthy work environment for nurses, "Commitment and Care: The Benefits of a Healthy Workplace for Nurses, Their Patients and the System" (Baumann, O'Brien-Pallas, Armstrong-Stassen, Blythe, Bourbonnais, Cameron, et al., 2001), was published in 2001. This Canada–wide study emphasized the importance of key attributes of the work environment in ensuring a satisfied and sustainable nursing workforce. This document serves as a guiding framework for leaders and includes the following recommendations to ensure a healthy nursing culture:

- Address staffing issues
- Reward effort and achievement
- Strengthen organizational structures
- Support nursing leadership and professional development
- Promote workplace health and safety
- Ensure a learning environment
- Promote recruitment and retention

A healthy work environment is essential in all work settings—even more so in a health care environment, where the safety of patients and clients is significantly affected by the overall health and well-being of the individuals and teams who provide care. A positive and healthy work culture results in reduced absenteeism, improved ability to attract and retain new employees, and high levels of staff satisfaction. When staff morale is high and when engagement and commitment to the organization is sustained, the setting becomes recognized as a workplace of choice. In a health care environment, employer savings associated with low absenteeism and turnover rates are then available to invest in additional strategies to improve the work environment and to advance patient or client care (Dugan, Lauer, Bouquot, Dutro, Smith, & Widmeyer, 1996; Lundstrom, Pugliese, Bartley, Cox, & Guither, 2002; Estabrooks, Midodzi, Cummings, Ricker, & Giovannetti, 2005; Agency for Healthcare Research and Quality, 2003).

Models available to assist employers in creating healthy and positive work environments are discussed next.

THE NATIONAL QUALITY INSTITUTE MODEL

The National Quality Institute (NQI; http://www.nqi.ca), together with Health Canada and in collaboration with health care professionals, developed criteria with which to evaluate the health status of a work environment. The criteria provide a framework to organizations to facilitate the development of a healthy environment. This framework is also used to identify workplaces that receive awards in recognition of meeting standards of a healthy work environment. The NQI model integrates three dimensions: organizational culture; physical environment and occupational health and safety; and health and lifestyle practices. Within this model is recognition that the individual, the organization, and the system each share accountability for a healthy work environment (National Quality Institute & Health Canada, 2006).

*Organizational Culture*

Organizational culture focuses on the patterns of relationships and communication that create a healthy culture, an essential of which is leadership that nurtures the ability of people to fully use their talents and resources. Seen as significant contributors to a healthy culture are recognition of staff, opportunities for personal and career development, and a work environment that is open to receiving input and feedback and transparent regarding its decisions and strategy (National Quality Institute & Health Canada, 2006).

*Physical Environment and Occupational Health and Safety*

The attribute of physical environment and occupational health and safety is linked with external legislation and directives that guide a safe workplace, but in addition, challenges workplaces to exceed these expectations. Many health care facilities pose safety challenges for staff. Not only are there physical work demands, but in many health care facilities, staff are exposed to infectious disease, radiation, chemotherapy, and other toxic substances—some known and some that may not yet be known (National Quality Institute & Health Canada, 2006).

*Health and Lifestyle Practices*

The dimension of health and lifestyle practices requires that workplaces enable and support healthy lifestyle behaviours and encourage good health practices among their employees. Examples include health promotion and illness prevention programs, healthy eating awareness, and fitness opportunities. The goal is to help staff balance work and life and to build this balance into the organizational culture (National Quality Institute & Health Canada, 2006).

RNAO HEALTHY WORK ENVIRONMENTS BEST PRACTICE GUIDELINES PROJECT

A framework more relevant to nursing was established upon a recommendation made in "Ensuring the Care Will Be There: Report on Nursing Retention and Recruitment in Ontario" (2000). The Ontario Ministry of Health and Long-Term Care provided funding to the Registered Nurses' Association of Ontario (RNAO; http://www.rnao.org) in 2003 to develop evidence-informed guidelines to facilitate the creation of healthy work environments and to thereby support the recruitment and retention of nurses. The Health Canada Office of Nursing Policy (a federal organization) partnered with the RNAO to establish these guidelines in part to address priorities identified by the Canadian Nursing Advisory Committee (2002). These best practice guidelines have been adopted by nursing organizations across Canada and internationally. The reader is invited to review the RNAO Web site (http://www.rnao.org) for more information on this project.

*Organizing Framework for the RNAO Healthy Work Environments Best Practice Guidelines Project*

To guide the development of best practices guidelines project, the RNAO established a conceptual model to describe the components and elements of a healthy work environment for nurses.

This framework conceptualizes a healthy work environment as a complex system that has multiple dimensions and components that interact with one another, and demonstrates the interdependence between the individual, the organization, and the external system (e.g., government, regulatory bodies). Since nurses function in a system mediated and influenced by these interactions, interventions to create and sustain a healthy work environment within this model focus on these dimensions and their interactions with each other. A healthy work environment is further described as "a practice setting that maximizes the health and well-being of nurses, quality patient/client outcomes, organizational performance, and societal outcomes" (Registered Nurses' Association of Ontario [RNAO], 2007a, p. 12). The achievement of a healthy work environment for nurses benefits all interprofessional team members, positively influences recruitment and retention, and results in positive patient care outcomes.

As a result of the development of this model, seven guidelines for a healthy work environment were initially identified and developed:

1. Developing and Sustaining Nursing Leadership
2. Collaborative Practice in Nursing Teams
3. Embracing Cultural Diversity in Health Care

4. Professionalism in Nursing
5. Workload and Staffing
6. Workplace Health and Safety of the Nurse
7. Prevention of Violence in the Workplace

As an example, the guideline *Professionalism in Nursing* (RNAO, 2007b) demonstrates the interacting attributes of knowledge, a spirit of inquiry, accountability, autonomy, advocacy, innovation and vision, collegiality and collaboration, and ethics and values. The guideline acknowledges that nurses succeed when they are in an environment that supports and values ethical reflection and discourse. Within the guideline, recommendations are made to ensure that systems and processes are in place in order to meet this standard, which would not be possible in isolation of all the components and attributes that make up a healthy work environment.

## Right to Be Protected From Harm

Health care environments can pose multiple risks to nurses and other employees. Some are in the form of exposure to agents such as disinfectants (e.g., glutaraldehyde or cidex), antineoplastic agents, anesthetic gases, radiation, electromagnetic fields, and so on (Charney & Schirmer, 1990). Exposure to infectious diseases is also a growing concern. Other risks are less tangible. Health care is a highly stressful environment predisposing nurses not only to the effects of their own personal stress but to the consequences of stress in others. Nurses may experience the effects of a disrespectful and nonsupportive work environment through the actions of their leaders, peers, or other team members. Nurses may also be at risk of physical harm from patients, who may be cognitively impaired due to their illness or treatment. They also interact with families under extreme stress, who cope and respond in varying ways. These multiple risks in the health care environment must be recognized, and interventions need to be put in place to minimize and manage these appropriately.

A number of strategies, including legislation and workplace standards and guidelines, exist to ensure a healthy and safe environment for nurses.

## Occupational Health and Safety

In an effort to ensure that working conditions are as safe and healthy as possible, all provinces have enacted occupational health and safety (OH&S) legislation. (See Alberta: *Occupational Health and Safety Act*, R.S.A. 2000, c. O-2; British Columbia: *Workers Compensation Act*, R.S.B.C. 1996, c. 492; Manitoba: *Workplace Safety and Health Act*, C.C.S.M. c. W210; New Brunswick: *Occupational Health and Safety Act*, S.N.B. 1983, c. O-0.2; Newfoundland and Labrador: *Occupational Health and Safety Act*, R.S.N.L. 1990, c. O-3; Northwest Territories and Nunavut: *Safety Act*, R.S.N.W.T. 1988, c. S-1; Nova Scotia: *Occupational Health and Safety Act*, S.N.S. 1996, c. 7; Ontario: *Occupational Health and Safety Act*, R.S.O. 1990, c. O.1; Prince Edward Island: *Occupational Health and Safety Act*, R.S.P.E.I. 1988, c. O-1.01; Quebec: *Occupational health and safety, An Act respecting*, R.S.Q. c. S-2.1; Saskatchewan: *Occupational Health and Safety Act, 1993*, S.S. 1993, c. O-1.1.) These statutes mandate the establishment of health and safety committees comprising representatives of management and nonmanagerial employees. The object of these committees is to identify and recommend solutions to potentially hazardous conditions in the workplace. Further, many provinces' statutes provide for the selection of OH&S representatives to inquire into and inspect hazardous working conditions, materials, substances, or unsafe equipment.

As with all employers, hospitals and other employers of health care professionals are legally obligated to provide safe working environments for their employees. In Ontario, for example, the *Health Care and Residential Facilities Regulation* (O. Reg. 67/93, s. 9), made under the *Occupational Health and Safety Act* (1990), requires employers of nurses and other health care professionals, among other things, to have written plans, policies, and procedures for such matters as infection control, proper hygiene, protection against biological and chemical hazards in the workplace, the use and wearing of personal protective equipment, and so forth. The same legislation exists in many other provinces, including Nova Scotia and New Brunswick.

In addition to this, the *Occupational Health and Safety Act* allows workers to refuse to work in circumstances in which "the physical condition of the workplace or the part thereof in which he or she works or is to work is likely to endanger himself or herself" (*Occupational Health and Safety Act*, 1990, s. 43(3)(b)). Despite this, a person employed in a hospital or health care facility does not have this right if the condition of the workplace "is inherent in the worker's work or is a normal condition of the worker's employment" or if "the worker's refusal to work would directly endanger the life, health or safety of another person" (*Occupational Health and Safety Act*, 1990, ss. 43(1), (2)). Thus, in a situation such as the SARS outbreak discussed earlier, a nurse working in a hospital providing care for such patients would not likely have a right to refuse to work because of the conditions since it is fairly certain that risk of infection and working with infected patients in a highly infectious environment is inherent in a nurse's work. This does not mean, however, that a hospital is absolved of its legal responsibility to provide a safe work environment and to have proper procedures and protocols in place to minimize the risk of infection in the workplace. Employees have essentially similar rights (with some minor differences) in all other provinces and territories except British Columbia, where there is no stated right to refuse to work. In British Columbia, however, a government official may order a work stoppage where he or she deems the workplace to be unsafe.

## Violence in the Workplace

One of the most serious contributors to moral distress and an unhealthy work environment is **workplace violence**. Nurses may experience many forms of violence in their work environments. Unfortunately, much of this violence may go unrecognized. The rights of nurses to be protected from harm in the workplace include having a violence-free work environment.

Nurses are at risk of violence from many perspectives. They work with seriously ill patients whose illnesses may predispose them to unintentional violence. They may encounter patients and their families who, owing to their personality or previous experiences, inflict physical or verbal abuse as a means of self-assertion. They may also experience violence in the form of disrespectful behaviour, bullying, or harassment from each other, their leaders, or other members of the team. There are a number of strategies individual nurses, leaders, and organizations (Braverman, 1999) can introduce to prevent these forms of violence and to manage them effectively if they occur.

Safeguards and protections organizations can put in place to reduce the risk of harm include:

- Assessing the workplace to determine areas of risk
- Ensuring prevention strategies are in place, including appropriate education to identify the potential for violence
- Ensuring employees have the knowledge and skills to defuse violent situations and to respond appropriately when assistance is needed

For example, the nurse visiting patients in their homes may be vulnerable owing to the isolated environment, and nurses in psychiatric and emergency departments, where patients may be cognitively impaired due to their illnesses and where families may be under immense stress, are at higher risk of violence. At the same time, employers have the responsibility to recognize and minimize the risk of harm to nurses regardless of where they work but especially in high-risk environments.

The Canadian Nurses Association and the Canadian Federation of Nurses Unions (CFNU) issued a joint position statement on workplace violence in 2007. It stated that it is the "right of all nurses to work in an environment that is free from violence" (Canadian Nurses Association [CNA] & Canadian Federation of Nurses Unions [CFNU], 2007, p. 1). The definition of *violence* set out in the statements is:

actual and attempted incidents of verbal, physical, psychological (including bullying) and sexual abuse, in circumstances related to work, that result in personal injury, either physical or psychological, or give reasonable cause to believe that risk of injury or detrimental impact on an individual's health exists. (CNA & CFNU, 2007, p. 1)

The statement also outlines the serious implications of workplace violence, including:

- Compromising patient safety
- Injury and emotional and psychological trauma
- Impact on retention, absenteeism, morale, productivity, and so on

The risk of violence in the workplace is influenced by many factors, including:

- The physical layout of the environment (e.g., nurses working in isolation)
- Aggressive management of patients (e.g., via restraint, seclusion, and medication) (Duxbury, 1999, 2002)

- Composition of nursing staff (number, age, experience, skill mix) (Owen, Tarantello, Jones, & Tennant, 1998)
- Whether patients are disoriented, have violent histories, or have engaged in, for example, substance abuse (Owen et al., 1998)

There are circumstances in which a nurse may be threatened or assaulted by a confused, disoriented, or delusional patient. Though nurses often understand that the behaviour of their patients may be a result of illness, response to treatment or medication, or sleep deprivation, workplaces should have in place strategies to prevent and neutralize violence and to access Security if this becomes necessary. When a high-risk patient is identified, a clear strategy for managing that patient needs to be determined. The nurses assigned to that patient must have the knowledge and experience to recognize signs of and implement tactics to prevent escalating aggressive behaviour. When faced with patients who are confused, agitated, or mentally ill, nurses must recognize that these violent behaviours may result from their illness, fear, or stress. Thus, nurses need the knowledge and skills to identify clients who are medically or psychiatrically predisposed to violence; to recognize the triggers that precipitate violence; and to devise and initiate appropriate strategies for prevention and effective management of violent behaviours if this becomes necessary.

Nurses who work in the community may be at further risk if they are sent alone to environments where there is known criminal or gang activity. Backup should be provided, and nurses should not be put in a position of danger without adequate support and security measures.

Unfortunately, violence in the workplace occurs most frequently between peers and in supervisor–employee relationships. Significantly underreported (Farrell, 1997, 1999; O'Connell, Young, Brooks, Hutchings, & Lofthouse, 2000), workplace violence may involve misuse of power and control (Deans, 2004; Farrell, 1999; MacIntosh, 2003) and may take the form of physical, psychological, or sexual abuse, harassment, bullying, or aggression. It may involve the interaction of people in different roles and power relationships (Deans, 2004) and is more likely to be verbal, passive, and have a top-down element (Burnazi, Keashly, & Neuman, 2005).

Most troubling is the extent of peer-to-peer violence, especially when it goes unrecognized and unreported, which is often the case. Nurse-to-nurse violence is well documented in the literature, begins early in nursing programs, and extends across all health care work environments. Bullying (e.g., passive–aggressive behaviour, personal diminishment) and incivility (e.g., rudeness, lack of respect, gossip) are the most common forms of violence in the workplace. Bullying includes behaviour toward others that is intimidating, lacking in respect, coercive, critical, and belittling. Incivility includes condescending and insulting behaviour, and ignoring or humiliating the victim (Pejic, 2005).

Targets of bullying behaviour are often competent, committed employees who are trying to do a good job. They do not always perceive the bullying event, but it tends to be recognized by other colleagues (Lewis, Coursol, & Herting, 2002; Lewis, M., 2006; Lewis,

M. A., 2006). Bullies themselves are often insecure, fearful, or jealous. They bully to protect themselves and are often unable to assess their own behaviour (MacIntosh, 2003). Bullying is most often found in organizations with a negative social climate and unsupportive leadership (Hansen, Hogh, Persson, Karlson, Garde, & Ørbæk, 2006).

As mentioned earlier, bullying behaviour is underreported. Causes for this include peer pressure not to report, lack of awareness that it constitutes violence, perception that it is part of the job, fear of being blamed for causing the violent act, and fear of job loss (McKoy & Smith, 2001).

Sustained exposure to workplace violence can have serious physical and psychological consequences (MacIntosh, 2003, 2005; McKenna, Smith, Poole, & Coverdale, 2003). Abused nurses report feeling unwanted or devalued, having thoughts about leaving their jobs, not wanting to go to work, having difficulty sleeping, experiencing anxiety and feelings of worthlessness, and being more critical of the organizational climate within which they work (Quine, 2003).

A recent review of 110 studies undertaken over 21 years comparing the consequences of **sexual harassment** and bullying at work concluded that though both can poison the work environment, the latter has the worse consequences:

> Victims of bullying, incivility or interpersonal conflicts are more likely to quit jobs, feel worse, and be less happy with their jobs and leaders than those who were sexually harassed. Society has deemed sexual harassment to be illegal and reaches out to victims in contrast to bullying and incivility leaving victims to fend for themselves. Bullying can be very subtle, making it difficult to deal with and punish. (Stephens, 2008)

RNAO BEST PRACTICE GUIDELINE: PREVENTING AND MANAGING VIOLENCE IN THE WORKPLACE

In 2008, the RNAO introduced the guideline *Preventing and Managing Violence in the Workplace*, making recommendations to government; researchers; accreditation bodies; academic settings; professional, regulatory and union bodies; organizations; individuals; and teams. These recommendations are aimed at preventing and managing all forms of violence in the workplace. The reader is encouraged to review this guideline at http://www.rnao.org.

Within the guideline, violence in the workplace is defined as:

> a multidimensional phenomenon involving the misuse of power and resulting in physical, psychological or sexual abuse of targets. Perpetrators of violence may not be known to the organization (type I) or may involve patient/client/family members (type II), present or past staff members (type III) or personal relationships (type IV). (RNAO, 2008, p. 14)

The intent of the guideline is to define and describe violence, identify strategies that help in the recognition and prevention of violence, and to monitor and evaluate outcomes associated with it. The guideline sets out a number of key recommendations to organizations for the prevention and management of workplace violence. These include:

- Ensuring policies and guidelines are in place to prevent, mitigate, and respond to workplace violence
- Undertaking risk assessments to identify the vulnerable areas and environments
- Ensuring staff awareness of what constitutes workplace violence
- Having reporting processes in place
- Following up on every incident
- Providing education to all staff (RNAO, 2008)

Since this culture seems to be pervasive in health care, nursing leaders in all settings need to address these problematic issues if nursing is to be sustained in the future and safe and ethical care is to be ensured for patients. If bullying behaviour exists among nurses, what then is the bully's approach to patients, clients, and families? How do we ensure a viable health care system in the future if we cannot ensure a safe and supportive environment for nurses?

An extreme example of violence toward a nurse led to a coroner's inquest when a nurse employed at a hospital in a major Canadian city was murdered. This provides a vivid illustration of the need for health care facilities and employers to follow up on disruptive and inappropriate behaviour and complaints brought forward by nurses and other employees. In this case, the nurse was murdered by her former partner, who had privileges as an anesthetist at the same hospital. It was revealed during the inquest into the nurse's death that numerous officials at the hospital were aware of the doctor's disrespectful conduct toward the nurse and others, yet they failed to take adequate steps to address his behaviour. The coroner's jury made numerous recommendations to ensure a safe and violence-free workplace. The Ontario legislature is also considering a private member's bill that would require all employers to implement policies to protect their employees from workplace harassment and violence. The bill, still at first reading stage as of this writing, would specifically require that employers prepare

> guidelines and processes for identifying, eliminating and dealing with incidents of workplace related harassment or violence including such guidelines and processes as may be prescribed and to develop and deliver regular harassment and violence prevention training for its workers, including those who exercise managerial functions and require workers to attend the training provided. (Bill 29, clause 49.2(c), (d))

Meanwhile, other provinces have already enacted such legislation. Nova Scotia, for example, has specifically enacted regulations pursuant to its *Occupational Health and Safety Act* (S.N.S. 1996, c. 7) that provide a positive duty on employers to protect employees from workplace violence (see N.S. Reg. 209/2007 made under the *Occupational Health and Safety*

*Act* (Nova Scotia)). This regulation specifically applies to (among other workplace settings) a "healthcare workplace," which is defined in the regulation as:

> a district health authority under the *Health Authorities Act* (such as a hospital or other health care facility), a nursing home, a home for the aged, a residential care facility under the *Homes for Special Care Act* or any other long-term-care facility, and a place where emergency health services or home care services are provided. (N.S. Reg 209/2007, s. 2(d))

It requires employers to conduct a violence risk assessment of the workplace and prepare a report on any such risk and the extent of the risk in that workplace. Where a risk of such violence is found, the employer must prepare and implement policies and procedures designed to minimize such risks and to provide for the reporting, documentation, and investigation of incidences of workplace violence. New Brunswick has enacted a regulation under its *Occupational Health and Safety Act* (R.S.N.B. c. 0-1.2) that establishes a code of practice to protect workers who work alone from risks arising from or in connection with their work (N.B. Reg. 92-133).

In the Ontario case, the coroner's jury found that the hospital had allowed a culture to exist in which the doctor could continue his outrageous and harassing conduct, which included throwing his computer across the room while a patient awaiting surgery was still conscious. The inquest raised concerns that there was not a plan to address his inappropriate behaviour. It also identified a pervasive culture of "physician dominance" that may lead to double standards by which inappropriate conduct by physicians may be left unchallenged at the expense of a poisoned and potentially unsafe work environment for nurses and other health care workers. The jury recommended, among other things, that hospitals be given the requisite authority over physicians working in their facilities to enable them to better manage any such disruptive behaviour. It also urged that labour legislation be amended to give the Ontario Ministry of Labour the authority to investigate workplace harassment and abuse claims.

## Moral Distress

To illustrate the significance of healthy work environments that support ethical practice, let us once again consider the notion of moral distress (discussed in detail in Chapter 2).

**Moral distress** is defined as the emotional and psychological pain that occurs when "one knows the right thing to do, but institutional constraints make it nearly impossible to pursue the right course of action" (Jameton, 1984, p. 6). Moral distress often arises in situations in which nurses are faced with moral uncertainties or dilemmas, and power imbalances exist within the team making the difficult ethical decisions. The Canadian Nurses Association describes *moral distress* as:

> situations in which nurses cannot fulfill their ethical obligations and commitments (i.e. their moral agency), or they fail to pursue what they believe to be the right

course of action, or fail to live up to their own expectation of ethical practice, for one or more of the following reasons: error in judgment, insufficient personal resolve or other circumstances truly beyond their control. They may feel guilt, concern or distaste as a result. (CNA, 2003, p. 2)

To minimize moral distress, the CNA encourages a climate of openness that encourages peer support, trust, respect, open communication, and facilitation of dialogue in which all team members are participants. Moral distress is minimized further in environments in which mentorship is provided, leaders are role models in accountability and disclosure of adverse events, nurses are provided with knowledge and tools to understand and address ethical challenges, and individual values and beliefs are respected. These are all descriptors of a healthy work environment.

Evidence suggests that certain types of situations in the workplace contribute to moral distress. These situations may include a lack of necessary resources, rule-oriented environments, conflicts of interest, and minimal support systems (Solomon, O'Donnell, Jennings, Guilfoy, Wolf, Nolan, et al., 1993). If issues of moral distress are not addressed in the workplace, the consequences may be serious: nurses may choose to leave the organization or, unfortunately, the profession. Distress may result in positive coping strategies (e.g., compassion and self-reflection) or negative coping strategies (e.g., negativity, despair, loss of integrity, or fractured relationships) (American Association of Critical-Care Nurses, 2006; Rushton, 2006). Those who remain in the workplace may lack trust, fail to collaborate with others, and experience or exhibit negative behaviour and disrespectful communication.

An ethical and healthy work environment can be achieved by leaders if attention is paid to important issues such as:

- Acknowledging and responding to moral distress in a respectful and compassionate manner
- Addressing practice environment issues, such as systems of care, supports, and resources
- Ensuring collaborative, respectful relationships with shared authority and responsibility
- Influencing the culture of the work environment by setting standards for norms and behaviours, ensuring effective communication processes, and introducing processes and frameworks for resolving ethical conflicts (American Association of Critical-Care Nurses, 2006; Rushton, 2006)

Nursing leaders should review the RNAO best practice guidelines and the *Code of Ethics for Registered Nurses*, and implement these practices and guidelines in their workplaces.

# Case Scenario

## WHY DO NURSES "EAT THEIR YOUNG"?

Lina is a new graduate in a small rural hospital. She grew up in the small town and was thrilled to graduate at a time when it had a rare nursing vacancy.

Initially excited about this opportunity, she soon found herself disappointed. Most of the nurses had worked there for many years and had developed strong friendships and affiliations. Not used to working with new graduates, they were surprised that Lina was not as clinically competent as they believed they were when they graduated from nursing school. As a result, they were highly critical of Lina and the modern theoretical approach to education she had experienced.

Lina felt isolated from the team. She was not included in breaks, her requests for help were ignored, and she felt the nursing care she gave was constantly monitored by the team.

She became extremely stressed and was having trouble sleeping at night. She was reluctant to confide in her mother since some of her coworkers were family friends, and the manager of the unit was good friends with most of the nurses.

Lina's stress and sleeplessness increased, and one day when she was unable to focus, she made a serious medication error. She was worried about reporting the error because she feared the consequences, but before she could confess it herself, one of the other nurses reported it to the manager.

In the background observing all of this was a member of the cleaning staff, Terri, who was also part of the local community. As a subordinate to the nurses, she had experienced some alienation and was sensitive to what Lina was experiencing. She wanted to bring forward her concerns to the manager but was fearful of the consequences.

### Issues
1. Does this scenario highlight a form of workplace violence?
2. What options are available to Lina and Terri?
3. What are the ethical issues involved?
4. Do you think this is an isolated incident?
5. What strategies would you use to improve your work environment when you graduate as a nurse?
6. As a student, have you been exposed to workplace violence? What types? How have you dealt with these incidences?
7. What would you do if you experienced bullying in your existing environment?

# Case Scenario

## A RISKY ENCOUNTER?

Casey is a visiting nurse in a major Canadian city. Her region is in a poor area of the city where there are known gangs. She is sent to the home of a young woman to ensure that her nutritional needs are being met. This young woman, Tricia, suffered major weight loss after undergoing serious abdominal surgery. Tricia lives alone, but each time Casey visits, a male neighbour is present. Casey is concerned since Tricia continues to lose weight, and, in spite of financial support, there is little evidence of food in the home. The neighbour is dominating and aggressive, and Casey finds him intimidating. She is worried about his influence on Tricia, concerned that her money is being used to support his drug habit (previously disclosed to Casey by Tricia), and is uncertain about next steps. She feels if she takes a stand on the issues to protect Tricia, she will be at personal risk.

### Issues

1. Do you think this is an unsafe work environment for Casey?
2. What support should she receive from her employer?
3. What strategies should Casey undertake to help Tricia while ensuring her own safety?

## Labour Relations and Collective Bargaining

Most nurses in Canada work in public hospitals and other health care facilities in which the employees are unionized. It is helpful for nurses to have a basic understanding of such labour relations concepts as union formation, collective bargaining, grievance procedures, arbitration, and the right to strike, since they will likely come across these matters at some point in their practice. An exhaustive study of labour law and labour relations is beyond the scope of this book. However, a brief review of the basics and some of the related procedures follows, in order to provide a general understanding of this subject.

Similarly, the field of occupational health and safety (OH&S) has grown widely in the past 30 years. Many provinces have enacted stringent OH&S statutes in an effort to ensure that working conditions of all employees (whether unionized or not) are made as safe and healthy as possible. This impetus has arisen from a better understanding of how the human body reacts to its environment and the hazards posed by toxic or dangerous substances or activities in the workplace (e.g., radiation, chemotherapy).

## Union Formation and Certification

Though it should be noted that not all health care settings are represented by a union, the extent of unionization across Canada is such that issues related to unionization should be addressed. In settings without unions, structures and processes are in place to ensure the appropriate input from and support for nurses. These often take the form of self-governance models or councils (Rotstein & Peskun, 2008; Manuel & Bruinse, 2005).

UNION ORGANIZATION

The recognition of labour unions in Canada and the concomitant rights of workers to organize and to bargain collectively with their employers, as in the rest of the industrialized world, came about as a result of a long struggle fraught with social unrest, strikes, and violence throughout the late nineteenth and early twentieth centuries. Gradually, unions and the principle of collective bargaining came to be seen as valid means to equalize the bargaining power of employees with that of the often large, wealthy, and powerful corporations who employed them. Unions, recognized as protectors of workers' interests, could ensure that those workers would receive fair wages and achieve better and safer working conditions. The right to unionize was constitutionally enshrined in 1982 in the *Canadian Charter of Rights and Freedoms* (1982, s. 2(d)), although such a right was recognized in Canadian law and labour relations statutes well before that time.

A **union** is a provincially certified group of employees, in most cases having a common employer. Unionized employees often work in common or related activities in the businesses or undertakings of these employers. The object of uniting is to provide bargaining influence, power, and leverage, by force of numbers, in negotiations pertaining to the terms of employment affecting each member (e.g., wages, hours of work, benefits, work scheduling, layoff and termination, disciplinary matters and procedures, seniority, and job security). Thus, with a common interest in the terms of their employment, the employees, through their union, negotiate the terms and conditions of the employment contract collectively for the benefit of all employees.

Most aspects of union certification and labour relations are governed by the provinces by virtue of the jurisdiction given to them by the Constitution (see Chapter 4 for more information on the legal system). All provinces have passed labour relations legislation dealing with union certification, procedures for collective bargaining, procedures for strike votes (in some cases), definition of unfair labour practices, and prohibition of strike breaking, as well as the establishment of labour relations boards, their duties and powers. (See British Columbia: *Labour Relations Code*, R.S.B.C. 1996, c. 244; Alberta: *Labour Relations Code*, R.S.A. 2000, c. L-1; Saskatchewan: *Trade Union Act*, R.S.S. 1978, c. T-17; Manitoba: *Labour Relations Act*, C.C.S.M. c. L10; Ontario: *Labour Relations Act, 1995*, S.O. 1995, c.1, sched. A; Quebec: *Labour Code*, R.S.Q. c. C-27; New Brunswick: *Industrial Relations Act*, R.S.N.B. 1973, c. I-4; Nova Scotia: *Trade Union Act*, R.S.N.S. 1989, c. 475; Prince Edward Island: *Labour Act*, R.S.P.E.I. 1988, c. L-1; Newfoundland and Labrador: *Labour Relations Act*, R.S.N.L. 1990, c. L-1.)

The federal government has also passed labour legislation to deal with labour relations issues arising from industries or activities that fall under federal legislative jurisdiction including labour relations in the three territories (*Canada Labour Code*, 1985). Examples of federally regulated industries include certain airline, postal, and telecommunications workers. Similarly, civil servants at both the provincial and federal levels are usually covered by separate legislation specifically applicable to such government employees.

Before it can be certified, the union must be formed. Where there is no existing union willing to apply for certification on behalf of a group of employees, those employees may themselves form a union. The question as to whether a union is properly constituted usually arises during certification proceedings before a provincial Labour Relations Board. This body is charged, as part of its overall duties under the labour statute, with reviewing the union's application for certification and ensuring that all procedural formalities have been met.

An overview of the formalities necessary to the formation of a union was provided by the Ontario Labour Relations Board (OLRB) in one of its decisions in 1977 (*Re Local 199 UAW Building Corp.*, 1977, p. 473). Similar considerations would apply in other provinces. The OLRB laid down the following requirements:

1. A constitution must be drafted wherein the purpose of the union (including the conduct of labour relations) must be stated and procedures for electing officers (e.g., president, secretary, treasurer) and calling meetings of the union must be set out.
2. A meeting of the employees (in whose interest the union is being formed) must be held for the purposes of discussing and approving the proposed constitution.
3. The employees attending such a meeting must be admitted as members of the union. (Membership cards may be issued.)
4. A vote of the members at this meeting must be taken to ratify (approve) the proposed constitution.
5. The officers of the union should then be elected according to the procedures laid out in the newly approved constitution.

At this point, an application for certification can be filed with the Labour Board.

CERTIFICATION

All provinces and the federal government have some form of **certification** process that must be passed before a union can represent the employees of a particular employer. The size and membership of the group of employees will usually be examined by the particular provincial Labour Board in order to determine whether it is appropriate for collective bargaining—that is, whether its members are truly employees and the group is of an appropriate size. Some provinces require that a specific percentage of all employees of an employer be members of the union. Others do not impose this requirement. In some provinces, a representation vote may have to be taken to determine the union's level of support among the employees of the employer.

Once certified, the union becomes the exclusive **bargaining agent** for its employees. That union alone is then authorized to negotiate a collective agreement on behalf of the employees in the **bargaining unit** (the specific group of employees of a specific employer or group of employers whom it was certified to represent).

The labour relations statutes do not apply to managerial employees, who are seen to represent employers. To allow managers to participate in union formation, membership, and activities would create a conflict of interest because managers are usually charged with executing the employer's administrative, disciplinary, and evaluative policies; in many cases, they negotiate the terms of a collective agreement with the unions as representatives of the employer. These activities are regarded as being inconsistent with the interests of workers in collective bargaining.

For example, a nurse manager whose duties are primarily administrative and managerial will not be covered by the collective bargaining scheme and provisions of the provincial labour relations statute. He or she is not permitted to participate in the formation of the union nor to be listed on the certification application as a union member and thus one of the employees represented.

Some provinces allow employees to refuse to join a union or to refuse to pay dues to a union on religious grounds. In such cases, the statutes provide that an amount equal to the union dues be paid by the dissenter to a charitable institution mutually agreed upon by the parties. In Manitoba, Saskatchewan, Ontario, and Quebec, an employee who is eligible for membership but is not, in fact, a member must still pay dues to the union. Such dues are usually deducted by the employer from the employee's paycheque and paid to the union.

In some provinces, closed shops are permitted. A **closed shop** is a place of employment that requires all employees to be members of the union as a condition of employment. This stipulation will appear among the terms of the collective agreement. Or the contract may simply provide that, while union membership is not mandatory (that is, the place of employment is an **open shop**), preference in hiring will be given to union members over nonmembers.

In some provinces, certification may be automatic upon the union's demonstrating that it has achieved a certain level of membership. Not all employees of an employer need be members of the union seeking certification. But if a large majority of them are, this may be sufficient, in some provinces, for automatic certification. In Alberta, for example, it is possible for an employer to voluntarily recognize a union as the bargaining agent for a group of employees without the union's being certified (see *Alberta Labour Relations Code*, s. 42).

DECERTIFICATION

A union may also lose its right to act as bargaining agent for a group of workers, or it may be dissolved. This is usually referred to as **decertification**. For example, a union can lose its rights by failing to negotiate a collective agreement in good faith within a certain period of time. A group of the union's members can then apply for a declaration from the provincial Labour Relations Board that the union no longer represents, and thus can no longer negotiate for, the employees in a given bargaining unit.

In some provinces, a minimum number of employees may have to consent to such declaration before the board may decertify the union. The union may also lose its certification if it fails to give the employer notice within a certain period of time of its desire to begin negotiations for a new collective agreement or to renew an existing agreement.

It is important for nurses who are members of labour unions to know that, in all cases, their employers are not free to give them individual advice if nurses are dissatisfied with the manner in which their union is representing them. At all times, nurses in such a situation have the right to consult with a labour lawyer. A legal professional can best advise the nurse or nurses on all appropriate courses of action and their legal rights.

## Collective Bargaining

**Collective bargaining** is a process whereby workers, through their union representatives, meet with their employers in order to negotiate the terms and conditions of employment applicable to each worker. It is a right that was not recognized historically in common law and was even prohibited in past times as a "conspiracy of persons in restraint of trade." Today, collective bargaining is fully recognized and promoted in the various labour relations statutes, both federal and provincial.

Under the laws of all provinces and the federal government, the parties to an expired collective agreement are obliged to negotiate a new contract when one of the parties serves the other with a notice to bargain for a new agreement (or, where there is no prior agreement and a union is newly certified, the first collective agreement). The notice begins the process of collective bargaining. In some provinces, a union can lose its certification and authorization to bargain for a specific bargaining unit if it does not serve such a notice and begin negotiation within a specified period of time. This will usually result in another union's being certified to represent the employees in the bargaining unit in place of the first union.

In collective bargaining, each side puts forth its desired terms and conditions for a new employment contract. Such terms may include wages; hours of work; work schedules; vacation pay; sick leave; pensions and other employee benefits; mechanisms for settling disputes that arise from the application, administration, interpretation, or alleged violation of the collective agreement (called grievance procedures); and employer and employee representation on the joint OH&S committee for the workplace.

Often, negotiations become mired in disagreement over one or more terms. These disputes, if not settled promptly, can lead to strike action by employees or a lockout of employees by an employer. Thus, the labour relations statutes contain procedures for appointing conciliators and mediators to assist the parties in resolving such disagreements and to negotiate a contract. A **conciliator** may be appointed at the request of either party to resolve outstanding issues, or, in some cases, the provincial Minister of Labour may choose to appoint a conciliator or mediator.

In all provinces, once a notice to bargain has been given, the employer cannot change the existing terms or conditions of employment, including wages, unless it has the permission of its board of directors and the union, or the provisions of the collective agreement permit it.

### THE COLLECTIVE AGREEMENT

The contract that emerges from the collective bargaining negotiations is called a **collective agreement**. In all provinces and at the federal level, the agreement must be effective for a minimum duration of one year and must be in writing, but it need not be embodied in a single document. For example, an exchange of letters, notes, and memoranda may constitute the collective agreement if the parties thereto set out the agreed-upon terms.

If the collective agreement expires before a new one is in place, the terms and conditions of the old agreement usually continue to apply provided that there is no evidence that the parties intended otherwise. Some contracts specify that they will continue after the expiry date until and unless either party notifies the other of its desire to terminate the agreement. In all provinces except Quebec and Nova Scotia, no employee is permitted to strike, nor may any employer lock out its employees, during the life of the contract. This is to preserve labour peace. This condition applies even after the agreement has expired and until a specified period has elapsed from the time a conciliator is appointed by the Minister of Labour (or other authorized person) to the time a conciliator's report is released to the parties. This is colloquially known as a **cooling-off period**.

## Grievance Procedures and Arbitration

Since workers are not permitted to strike during the currency of a collective agreement, nor employers to lock out workers, there must be a means of resolving disputes arising from the application, administration, interpretation, or alleged violation of the terms of the agreement. Without it, labour tensions might build to an explosive point. The violence of past labour disputes has shown the necessity and desirability of having effective and timely dispute resolution procedures in place before matters get out of hand. Indeed, all provincial labour statutes except Saskatchewan's require that collective agreements contain procedures for settling management–labour disputes. If they do not, the legislation deems certain provisions to be part of the agreement.

Such grievance procedures will be negotiated as part of the terms of the collective agreement. Many agreements provide relatively informal mechanisms for the presentation of a grievance. As well, many workplaces have grievance committees, which consist of employee representatives, and employer representation.

For example, suppose a nurse is asked by her supervisor to work an additional hour beyond what the contract requires. The request may possibly result from the supervisor's misunderstanding of the terms of the collective agreement. The nurse refuses to work and is disciplined. She may then choose to file a grievance against that supervisor.

Some hospitals have hospital association committees comprising members of the hospital's management and nonmanagerial nurse employees. They meet on a regular basis to review any grievances in an attempt to resolve them in an informal, cooperative setting before they become adversarial and part of a formal grievance process. If informal mechanisms fail, however, grievance procedures are implemented.

The following grievance procedures are not necessarily followed uniformly across Canada but are fairly common in many labour relations settings. They usually involve a progressive three-step process.

### STEP 1: WRITTEN SUBMISSION

In the event that the nurse's grievance is not settled satisfactorily after it is brought to the supervisor's attention, then, within a specified time, the grievance must be submitted in writing to the immediate supervisor for a response. Failing a settlement, it then must be filed within a specified time to the director of nursing for resolution. If it is still not settled, the procedure provides that it be submitted to the hospital administrator or other authorized hospital official within a set period of time for a meeting.

### STEP 2: MEETING WITH THE GRIEVANCE COMMITTEE

The administrator, the person who filed the grievance, the grievance committee, and a representative of the union meet. Within a specified time, the hospital must then make a decision as to how it will deal with the grievance. Thus, the procedure provides for the grievance's being submitted to a progressively higher authority as long as it remains unsettled. (In many hospitals, this procedure is managed through the human resources department.) The collective agreement will also provide that any settlement reached through these procedures is binding on the parties.

### STEP 3: BINDING ARBITRATION

If the decision rendered by the hospital administrator does not settle the issue, then the matter is submitted to binding arbitration.

*Binding arbitration* is a procedure mandated by the labour relations statutes of many provinces. Usually, the parties have a specified time from the rendering of the hospital administrator's decision to have the matter submitted to binding arbitration. At that time, the party requesting arbitration will nominate a person to be part of a three-member arbitration board.

The party to whom the notice is given then has a specified time in which to nominate a second person to that board. If a nomination is not forthcoming, the party who served the notice may request that the Minister of Labour nominate a second person.

No person who has been involved in attempting to negotiate or settle the grievance prior to its submission to arbitration may sit on the arbitration board. These two persons choose a third person to chair and complete the board. If they cannot agree, then the minister appoints a chair.

Recent years have seen disputes over workloads and the right of nurses to refuse to provide services once the number of patients placed in their care exceeds their ability to provide adequate care. In *Re Mount Sinai Hospital and the Ontario Nurses' Association* (which was discussed earlier in this chapter), the nurses refused to care for an additional patient assigned to their unit. The nurses were disciplined, and the disciplinary measures were upheld upon arbitration under the collective agreement. The arbitration board felt that the nurses had not had just cause under the circumstances to refuse to care for the additional patient. Such a situation is now addressed in the professional responsibility clause of most collective agreements.

Under the "obey and grieve" rule, mentioned earlier, a nurse who believes that he or she is being given a workload so large as to preclude proper patient care may file a complaint in writing to the hospital association committee within a certain period of time after having been assigned the large workload. The complaint, if unresolved, proceeds to an assessment committee hearing, whose members are chosen by both the hospital and the nurses' union. The committee then investigates the matter and holds a hearing to determine whether or not the complaint is well founded. It then reports its findings to the parties to the hearing and makes recommendations in an attempt to resolve the situation. In this way, the professional integrity of nurses is maintained, and they are permitted some control over their workload and the number of patients in their care. Thus, their ability to deliver effective, efficient, and proper nursing care is maintained.

A matter may be submitted to arbitration only after all preliminary grievance procedures have been exhausted. A majority of the provincial Labour Relations Board determines the issue. All time limits for the giving of notice must be strictly observed; if notice that a party wishes the matter submitted to binding arbitration is not given within a specified time, the grievance is deemed to have been abandoned. Alternatively, the parties may agree that the matter be settled by a single arbitrator.

Thus, through arbitration, every attempt is made to resolve disputes arising out of the collective agreement. This procedure has been referred to as the quid pro quo—that is, something in return for the fact that the right to strike or to lock out is suspended during the life of the agreement.

There are a number of cases involving nurses disciplined for unprofessional conduct. In many of these, the nurse grieved the matter according to the union's collective agreement.

In *Re Ontario Cancer Institute and Ontario Nurses' Association (Priestley)* (1993), a nurse was discharged after striking a terminally ill patient. The nurse, through her union, brought a grievance against her hospital employer for unjust discharge. The union argued that the patient had provoked the nurse. Although there were no witnesses to the incident, the nurse had admitted the act to two colleagues and said that "it felt good" (*Re Ontario Cancer Institute and Ontario Nurses' Association (Priestley)*, 1993 p. 129).

The evidence presented at the hearing suggested that patient load had been very heavy in the unit for some months and that stress levels among staff were high. The patient struck by the nurse required the most attention in the unit and was very demanding of the nurses' time and attention. He had had a tracheotomy and was often confused, restless, and incontinent. The nurse admitted to striking the patient hard across the legs because she had become frustrated with his restless behaviour the night before. In finding that the nurse's discharge was justified, the arbitrator stated, in part:

> I heard much evidence about what a difficult and heavy care patient [the patient] was. I accept that evidence.... However, the actions of a patient who is terminally ill and not in control of his mental or physical faculties cannot constitute provocation that would excuse a health care professional's physical retaliation. (*Re Ontario Cancer Institute and Ontario Nurses' Association (Priestley)*, 1993, pp. 135–136)

The arbitrator declined to interfere with the hospital's decision to discharge the nurse.

Similarly, in *Vancouver General Hospital (Health and Labour Relations Assn.) and British Columbia Nurses Union* (1993), a nurse was discharged for continuing to feed a patient in an inappropriate manner despite having been shown the correct way by an occupational therapist. She had previously been suspended for improperly responding to a patient's seizure because she was in a hurry to go home. In the second incident, which led to her dismissal, the nurse attempted to feed milk to a patient who was improperly positioned and already had food in her mouth. There was great risk of aspiration to the patient. Moreover, the patient was drowsy following surgery and insufficiently alert to be fed orally. The arbitrator held that the hospital had just cause for disciplinary action, given the nurse's record.

## Right to Strike

Traditionally, common law did not recognize the right of employees to refuse to work. Today's statutes usually distinguish between a lawful and an unlawful strike. The same distinction applies to a **lockout**, a practice whereby an employer shuts out or refuses to continue to employ union employees as a means to pressure and influence them during negotiations for a collective agreement. It, like the strike, is a coercive tactic.

In most provinces, during the life of a collective agreement, employees may not strike, nor may an employer lock out employees. Even after the expiration of the agreement, employees and employers must wait for the passage of the cooling-off period before a lawful strike or lockout can occur.

Once the collective agreement has expired, its terms can be continued while the parties negotiate a new agreement. However, if no agreement is reached, in some provinces, the provincial Minister of Labour may be requested or may decide to appoint a conciliation board in an attempt to settle outstanding issues and to effect a new collective agreement. Such board or conciliator (if one person is appointed) must file a report on the results (or lack thereof) of any conciliation efforts to the Minister of Labour, who then releases the report to the parties.

Once a specified period has elapsed after the report's release or, if no conciliator has been appointed, after the minister has notified the parties that he or she considers it inappropriate to appoint a conciliator, the union may then lawfully call a strike. Similarly, the employer may lawfully lock out employees.

Certain activities during the life of the collective agreement may or may not constitute a strike according to the applicable labour relations statute. Employees may vote to work to rule (i.e., to work only as much as is demanded by the terms of their employment) as a form of protest; for example, they may refuse to work overtime when requested to do so. If such conduct has the effect of stopping all work in order to pressure an employer to accede to union demands, it may be deemed a strike by the provincial Labour Relations Board. However, a refusal to work because of hazardous working conditions would likely not be deemed a strike, as it is not intended to affect collective bargaining but rather to avoid potentially serious injury to workers.

In most provinces, nurses and other hospital employees are not legally permitted to strike. While this provision may not affect nurses who are not employed at hospitals (which are defined in detail in the statutes), any nurse working at an institution that falls within the definition of a hospital would be prevented from going on strike. (See, for example, Alberta: *Hospitals Act*, R.S.A. 2000, c. H-12; Ontario: *Hospital Labour Disputes Arbitration Act*, R.S.O. 1990, c. H.14, s. 11(1), as amended.) Similarly, hospitals are not permitted to lock out their employees at any time. These provisions are designed to ensure that vital hospital services are not compromised, nor services to the public diminished, as a result of labour disputes. This is not to say that nurses are not permitted to form unions and to bargain collectively; however, different dispute resolution procedures may apply, and employees will not be permitted to strike to enforce collective bargaining rights.

Strike breaking—that is, the use of strong-arm, threatening, or other such tactics by an employer in an effort to pressure striking employees to abandon a lawful strike or to yield in contract negotiations—is prohibited in all provinces.

Depending on the province, a strike vote among employees may be required before a strike can begin. If a strike vote is held, all employees in the bargaining unit may vote. Voting is usually by secret ballot. A vote may also be held to ratify an agreement concluded between management and the union's negotiators. Nurses have initiated strike action in the past. For example, in late 2000, nurses in Saskatchewan went on strike in support of a demand for a pay raise beyond what the provincial government was willing to offer. The government ordered them back to work via legislation, but the nurses continued their strike in defiance of the legislation ("Striking nurses reject gov't offer," 2000). In response, Saskatchewan eventually enacted the *Public Service Essential Services Act*, which provides that certain public services, such as nursing in hospitals, are declared to be essential services. Public-sector employers, such as hospitals and health care authorities that provide such services, are required to enter into an essential services agreement with their unionized employees, including nurses, to set out which services are deemed to be essential and to provide for a certain number of unionized employees (including nurses) who must continue to provide services in the event of a strike. Many other provinces have enacted similar legislation. The effect of this legislation is that now nurses' right to strike is very limited in most provinces.

## Unfair Labour Practices

All provinces have prohibited unfair management tactics, which in previous times were used by employers to pressure workers into returning to work or to induce employees to accept certain terms and conditions of employment. For example, it is illegal for an employer to discipline a worker for taking part in a lawful strike or in lawful union activities, such as encouraging new employees to join the union. Similarly, employers are prohibited from participating in or funding the creation of a union. Such prohibition is intended to avoid conflict of interest.

It is likewise illegal for an employer to discriminate in any way against employees because they either are or are not members of a union; to discipline them for exercising their rights under a labour relations statute; to use any form of intimidation against them for participating in union activity; or to induce them to join a particular union. Another illegal labour practice is the "yellow dog" contract, by which it is made a condition of a person's employment that he or she will not join a union or participate in any union activities.

If an employee alleges that an employer has engaged in an unfair labour practice, the employee can bring the matter to the attention of the union representative. The matter may be taken up as a grievance by the union, or, if it is serious enough, it may be reported to a labour inspector appointed by the provincial Labour Relations Board. The Labour Boards of most provinces are given wide powers to order employers to cease and desist from engaging in such practices.

## Professional Accountability and the Influence of Unionization

Nurses are accountable to their profession, their regulatory body, their patients or clients, and their employers. These multiple accountabilities can at times pose conflicts for the nurse. Nurses in some settings have another dimension added to these complex relationships: that of a union or collective bargaining unit.

A situation that occurred in Toronto in the mid-1970s illustrates the conflict that can arise between nurses' rights as employees and union members under a collective agreement and their duties and responsibilities as professionals. In *Re Mount Sinai Hospital and the Ontario Nurses Association* (1978), the staff of the Mount Sinai Intensive Care Unit was informed one evening of the urgent need to admit a patient with cardiac problems from the emergency department. This occurred during the night shift, when the ICU was already working at maximum capacity. The nurses informed Admitting that they could not handle another patient. They claimed, further, that they were not obliged to take such an additional patient under the terms of the union's collective agreement with the hospital. The medical staff, despite the nurses' refusal to help, brought the patient to the unit. Though told by their supervisor to accept this patient, none of the nurses on the night shift assisted the admitting resident, who was required to care for this very ill patient by himself for the duration of the night.

As a result of their refusal to care for the additional patient, the nurses were disciplined and suspended for three tours of duty. They grieved the matter, following grievance and arbitration procedures set out in their respective collective agreement, and the issue was passed on to an arbitrator. The arbitrator ruled in favour of the hospital and found that the nurses had been insubordinate, as they had refused a direct order by their supervisor to provide care. They were not entitled, under the collective agreement, to refuse such an order.

Quite apart from the labour aspect, this case raises ethical concerns regarding standards of care. For example, the nurses had not re-evaluated the allocation of their resources. They had not reassessed their workload and staffing, nor had they tried to determine whether some patients in their unit could be discharged to make room for the new admission. As they had not even tried to restructure their assignments to accommodate the patient, they violated the principles of beneficence and nonmaleficence. Further, they had not accorded the patient justice, fairness, or equity.

The rule that evolved from this case is now termed the "obey and grieve" rule. It provides that, even if a nurse employee has a legitimate grievance under the terms of a collective agreement or with respect to workload or working conditions, he or she must obey the orders of the supervisor and provide needed care, and then grieve the matter to the union if he or she feels there is a legitimate complaint. There is plenty of opportunity for such complaints to be heard and adjudicated upon at a more appropriate time, using the collective agreement's grievance procedures. In the present moment, however, the rights and needs of the patient must come first, and the fact that a nurse has a complaint must not be permitted to interfere with proper patient care. This approach is further supported in the Canadian Nurses Association code of ethics:

> When resources are not available to provide ideal care, nurses collaborate with others to adjust priorities and minimize harm. Nurses keep persons receiving care, families and their employers informed about potential and actual changes to delivery of care. They inform employers about potential threats to safety." (CNA, 2008, p. 10)

The employee, during regular hours of work, has an accountability to the employer. There are ample mechanisms to protect the employee's rights should these be violated by the employer, but the patient's care is paramount, especially given the fact that the health care facility is under a legal duty to provide competent and proper nursing care once a patient is admitted. This implies a corresponding right of the employer to discipline the employee and even to terminate the employment of a nurse who repeatedly fails to work to proper nursing standards. The employee in such a situation has the right to grieve or, if not unionized, to have recourse in the courts in an action for wrongful dismissal.

## Summary

This chapter has explored the rights of nurses as professionals, individuals, and employees. The varied contexts within which nurses engage in practice (e.g., the community, long-term care, acute care, education) may pose varying ethical and legal challenges that have an impact on their values, beliefs, and well-being. While nurses have the right to respect and should be able to practise in a safe work environment free from harm, harassment, or abuse, the reality is that some will face such difficult situations. It is important that nurses have the knowledge and skills to address these challenging issues and to know where to seek support and guidance when necessary.

Employers have an obligation to represent the interests and rights of nurses. They must be aware of the risks to nurses and ensure that appropriate prevention strategies are in place. They must also be prepared to respond appropriately if nurses are harmed as a result of these risks. When this obligation is not fulfilled, then the collective agreement and collective bargaining rights of nurses who are unionized may provide protection and a mechanism for dealing with some situations. In other cases, the advice of a competent legal professional may be required.

Nurses should be aware of their rights and the responsibilities and obligations of their employers, with respect to working conditions. The nurse has the right to a safe and violence-free working environment. If nurses' rights are not protected in an environment based on mutual respect, then they will be unable to deliver high-quality care to patients and clients consistent with the standards of their profession.

# Critical Thinking

The following case scenarios are provided to facilitate reflection, discussion, and analysis.

## RIGHT OR PRIVILEGE?

Carmen, a nurse in a busy Critical Care Unit, is scheduled to work nights on a weekend when she is invited to attend an informal university class reunion. She knows that it is too late to ask for the weekend off, and that none of her colleagues is likely to willingly switch shifts with her on such short notice. As she has taken little sick leave, she decides to call in sick. Carmen believes that she is entitled to this time, and that this is a legitimate reason to take the weekend off.

That night, a number of emergency patients are admitted to the unit. Owing to Carmen's absence, the nurses on duty must take on a double assignment of patients. One of the nurses, aware of Carmen's reason for calling in sick, is so upset that the following Monday, she discloses this information to the nurse manager.

### Questions

1. Is Carmen entitled to take this time off? If not, what disciplinary action may ensue?
2. If the manager chooses to discipline Carmen, can Carmen grieve the matter?
3. What ethical principles, if any, did Carmen breach?
4. How could this situation have been prevented?

## SAFETY IN THE WORKPLACE?

Connie, a public health nurse, is assigned to a young single mother, Sheryl, and her 8-month-old son, Sean. This family receives welfare and lives in a subsidized housing unit.

During one of Connie's regular visits, Sheryl's estranged boyfriend arrives. He has been drinking and becomes belligerent toward Sheryl. When Connie—concerned about her clients' safety—intervenes, the boyfriend turns his aggression on her, hitting her on the head. Connie falls and strikes her head on the edge of a coffee table, sustaining a serious injury.

Although Connie recovers physically, her mental capacity is such that she can never practise nursing again.

continued on following page >>

**Questions**

1. What obligations did Connie's employer have to ensure a safe working environment?
2. What responsibilities does the employer have with respect to Connie's permanent disability?
3. What charges can be laid against the boyfriend?
4. What obligations did Connie's employer have to educate her with respect to such potentially violent and dangerous situations?
5. How could this situation have been prevented?

## RIGHT TO STRIKE?

Andrew is an RN in a long-term care facility. Recently, contract discussions between his union and the facility have broken down. Neither side is willing to compromise, and the staff has voted to strike. A plan is in place for a minimal number of nurses to be available in emergencies.

Andrew is concerned about the strike decision. He worries about his patients in the Geriatric Unit. Knowing how difficult and confusing the strike will be for them, he decides to cross the picket line and go to work. As he enters the building, Andrew is heckled by some of his colleagues.

**Questions**

1. What are Andrew's rights and responsibilities in this situation?
2. Is the behaviour of the nurses on the picket line justifiable?
3. What would you do in Andrew's place?
4. How could this situation have been prevented?

**Discussion Points**

1. As a nurse, do you have rights that may supersede those of your patients or clients? What rights may at times be in conflict?
2. Do nurses give up certain rights when they assume their professional role?
3. Have you ever experienced violence in the workplace? Was anything done about it? If it happened now, what would you do?
4. What role should unions play in establishing rules that govern professional practice and conduct?
5. What mechanisms are in place in your facility to ensure the appropriate balance between caregiver and patient rights?

# References

## Bills

Bill 29, *An Act to amend the Occupational Health and Safety Act to protect workers from harassment and violence in the workplace*, 1st session, 39th Legislature, Ontario (2008).

## Statutes

*Canada Labour Code*, R.S.C. 1985, c. L-2 (Canada).

*Charter of Rights and Freedoms*, Part I of the *Constitution Act, 1982*, being Schedule B to the *Canada Act 1982* (U.K.), 1982, c. 11.

*Hospitals Act*, R.S.A. 2000, c. H-12 (Alberta).

*Hospital Labour Disputes Arbitration Act*, R.S.O. 1990, c. H.14 (Ontario).

*Industrial Relations Act*, R.S.N.B. 1973, c. I-4 (New Brunswick).

*Labour Act*, R.S.P.E.I. 1988, c. L-1 (Prince Edward Island).

*Labour Code*, R.S.Q. c. C-27 (Quebec).

*Labour Relations Act*, C.C.S.M., c. L10 (Manitoba).

*Labour Relations Act*, R.S.N.L. 1990, c. L-1 (Newfoundland and Labrador).

*Labour Relations Act, 1995*, S.O. 1995, c.1, sched. A (Ontario).

*Labour Relations Code*, R.S.A. 2000, c. L-1 (Alberta).

*Labour Relations Code*, R.S.B.C. 1996, c. 244 (British Columbia).

*Occupational health and safety, An Act respecting*, R.S.Q. c. S-2.1 (Quebec).

*Occupational Health and Safety Act*, R.S.A. 2000, c. O-2 (Alberta).

*Occupational Health and Safety Act*, R.S.N.L. 1990, c. O-3 (Newfoundland and Labrador).

*Occupational Health and Safety Act*, R.S.O. 1990, c. O.1 (Ontario).

*Occupational Health and Safety Act*, R.S.P.E.I. 1988, c. O-1.01 (Prince Edward Island).

*Occupational Health and Safety Act*, S.N.B. 1983, c. O-0.2 (New Brunswick).

*Occupational Health and Safety Act*, S.N.S. 1996, c. 7 (Nova Scotia).

*Occupational Health and Safety Act, 1993*, S.S. 1993, c. O-1.1 (Saskatchewan).

*Safety Act*, R.S.N.W.T. 1988, c. S-1 (Northwest Territories and Nunavut).

*Trade Union Act*, R.S.N.S. 1989, c. 475 (Nova Scotia).

*Trade Union Act*, R.S.S. 1978, c. T-17 (Saskatchewan).

*Workers Compensation Act*, R.S.B.C. 1996, c. 492 (British Columbia).

*Workplace Safety and Health Act*, C.C.S.M. c. W210 (Manitoba).

## Regulations

*Health Care and Residential Facilities Regulation*, O. Reg. 67/93 (Ontario).

N.S. Reg. 209/2007 made under the *Occupational Health and Safety Act* (Nova Scotia).

N.B. Reg. 92-133 made under the *Occupational Health and Safety Act* (New Brunswick).

## Case Law

*Re Local 199 UAW Building Corp.*, [1977] O.L.R.B. Rep. July, 472.

*Re Mount Sinai Hospital and the Ontario Nurses' Association,* (1978), 17 L.A.C. (2d) 242 (Ont. Arb.).

*Re Ontario Cancer Institute and Ontario Nurses' Association (Priestley)* (1993), 35 L.A.C. (4th) 129 (Ont. Arb.)

*Vancouver General Hospital (Health and Labour Relations Assn.) and British Columbia Nurses Union* (1993), 32 L.A.C. (4th) 231 (B.C.).

## Coroner's Inquests

*Verdict of Coroner's Jury serving on the inquest into the deaths of Lori Dupont and Dr. Marc Daniel.* (December 11, 2007). Retrieved January 19, 2009, from http://www.mcscs. jus.gov.on.ca/stellent/groups/public/@mcscs/@www/@com/documents/webasset/ ec063542.pdf

## Texts and Articles

Agency for Healthcare Research and Quality. (2003, March). The effect of health care working conditions on patient safety (Summary). *Evidence Report/Technology Assessment: Number 74.* AHRQ Publication No. 03-E024. Rockville, MD: Author.

American Association of Critical-Care Nurses. (2006). *The 4 A's to rise above moral distress toolkit.* Aliso Viejo, CA: Author.

Baumann, A., O'Brien-Pallas, L., Armstrong-Stassen, M., Blythe, J., Bourbonnais, R., Cameron, S., et al. (2001). *Commitment and care: The benefits of a healthy workplace for nurses, their patients and the system—A policy synthesis.* Ottawa, ON: Canadian Health Services Research Foundation and The Change Foundation.

Braverman, M. (1999). *Preventing workplace violence: A guide for employers and practitioners.* Thousand Oaks, CA: Sage Publications, Inc.

Burnazi, L., & Keashly, L., & Neuman, J. H. (2005, August). *Aggression revisited: Prevalence, antecedents, and outcomes.* Paper presented at the Academy of Management Annual Meeting, Honolulu, HI.

Canadian Nurses Association. (2003, October). Ethical distress in health care environ-ments. *Ethics in Practice for Registered Nurses* (Newsletter). Ottawa, ON: Author.

Canadian Nurses Association. (2008). *Code of ethics for registered nurses.* Ottawa, ON: Author.

Canadian Nurses Association & Canadian Federation of Nurses Unions. (2007). *Workplace violence.* Joint Position Statement. Retrieved January 20, 2009, from http://www. nursesunions.ca/media.php?mid=676

Canadian Nursing Advisory Committee. (2002). *Our health, our future: Creating quality workplaces for Canadian nurses.* Ottawa, ON: Advisory Committee on Health Human Resources.

CBC News. (2000, November 10). Striking nurses reject gov't offer. Retrieved January 21, 2009, from http://www.cbc.ca/canada/story/1999/04/16/sk_nurseII990416.html

Charney, W., & Schirmer, J. (1990) Essentials of modern hospital safety. Chelsea, MI: Lewis Publishers, Inc.

Deans, C. (2004). Nurses and occupational violence: The role of organisational support in moderating professional competence. *Australian Journal of Advancing Nursing, 22*(2), 14–18.

Dugan J., Lauer, E., Bouquot, Z., Dutro, B. K., Smith, M., & Widmeyer, G. (1996). Stressful nurses: The effect on patient outcomes. *Journal of Nursing Care Quality, 10*(3), 46–58.

Duxbury, J. (1999). An exploratory account of registered nurses' experience of patient aggression in both mental health and general nursing settings. *Journal of Psychiatric and Mental Health Nursing, 6*(2), 107–114.

Duxbury, J. (2002). An evaluation of staff and patient views of and strategies employed to manage inpatient aggression and violence on one mental health unit: A pluralistic design. *Journal of Psychiatric and Mental Health Nursing, 9*(3), 325–337.

Estabrooks, C. A., Midodzi, W. K., Cummings, G. G., Ricker, K. L., & Giovannetti, P. (2005). The impact of hospital nursing characteristics on 30-day mortality. *Nursing Research, 54*(2), 74–84.

Farrell, G. (1997). Aggression in clinical settings: Nurses' views. *Journal of Advanced Nursing, 25*(3), 501–508.

Farrell, G. (1999). Aggression in clinical settings: A follow-up study. *Journal of Advanced Nursing, 29*(3), 532–541.

Hansen, A. M., Hogh, A., Persson, R., Karlson, B., Garde, A. H., & Ørbæk, P. (2006). Bullying at work, health outcomes and physiological stress response. *Journal of Psychosomatic Research, 60*(1), 63–72.

Jameton, A. (1984). *Nursing practice: The ethical issues.* Englewood Cliffs, NJ: Prentice-Hall.

Lewis, J., Coursol, D., & Herting, K. (2002). Addressing issues of workplace harassment: Counseling the targets. *Journal of Employment Counseling, 39*(3), 109–116.

Lewis, M. (2006). Organisational accounts of bullying: An interactive approach. In J. Randle (Ed.)., *Workplace Bullying in the NHS* (pp. 25–46). Oxford, England: Radcliffe Publishing.

Lewis, M. A. (2006). Nurse bullying: Organizational considerations in the maintenance and perpetration of health care bullying cultures. *Journal of Nursing Management, 14*(1), 52–58.

Lundstrom, T., Pugliese, G., Bartley, J., Cox, J., & Guither, C. (2002). Organizational and environmental factors that affect worker health and safety and patient outcomes. *American Journal of Infection Control, 30*(2), 93–106.

MacIntosh, J. (2003). Reworking professional nursing identity. *Western Journal of Nursing Research, 25*(6), 725–741.

MacIntosh, J. (2005). Experiences of workplace bullying in a rural area. *Issues in Mental Health Nursing, 26*(9), 893–910.

Manuel, P., & Bruinse, B. (2005, November 17–18). A registered nurses' council: Cultivating a healthy community for nurses. 5th Annual International Healthy Workplaces in Action Conference, Toronto, ON.

McKenna, B. G., Smith, N. A., Poole, S. J., & Coverdale, J. H. (2003). Horizontal violence: Experiences of registered nurses in their first year of practice. *Journal of Advanced Nursing, 42*(1), 90–96.

McKoy, Y., & Smith, M. H. (2001). Legal considerations of workplace violence in health-care environments. *Nursing Forum, 36*(1), 5–14.

National Quality Institute and Health Canada. (2006). Healthy workplace progressive excellence program. Toronto, ON: National Quality Institute.

O'Connell, B., Young, J., Brooks, J., Hutchings, J., & Lofthouse, J. (2000). Nurses' perceptions on the nature and frequency of aggression in general ward settings and high dependency areas. *Journal of Clinical Nursing, 9*(4), 602–610.

Owen, C., Tarantello, C., Jones, M., & Tennant, C. (1998). Violence and aggression in psychiatric units. *Psychiatric Services, 49*(11), 1452–1457.

Pejic, A. R. (2005). Verbal abuse: A problem for pediatric nurses. *Pediatric Nursing, 31*(4), 271–279.

Quine, L. (2003). Workplace bullying, psychological distress, and job satisfaction in junior doctors. *Cambridge Quarterly of Healthcare Ethics, 12*(1), 91–101.

Registered Nurses Association of Ontario and the Registered Practical Nurses Association of Ontario. (2000). *Ensuring the care will be there: Report on nursing recruitment and retention in Ontario.* Toronto, ON: Author.

Registered Nurses' Association of Ontario. (2007a). *Embracing cultural diversity in health care: Developing cultural competence.* Healthy work environments best practice guidelines. Toronto, ON: Author.

Registered Nurses' Association of Ontario. (2007b). *Professionalism in nursing.* Healthy work environments best practice guidelines. Toronto, ON: Author.

Registered Nurses' Association of Ontario. (2008). *Preventing and managing violence in the workplace.* Healthy work environments best practice guidelines. Toronto, ON: Author.

Rotstein, M., & Peskun, C. (2008, November 21). RN council as a forum to promote healthy work environments. 7th International Healthy Workplaces in Action Conference, Toronto, ON.

Rushton, C. H. (2006). Defining and addressing moral distress: Tools for critical care nursing leaders. *AACN Advanced Critical Care, 17*(2), 161–168.

Solomon, M. Z., O'Donnell, L., Jennings, B., Guilfoy, V., Wolf, S. M., Nolan, K., et al. (1993). Decisions near the end of life: Professional views on life-sustaining treatments. *American Journal of Public Health, 83*(1), 14–23.

Stephens, L. (2008, March 8). Workplace bullies most poisonous: Even sexual harassment takes second place to the harm done by on-the-job bullying. *Toronto Star,* p. L11.

University of Toronto Joint Centre for Bioethics. (2008). *Ethics and SARS: Learning lessons from the Toronto experience.* A report by a working group of The University of Toronto Joint Centre for Bioethics. Toronto, ON: Author. Retrieved September 2008 from http://www.yorku.ca/igreene/sars.html

# Chapter 12

## Ethical Issues in Leadership, the Organization, and Care

### Learning Objectives

The purpose of this chapter is to enable you to understand:

- The evolving challenges in the health care sector
- The important ethical issues facing nursing leadership and health care organizations
- The complexities of the diverse Canadian landscape and how they influence nursing practice
- The contribution of nursing within an interprofessional practice model and the advantages of the interprofessional approach
- The critical importance of patient- and family-centred care

## Introduction

THIS CHAPTER EXPLORES SOME of the ethical considerations that may not necessarily involve individual patient issues but that have significant influence on the outcomes of care. These ethical issues include leadership behaviour and values, and the strategy, processes, and operations of an organization. A moral organizational climate is essential in order to ensure support for those at the clinical level who deal with the complex and challenging ethical issues related to direct patient care. Supportive and ethical leaders enable a healthy and open culture that supports the ethical practice of nurses and ensures that the needs of patients and clients are met. Leaders also influence approaches to care from the perspective of how teams are organized, how they interact with each other, and how they work toward common patient and family outcomes.

## Leadership and Organizational Ethics

Nursing leaders must be aware of the ethical challenges nurses face in day-to-day practice and also appreciate their role as leaders in ensuring ethical leadership and organizational practices.

Leaders must understand how:

- An organization's structure and culture influence ethical decision making
- To identify the ethical dimensions of decisions and challenges within the organization
- To identify and address the ethical issues related to allocation of resources
- To address human resources, diversity, and privacy issues from an ethical perspective
- To ensure their leadership practices are value-based and meet high ethical standards
- To support teams in addressing moral challenges in order to prevent moral distress

### Organizational Ethics

In any organization, how business is conducted matters. This is especially true in health care. Table 12.1 summarizes the key ethical issues and practices that are relevant to organizations. Beyond these elements, in the health care sector, there is the added dimension of responsibility for a vulnerable client population and the complex clinical ethics issues that arise. Organizational and clinical systems and processes must meet the same ethical standards as does practice since these systems and processes have a strong impact on the practice environment and the care patients receive (Piette, Ellis, St. Denis, & Sarauer, 2002).

Over the past few decades, health care organizations have focused primarily on clinical, not organizational, ethics. Organizations, Brodeur (1998) suggests, should first have assessed the ethical organizational life and infrastructure of the total organization, which he asserts is necessary to support ethical standards in the clinical and practice environment. Instead, health care organizations focused their ethics agendas on such specific clinical ethical issues as those surrounding death and dying, organ transplantation, and informed

---

**Table 12.1: Ethical Organizational Practices**

In any organization, sound ethical practices need to exist, with respect to:

- Human resources policies that pay attention to
  - Recruitment and retention
  - Equitable compensation
  - Labour relations
  - Performance improvement and, when necessary, progressive discipline
- Ensuring a healthy work environment (as discussed in Chapter 11)
  - That is safe and supportive
  - In which there is mutual respect and opportunities for advancement
- Leadership practices and organizational structures that ensure
  - Support and mentorship for staff
  - Succession planning
- The prevention of negative outcomes, such as moral distress, which are managed through
  - Processes by which ethical issues are identified and addressed
  - Education and awareness
  - Counselling
  - Transparency
  - Appropriate management of conflict
  - Processes to ensure a respectful work environment
- Issues regarding human rights, which are managed through
  - Establishing human rights as a priority
  - Ensuring equity and fairness
  - Ensuring just processes and procedures are in place
  - Providing accommodation for illness and disability

Extracted from Piette, M., Ellis, J.L., St. Denis, P., Sarauer, J. (2002). Integrating ethics and quality improvement: Practical implementation in the transitional/extended care setting. *Journal of Nursing Care Quality, 17*(1), 35–42.

---

consent (Sashkin & Williams, 1993; Worthley, 1999). This is understandable given the complex clinical ethics issues health care has faced; however, this has been challenging within cultures in which the norms and values of the total organization have been unclear. For example, if clinical staff members perceive that the organization's approach to recruitment or resource allocation is not guided by ethical principles or frameworks, that organization will find it difficult to implement standards with respect to the ethical care of patients.

There is now an emerging interest in addressing **organizational ethics** and in ensuring that ethical standards are met in leadership and in organizational structures and processes, which might include the organization's recruitment practices, the support that staff receives from leaders, how resources are allocated and used, how issues of diversity are addressed, and how employees are supported through times of extensive organizational change (Sashkin & Williams, 1993; Worthley, 1999).

The field of organizational ethics deals with those values that establish standards and influence how the organization is perceived both internally and externally (Lozano, 2003). That is, the ethical culture of an organization influences its image and reputation, establishes (or not) the legitimacy of its role in society, and clarifies what it stands for (Seeger, 2001). An organization's culture intersects with its ethics at the point of its organizational values, those underlying assumptions and guidelines of organizational life (Seeger, 2001). An ethical culture or climate is one in which all persons within the organization share common values and beliefs; in which there is trust, respect, openness, and transparency; in which all team members participate; in which there is accountability; and in which leaders are role models. In an ethical culture, the ethics and values of an organization inform all of its actions and decisions (Clegg, Kornberger, & Rhodes, 2007).

Values shape the structure of an organization, its practices, formal statements, and policies. In many organizations, the mission defines its purpose, the goal of which is to achieve excellence, the "good." For a true ethical culture, all persons within the organization must share common values. The influence of leaders, though important, it is not enough. Not only leaders but followers shape an ethical culture. One or the other can negatively shape the culture; therefore, both must embrace common and sound ethical practices (Grosenick, 1994). Hence, ethical organizational practices are those that are collaborative and sustained by qualities that enable effective teamwork and collaboration (Parsons, Clark, Marshal, & Cornett, 2007).

Trust and a sense of fairness are instrumental to an ethical organization. Williams (2006) suggests that "trust is the adhesive that binds its members" and that "fairness is an essential ingredient in trusting relationships regardless of roles" (p. 30). Evolving evidence demonstrates the importance of trust in ensuring nurse satisfaction and commitment to the organization (Laschinger, Finegan, Shamian, & Casier, 2000). Trust is the "positive expectations individuals have about the intent and behaviours of multiple organizational members based on organization roles, relationships, experiences, and interdependencies" (Shockley-Zalabak, Ellis, & Winograd, 2000, p. 37). Organizational trust-building behaviours are those that nurses and other employees will judge as fair—for example, how decisions are made (Williams, 2006). When one has input throughout an open and transparent consultation process, this will be deemed a fair process even if the decision does not coincide with the wishes of all involved.

Shockley-Zalabak, Ellis, and Winograd (2000) have developed a model of organizational trust that considers five key dimensions that result in great employee satisfaction and the perception that the organization is effective. These dimensions include leaders having concern for employees, an open and honest culture, employee connection or engagement with the organization, meaningful relationships between leaders and employees, and reliability and competence (Shockley-Zalabak et al., 2000).

Fairness and justice have a strong role in ensuring organizational trust. Williams (2006) suggests that organizational justice has two components: distributive and procedural justice. **Distributive justice** relates to outcomes such as allocation of resources, salaries, benefits, and work conditions, whereas **procedural justice** refers to the perception that processes have been fair and inclusive regardless of the outcome. For example, when key decisions are made, are the significant stakeholders included? In what manner are they involved? Is the process open and transparent (Williams, 2006)?

Renz and Eddy (1996) propose a model that can guide organizations in creating a sound ethical culture and a strong ethics infrastructure. A summary of the model, which is based on four key building blocks, follows.

## Creating an Ethical Culture

### Link Values to Mission and Vision

The strategy is to build the values, mission, and vision of the organization into the ethical framework. It is important to engage employees by encouraging their involvement in the development and design of the framework by using approaches such as retreats and focus groups. These approaches can also encourage team-building and sharing of perspectives, which would contribute to a shared commitment to the values, mission, and vision of the organization.

### Facilitate Communication and Learning About Ethics

This strategy would include the communication of the framework (i.e., values, mission, and vision) through multiple processes, such as placing statements in highly visible areas, offering education sessions that encourage interaction, role-playing, and value clarification. These types of sessions should occur on a regular basis and not be restricted to the launch of such an initiative.

### Create Structures That Support an Ethical Environment

An ethical environment is enhanced through the establishment of multiple processes and venues in which ethical issues can be addressed (e.g., creating ethics committees, introducing roles such as executive champion and ethicist, and building ethics into quality and performance-management processes).

### Monitor and Evaluate Ethical Performance

Implementation alone will not create a successful ethical culture; processes must be in place to constantly evaluate the effectiveness of these strategies. Such processes may include evaluating outcomes, eliciting regular feedback from employees, and reviewing the framework on a regular basis.

It takes time to change a culture, and effort to sustain this change. Change and sustainability are influenced by trust, respect, transparency, and open communication. In an ethical culture, all members, leaders, and followers participate. An ethical culture ensures the development of leaders who engage their teams in decision making and share with them accountability for outcomes (Keatings, 2005).

## Ethical Leadership

Leaders are instrumental in the creation of an ethical climate that is transparent, supports a healthy work environment, and promotes successful interprofessional collaboration. Nursing leaders must:

- Not only meet the ethical standards of the profession but also be ethical leaders and role models
- Ensure a climate and culture that support high standards of ethical nursing practice
- Model and advance a humanistic culture that is sensitive to the needs of staff, patients, and families
- Ensure processes are in place to address the ethical challenges and concerns of their employees (Brown, 2003)

Health care leaders must model ethical behaviour if they expect ethical care of patients and clients. Through their actions and approaches, leaders can demonstrate desired attributes such as compassion, flexibility, openness, and engagement.

Leaders ensure that challenging ethical issues and ethics in general are discussed regularly, possibly during rounds or team meetings (Brown, 2003). Leaders reward and recognize good practice and encourage ongoing advancements in care.

At the same time, nurses share accountability with leaders in ensuring sound ethical practice, a healthy work environment, and staff satisfaction in order to create a culture and climate conducive to positive patient care outcomes. The leader is responsible for supporting his or her employees, and employees are responsible for supporting each other and their leader. Without this shared accountability and support, an ethical climate will not be achieved (Kupperschmidt, 2004)

In order to be effective, nursing leaders must understand the key principles of leadership practices. The Canadian Nursing Advisory Report Committee (2002) made important recommendations related to nursing leadership. These recommendations make it explicit that leaders must have an appropriate span of control in order to sustain ongoing contact with their staff, that resources should be in place to support the nurse leader, and that succession planning strategies need to ensure the development of future nurse leaders. Also, new leaders need appropriate orientation, education, and mentorship in order to transition effectively to their new role (McGillis-Hall & Donner, 1997).

In summary, nursing leaders are instrumental in ensuring the engagement of staff through the development of trusting relationships, collaboration, transparency, the provision of opportunities for professional advancement, and consistency in the approach to addressing ethical challenges. Through these means, leaders contribute to positive outcomes for the patient, client, and family. The culture of an organization is also significantly influenced by nursing leaders, who must foster trust and a sense of fairness and shared responsibility. Nurses manage relationships with patients and clients and ensure that these relationships are ones of respect, transparency, and trust; these same principles apply to the relationships between the nurse leader and his or her team, and between the team and the individual professional (Kupperschmidt, 2004).

Consider the following case scenarios.

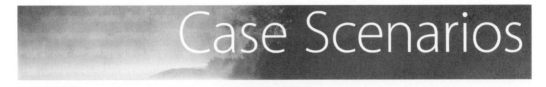

## WHEN LIFE INTERSECTS WITH WORK

Seonag, a nurse in a rehabilitation setting, is experiencing stress at home, which is influencing her work. She is involved in a common-law relationship, and her partner is threatening to leave her. Seonag has a 4-year-old daughter from a previous relationship and is worried she will not be able to care for her on her own. Having been distracted for the past few weeks, she has made three recent medication errors. Her manager has spoken with her about this and told her that her performance must improve, or she may be subject to disciplinary action, up to and including discharge.

### Issues

1. What responsibility do leaders have to understand the stresses their staff may be experiencing?
2. Do you think stress has an impact on patient safety?
3. How might Seonag be supported? What are her responsibilities as a nurse?

## PLEASE KEEP ME SAFE!

Hayden is a manager for a home nursing agency. His portfolio is in an urban area that has the highest crime rate in the city. Recently, nurses in the agency have been expressing concerns regarding their safety, especially when they work evenings. One of Hayden's staff members makes a recommendation that the agency supply the nurses with tracking devices so they could be located if an emergency situation arose. Hayden takes this to his director, who says it is an expensive and foolish proposal. The director notes that not one nurse has experienced a problem in recent months.

continued on following page >>

### Issues

1.  What responsibility does this leader have to ensure the safety of his staff?
2.  How does the safety of the nurse correspond with his or her obligations to clients?
3.  Are there mechanisms in place to ensure that the needs of the nurses and the clients are met?

## PEER RESPONSIBILITY?

Raj is a critical care nurse who has just returned to work after recovering from a work-related back injury. She is returning to modified duties and is not allowed to turn or lift patients. Her manager has developed a plan that involves assigning two other nurses to assist with caring for Raj's patients. Some of Raj's colleagues have become irritated with this situation and have stopped talking to her. Raj is feeling very uncomfortable, and her stress increases when she hears that the nurses have complained to her manager and are threatening to refuse to help her.

### Issues

1.  How should the leader of this area manage this challenge?
2.  How should the leader support Raj?
3.  Is Raj experiencing bullying behaviour?
4.  What are the responsibilities of nurses in ensuring support for their peers?

## Leadership Areas of Influence

### Nursing Resources

Nursing and nursing leaders of today face many challenges. Of paramount importance are those issues related to ensuring there are enough nurses to meet the current and future needs of patients and clients. Therefore, over the past few decades, nursing retention and recruitment have been at the forefront of the agenda of nursing leaders across the country.

Canada is one of a number of countries worldwide facing a potential crisis with regard to the availability of nurses. Over the past few years, a number of studies have made predictions on the future of nursing resources and have offered strategies to prevent or mitigate the possibility of severe shortages. Nursing leaders have a significant role in ensuring the success of these mitigating strategies (Baumann, Blythe, Kolotylo, Underwood, 2004; Tomblin Murphy, Maaten, Smith, Butler, 2005).

While, historically, there have been fluctuations in the nursing labour market, there are a number of existing and anticipated demographic changes that make the possibility of a future nursing shortage different from those of the past. Nursing shortages in the past were, in large measure, brought on by institutional efforts to cut costs during periods of higher staffing ratios and fiscal constraints. These efforts resulted in massive layoffs, the loss of full-time positions, casualization of the nursing workforce, increased use of unregulated health care workers, fewer nursing student positions, closure of nursing education programs, and cutbacks in numbers of students accepted into nursing programs (Baumann et al., 2004; Tomblin Murphy et al., 2005). It is imperative that nursing leaders and nurses institute strategies to improve the culture of health care so as to retain and engage nurses in the workplace and the profession. Still, looking ahead, demographic trends are emerging that promise new challenges to nursing and health care delivery.

The aging of the general population in Canada is having two important consequences for nursing. First, an aging population will create a growing demand on health care services. Second, an aging population means there are fewer young people in the overall population and an ever-shrinking number of people entering the profession. We thus have two considerable and opposing pressures being simultaneously exerted on the nursing labour market (Baumann et al., 2004; Tomblin Murphy et al., 2005).

Beyond the impact of demographics, advances in technology have meant that lives that would have previously been lost are being saved. That same technology, however, has resulted in an ongoing need for specialized education for nurses. In many cases, the development of new technology has meant a considerable increase in the workload of the frontline nurse as well as nurse educators, particularly those in critical-care and acute-care settings. As care is moved to the community, there are increasing demands on that sector.

Also linked to advances in technology is the tremendous growth in information industries and therefore a society that is increasingly informed about the availability of new treatments and technology. This, paired with a steady increase in prosperity, has led to higher expectations being placed on the health care system and its capacity to meet the health care needs and demands of the population. Whether influenced more by social and cultural changes or changes in technology, women, in particular, now have a much greater pool of careers from which to choose than ever before (Baumann et al., 2004; Tomblin Murphy et al., 2005).

The same studies that have examined trends in the nursing labour market and predicted possible outcomes have also produced a number of strategies designed to address the concerns already outlined. Those strategies include the following:

- Create a stable supply of nurses through a pan-Canadian approach to nursing education in collaboration with the provincial, territorial, and federal governments to prepare the number of qualified graduates needed. Enhance data collection to help predict future trends and health care human resources needs.
- Use a health care human resources planning framework based on population health care needs to plan for nursing resources.
- Use evidence-informed practices to inform staffing decisions, including retention and recruitment decisions. Implement effective and efficient mechanisms to address workload issues and improve patient, nurse, and system outcomes.
- Create work environments that influence positive patient, nurse, and system outcomes.
- Improve and maintain the health and safety of nurses.

- Develop innovative approaches to expand clinical experiences in nursing education. Newly graduated nurses need adequate clinical preparation to ensure quality of patient care, to avoid excessive strain on existing mentoring and teaching resources, and to help make the transition from student nurse to independent practitioner a positive experience.
- Maximize the ability of nurses to work to their full scope of practice. There is also a need to create and enhance opportunities for nurses to have meaningful involvement in decision making at various levels in health care organizations, especially when those decisions influence nursing and patient care (Baumann et al., 2004; Tomblin Murphy et al., 2005).

There is a longstanding pattern of nursing shortages and excesses. When there are cutbacks, young people become reluctant to enter a profession because they perceive limited employment opportunities. With the globalization of health care, there are also greater risks of losing Canadian-educated nurses to other countries. One strategy for recruitment used by some countries is to recruit internationally educated nurses. Since this strategy is utilized in many countries, including Canada, the International Council of Nurses (ICN) believed it was important to establish a policy on ethical recruitment. This position statement is endorsed by the Canadian Nurses Association and can be found on its Web site at http://www.cna-nurses.ca/CNA/documents/pdf/publications/psrecruit01Jan_2007_e.pdf

## Ethical Recruitment of Nurses

As evident in the statement from the ICN, philosophically and ethically, nursing associations do not support the recruitment of nurses from developing countries—those countries that can little afford to lose what resources they have. However, internationally educated nurses who decide to immigrate to Canada should be welcomed and supported in their transition to health care in Canada. There are considerable challenges that prevent or delay internationally educated nurses from integrating in a timely and fairly seamless way into the nursing profession in Canada.

## Internationally Educated Nurses (IENs): Migration Versus Recruitment

There are many complex ethical issues related to nursing migration (the movement of nurses from one country to another). Some of these issues relate to the aggressive recruitment of nurses from developing countries or those with shortages, and the transition of nurses who make a choice to immigrate to Canada (Griffith, 2001; McGuire & Murphy, 2005; Yi & Jezewski, 2000).

Consider the following scenarios, adapted from *Nurses on the Move: Migration and the Global Health Care Economy* (Kingma, 2006). The first story illustrates some of the factors that would "push" a nurse to immigrate to another country.

### Fatima's Story

Fatima, a member of a minority ethnic community in her home country, was frequently the butt of intolerable discriminatory remarks and actions from her colleagues and hospital leadership. After 11 years as a nurse, she was never able to secure full-time status. In spite of many efforts to advance her qualifications through continuing education courses, her applications were consistently ignored. Yet, the country was suffering a desperate shortage of nurses. This made her position even more untenable. Ultimately, she moved to Europe, and her career aspirations were fulfilled. "The decision to move was mine, and I would do it again," says Fatima.

Source: Adapted from Kingma, M. (2006). *Nurses on the move: Migration and the global health care economy* (pp. 9–10). New York: ILR/Cornell University Press.

Other nurses tell of the "pull factors," when aggressive recruitment agencies offer major financial and transition incentives, which in some instances disappear upon their arrival to the new country. Stories include those of nurses being forced to work in less than attractive clinical areas, accept cuts in pay, and cope with relentless processes and expenses associated with securing registration or licensure. Paradoxically, when incentives do materialize, they often experience the abuse of local nurses who perceive reverse discrimination since the perks are given only to the migrant nurse (Kingma, 2006).

The following story illustrates some of the factors that would "pull" a nurse to immigrate to another country.

### Vicki's Story

Vicki faced many economic and social challenges in her country. A recruitment agency convinced her that she would experience a better personal and professional life in a developed country. She was offered the opportunity to work in a private nursing home in the heart of a cosmopolitan city for an annual salary equivalent to $35,000. She was also told her expenses would be covered. When she arrived, not only were her expenses not covered but she was asked to sign a contract for an annual salary of about $26,000 and to give up her passport. Also, her place of employment was 100 miles from the city she had expected to be living in.

Source: Adapted from Kingma, M. (2006). *Nurses on the move: Migration and the global health care economy* (p. 10). New York: ILR/Cornell University Press.

Numerous business opportunities have arisen out of nursing migration. Not only has there been a proliferation of aggressive international recruitment agencies, but private education programs have been established primarily for preparing nurses for migration. The issue is much more complex as some countries produce and export nurses for their economic advantage, since nurses send remittances back to the home country to support their families. Other countries have excess unemployed nurses while patients fail to receive the care and resources they need. Further, in some countries, nurses are affected by the political climate and are forced to leave to protect their personal safety (Kingma, 2006).

Nurses choose to leave when they are not respected as professionals and when they are not appropriately compensated and therefore unable to provide sufficiently for themselves and their families. These are not simple issues but serious ethical challenges that nursing leaders need to address.

At the root of these push/pull factors is whether the international community is ready to address the conditions that push or pull nurses away. Of global concern is the tendency to utilize short-term solutions, such as migration, when the core issue is attracting and retaining nurses within a positive environment, one in which they feel satisfied with the care they are able to provide (Kingma, 2006).

These case scenarios illustrate that, on the one hand, it would seem unethical to engage in aggressive recruitment strategies to lure nurses from developing countries where shortages already exist. On the other hand, nurses should have a right to choose to leave an unsupportive environment in which their career aspirations are not fulfilled and their personal freedom is limited.

Many nurses from the international community choose to immigrate to Canada and are then faced with significant challenges to becoming registered in the profession here. For some, this process can take years. Nursing regulatory bodies in Canada need to review the transition processes to ensure a streamlined journey for the migrant nurse. This starts with the review of qualifications, continues with the delivery of education programs that enable them to meet Canadian standards and competencies, and concludes with the process of registration. For many, the process is very bureaucratic and time-consuming. As a profession, nursing has the ethical responsibilities to respect these nurses and to enable them to function in the Canadian health care sector (McGuire & Murphy, 2005).

Further challenges exist when the internationally educated nurse enters the clinical setting. These nurses need support and mentoring during this difficult transition. Beyond the normal orientation to a new clinical environment, they are transitioning to a new culture, adapting to a new language (Canadian health care jargon), and may be experiencing a new model or approach to the delivery of care. The scope of practice of Canadian nurses may be broader or narrower, depending on their country of origin. These nurses need to understand the Canadian health care environment and the challenges faced by nurses within this culture and system. Nurses educated in Canada working with internationally trained nurses have the opportunity to welcome a new perspective and to learn about different cultures and traditions. Nurses educated in other countries with a diverse cultural and ethnic perspective are therefore a positive addition to the multicultural model, which values diversity in a rich and vibrant Canadian community (Griffith, 2001; McGuire & Murphy, 2005; Yi & Jezewski, 2000).

Consider the following scenario.

# Case Scenario

## AN ETHICAL CULTURAL TRANSITION?

Malle emigrated from Estonia to Canada five years ago. She applied for registration in one of the provinces shortly after she arrived. Even though she had 10 years of experience in pediatrics in her own country, including 2 years as a nurse manager, it took her 5 years to become registered in Canada. She applied for a pediatric nurse position in a local community hospital. Things did not go well. She was given the same orientation as all new nurses but was confused about the "jargon" and the interaction of the nurses with the rest of the team. For example, she wasn't used to challenging the physicians or making suggestions to the team regarding the care of her patient. Since she had not been working for some time, she had misgivings about her competence, especially since technology had advanced since she had last practised. Her preceptor was frustrated with her, and Malle worried about what she would do.

### Issues

1. What support policies and process should the health care institution have in place to help internationally educated nurses such as Malle?
2. Should there be a unique orientation for IENs? Can the system afford this?
3. What strategies might leaders introduce to facilitate the recruitment and transition of IENs?

## Ethical Issues Associated With Diversity

Within the climate of the diverse Canadian community, it is imperative that nurses have the knowledge and skills to be able to provide culturally competent and culturally congruent nursing care. Whether in their homes, the community, hospitals, or nursing homes, nurses are exposed to patients and clients from multiple backgrounds and cultures. They engage with people and communities who live and interpret their worlds in many different ways (Arnold & Bruce, 2006). It is clearly not possible for nurses to be knowledgeable about the cultural background and values of all the patients and clients they care for. However, nurses should undertake a comprehensive cultural assessment of their clients and their families in an effort to understand their unique values and perspectives in order to design a strategy for care most consistent with their values and beliefs (Andrews & Boyle, 2002).

Since individuals and groups use their basic beliefs and values to guide their actions (Andrews & Boyle, 2002), it is important for nurses to understand these in order to understand the culture within the context of health and illness. For many cultures, ethical decisions are grounded in both religious beliefs and cultural values. It is important to be cautious that the assumptions of the dominant cultural values of Western society are not imposing on the various perspectives of other cultures (Andrews & Boyle, 2002).

Various cultures view their reality or world from many different perspectives. This is known as a culture's **worldview**, which is a comprehensive framework of basic beliefs and values that individuals, groups, and communities use to guide their actions (Uys & Smit, 1994). In a sense, it is the lens through which they interpret and clarify the reality of their everyday lives. Without an understanding that these various views exist, the nurse and other team members may not be aware of these differences and therefore may not be able to address the needs of that patient and family. When the unique cultural perspectives of patients and families are not understood or addressed, those with different worldviews can be left feeling frustrated, dominated, and oppressed (Uys & Smit, 1994).

Following are illustrations of varying worldviews, especially with respect to health care. They are offered as examples about how values and the interpretation of these values influence perspectives. These illustrations demonstrate the importance of undertaking individual cultural assessments, as it is not possible for nurses to know the complexities of every culture. Through a cultural assessment, nurses can learn and understand the values and beliefs of each patient, client, or family.

### Worldviews: Cultural Perspectives

#### Chinese Health Care Culture

Within the Chinese culture, holism and caring permeate every aspect of health care. Illness is viewed as a state of disharmony between the individual and the natural and social environment. Traditionalists in the Chinese culture believe that both caring and curative processes are necessary to enable the person's harmony to be restored and that the manner in which the sick person is cared for is important to a therapeutic environment. It is the moral duty of the family to provide care for family members who are sick. The family is considered to be the basic social unit through which a person learns appropriate ways of relating to others, and how a person treats his or her family is an important indication of his or her integrity (Wong & Pang, 2000). Consider the following norms within traditional Chinese culture and how they might influence health care:

- Children are required to obey their parents, protect them, bear their burdens, and try their best to help them lead a good long life.
- Families (not the individual) take charge of treatment decisions.
- Family members accept a moral duty to take care of their sick relatives. This is grounded in the Confucian ethical system of role relationships.

#### Aboriginal Communities

In Aboriginal languages, there is no direct translation corresponding to the Western concept of *health*. Instead, there are the concepts of the individual living in harmony with nature and of a

continued on following page >>

complex, dynamic process that has to do with social relationships, land, and the identity of the individual and his or her role within the community.

Through the oral tradition of Aboriginal cultures, stories are passed across generations, enabling a transfer of cultural experiences that embed values and beliefs. These stories have major significance as they reflect the entire historical range of Aboriginal human experience and provide an orientation to life and reality. They are often shared through fables that have animals as their characters. Within the fables, metaphors are used to illustrate the values and norms of the culture and hence to influence thinking and behaviour.

Aboriginals view themselves in terms of "self in society" rather than "self and society." They place a stronger focus on the family and the community, which has implications for their views of informed consent and decision making regarding care. An individual would want to con-sult with family members or community elders before making a decision regarding his or her course of treatment (Arnold & Bruce, 2006; Uys & Smit, 1994).

### Hinduism and Sikhism

Though unique in many ways, Hindu and Sikh cultures traditionally approach morality similarly, emphasizing duty over rights. They also share a belief in rebirth (reincarnation) and the concept of karma, in which actions of past lives influence the experience of present and future lives. The fundamental idea of karma is that each person is repeatedly reborn so that his or her soul may be purified and ultimately join the divine cosmic consciousness. The moment of conception marks the rebirth of a fully developed person who has lived many previous lives.

Though different from one another, in many respects, these cultures share values related to purity, and have a holistic view of the person that affirms the importance of family, culture, the environment, and the spiritual dimensions of life (Coward & Sidhu, 2000). Both cultures share the belief that for each person "birth and death are repeated in a continuous cycle" (Coward & Sidhu, 2000, p. 168). For example, in this belief system, the termination of a fetus would send that "soul" back into the karmic cycle of rebirth. This belief is significant, as it may influence decision making and the application of ethical principles in these circumstances. For instance, the issues that may challenge an expectant mother from a Western society may not be at play in these cultures as they would be assured that the soul would have the opportunity for future rebirth. These beliefs would also influence views on end-of-life choices, such as withdrawal of treatment.

### Questions for Discussion

1. How would these cultural differences influence your nursing practice? Should they influence practice?
2. What have you observed in practice when families from various cultures have views on consent that differ from the Canadian "norm"?
3. When a conflict of values exists and there are risks to the patient because of them, how should this conflict be resolved?

As noted earlier, in many cultures, the ethical agent may be neither the patient nor the family but the leader of the community. The individual is seen not as autonomous but, rather, as integrated with his or her extended family, caste, and environment. In some cultures, males are dominant, while in others, the women are matriarchs, leading the family. Nurses need to be respectful of these varied values and cultures in order to ensure optimal, ethical decision making that is not imposed on by dominant Western thinking. Nurses in all circumstances must:

- Understand the concepts that are important to the patient's culture
- Involve the family
- Respect modesty and purity concepts
- Use interpreters who understand the culture and the health care issues when necessary
- Consider traditional medicine (of that culture) as a complement to Western medicine
- Understand when cultures use a duty-based versus rights-based approach (as discussed in Chapter 2) to ethical decision making
- Be respectful of diverse cultural and religious assumptions regarding human nature, purity, health and illness, life and death, and the status of the individual

## How Does Diversity Influence Nursing Practice?

Clearly, patients and families who come from diverse cultural backgrounds are at risk not only because there may be language barriers but also because there may not be a shared understanding of what is meaningful to them. Illness and associated stressors compound these challenges of language and comprehension (Andrews & Boyle, 2002). To ensure culturally safe care, there needs to be a balance of power between providers and clients, as well as an acknowledgement of the social, political, and economic factors that influence and shape individual and collective attitudes. This is possible when nurses understand the health beliefs and practices of different cultural groups. As role models, nurses should engage in actions that respect and empower the cultural identity and well-being of individuals, families, and communities.

To address the gaps in health care delivery and health status among diverse groups, it is therefore important for nurses first to understand and reflect on the assumptions of the dominant Western cultural values that underlie health policies, research, and interactions (Racine, 2003; Andrews & Boyle, 2002).

In a country as diverse as Canada, it is impossible for nurses to be knowledgeable about all cultures. However, in order to provide culturally competent nursing care, nurses should perform assessments that include the exploration of a patient's or family's culture, their values, and what is meaningful to them regarding care and involvement of the family. A comprehensive cultural assessment is the foundation for culturally competent nursing care.

Health care institutions can also implement programs to encourage diversity in their workforces. Many will seek to hire nursing professionals from among visible or ethnic minorities to diversify the makeup of their health care teams. Such programs are encouraged by most government policies and are constitutionally protected by section 15 of the *Charter of Rights and Freedoms*, which protects reverse discrimination programs designed to provide advantages to traditionally disadvantaged ethnic or minority groups.

To be culturally competent, nurses should adjust their approach based on the culture of the patient or client and his or her family. Nurses do this by listening and by not making assumptions or judgements. Essentially, culturally competent nurses listen to a person's story.

# Case Scenario

## WHOSE BEST INTERESTS?: WHEN CULTURAL PERSPECTIVES CLASH

A 15-year-old Aboriginal adolescent has been transported from northern Manitoba to an acute-care facility in Winnipeg. He sustained serious injuries in a hunting accident when he tripped over brush and severely injured his right arm. Not sure that they can save the arm and worried about sepsis and gangrene setting in, the team members think it is in the patient's best interests to have it amputated. The problem is that doing so will significantly affect his future livelihood since hunting was to be a major source of his income. He and his family are reluctant to make this decision and ask for a meeting of tribe elders. Five leaders arrive at the hospital and ask that the team tries its best to save the arm.

### Issues
1. What are the rights of this young man? What are his best interests?
2. Hospital policy states that the substitute decision maker is the patient's next of kin—in this case, his parents. How would you manage this different view of consent?

## Interprofessional Practice (IPP)

**Interprofessional practice** has emerged as a health care priority in Canada. It is defined as the continuous interaction of two or more professions that are organized with a common goal of solving or exploring mutual issues with the best possible collaboration with the patient and family (Nicholas, Fleming-Carroll, & Keatings, submitted 2007). There has been a longstanding recognition of the need for teamwork in clinical practice, and finding new ways to ensure delivery of interprofessional care has been raised as an imperative for best practice (Sicotte, D'Amour, & Moreault, 2002; Curran, 2004).

Changes in the health care sector over the past two decades have been driven by an increasing emphasis on measurable outcomes, best practices, continuity of care, and cost containment. Patients and clients present with multifactorial problems and feel the impact of social determinants of health (e.g., poor nutrition, limited education, poverty), which require an interprofessional approach to care. This approach helps to ensure good communication, cooperation, coordination, collaboration, and integration for the purpose of exchanging ideas, expertise, theories, and perspectives. There is immense value in obtaining input from all professional team members who may define or explain a situation in different but qualitatively important ways.

Historically, there have existed many challenges to interprofessional collaboration. These have included the perceived uniqueness of each profession and its professional self-interest versus sharing knowledge and scope. There is a growing acceptance that scopes of practice do overlap but that each professional discipline has a distinct expertise to offer in order to achieve the best outcomes for patients and clients.

Hewison and Sim (1998) propose that professionals evolve through these levels of team functioning:

- **Unidisciplinarity**: Feeling confident and competent in one's own discipline.
- **Intradisciplinarity**: Believing that you and fellow professionals in your discipline can make an important contribution to care.
- **Multidisciplinarity**: Recognizing that other disciplines also have important contributions to make.
- **Interdisciplinarity**: Willing and able to work with others in the joint evaluation, planning and care of the patient.
- **Transdisciplinarity**: Making the commitment to teach and practise with other disciplines across traditional boundaries for the benefit of the patient's immediate needs (Hewison & Sim, 1998, p. 311).

Within one profession, though each member may have a unique perspective, there are usually some shared views and perspectives. At the same time, if team members within the same profession have various areas of expertise, they may offer different opinions regarding care. Further, when several professions are involved, each offers an approach or perspective influenced by the knowledge and expertise of that discipline.

Multidisciplinary teams focus on the same patients and may understand the contribution of each member of the team; however, the care can be fragmented as each member may be contributing his or her component of care in isolation from other team members. This may result in confusion for the patient and family.

In an interprofessional model, professionals from within each discipline share their views and perspectives in pursuit of a common set of objectives and a shared plan for the patient and family.

Interprofessional teams consult with each other, coordinate care as a team, and negotiate the role each member will play with respect to the care of the patient. *Coordination,* essential to interprofessional practice, is the integration of the team members' plans and action, and requires effective communication and common decision-making processes. *Collaboration*, also essential to interprofessional practice, is the process through which team members make decisions together and reach consensus on moving forward with a plan (Parsons, Clark, Marshal, & Cornett, 2007). This also implies shared responsibility and accountability for outcomes (Lessard, Morin, & Sylvain, 2008).

Although nursing values interprofessional collaboration, this does not mean that the profession should surrender its own identity. The success of interprofessional collaboration is dependent upon connecting each profession's shared value base, yet still maintaining each one's unique identity and skills.

Interprofessional collaboration requires different professions to learn from and about each other in order to provide efficient patient-focused delivery of health care. At the same time, the integrity of each profession must be maintained (Irvine, Kerridge, McPhee, & Freeman, 2002; Irvine, Kerridge, & McPhee, 2004).

In summary, interprofessional practice is conceptualized as the health care team's "sharing" in the delivery of patient and family-centred care. Within the vision of IPP, the health care team is viewed as a means for integrating knowledge and finding solutions to complex health problems, rather than working in isolation. The values of the team complement each other. They share decision-making data, planning, interventions, and care philosophies (Cowan, Shapiro, Hays, Afifi, Vazirani, Ward, et al., 2006).

## Shared Ethical Challenges of Interprofessional Teams

Emerging studies suggest that patients experience positive outcomes when professional members of the health care team work and learn together (Zwarenstein & Reeves, 2000; Walsh, Brabeck, & Howard, 1999). This is especially true when the team faces complex ethical issues and challenges. Collaboration and open discussion among team members are essential to ensuring that ethical issues are addressed (Kenny, 2002). The interprofessional team must enter into negotiations with one another when facing ethical decisions, as these issues are not isolated to one discipline (Botes, 2000) but involve all team members who are caring for that patient or client and family. As with all aspects of patient care, there is greater value when the team listens and learns from one another in order to understand the lens through which each profession views the issue or problem. Morality and ethics within the health care setting cannot be isolated to individual team members or disciplines. Together, the team has a greater influence on ethical practice and will be more likely to effect the best outcomes for patients and families.

There are various methods of encouraging team learning and facilitating team approaches to ethical discourse. Understanding one another's individual and professional values can be done through the narrative, as discussed in Chapter 2. As a tool, the narrative, or sharing of stories, helps both the individual and each profession as a whole to engage in moral reflection. It also offers a framework to facilitate understanding of the individual and professional lenses through which the issue is viewed (Verkerk, Lindemann, Maeckelberghe, Feenstra, Hartoungh, & de Bree, 2004).

Verkerk et al. (2004) offer a process whereby teams learn and understand each other's ethical perspectives. The initial phase of the model encourages shared decision-making regarding ethical choice and action:

1. Team members support each other in attaining "a heightened moral sensitivity to the vulnerabilities, values, and responsibilities they encounter in their work—a sensitivity acquired by identifying and developing a point of view that can be used as a touch-stone for the decisions about the best way of proceeding" (Verkerk et al., 2004, p. 32).
2. Team members support each other "to understand that they are a part of a practice that involves multiple perspectives and positions" (Verkerk et al., 2004, p. 32), thereby acknowledging that individuals may have different views and perspectives, all of which may have merit.
3. Team members support each other to "appreciate that they are participants in a socially shared practice" (Verkerk et al., 2004, p. 32) that requires collective action and decision making.

Through the process outlined above, the team becomes committed to a collaborative and supportive approach to ethical decision making. Verkerk et al. then provide a guide through which the perspectives of the various professionals involved are shared so that collectively they can decide on a plan and clarify their respective responsibilities as negotiated by the team (Verkerk et al., 2004):

1. The team members offer their initial reaction to the story.
2. The team members are guided to critically examine the moral particulars of the story.
3. The team members map out their professional responsibilities with respect to the situation.

This model serves to create a clearer understanding of the various perspectives of one's fellow professionals. Through this process, learning occurs and greater clarity about the roles of the team and its individual members is achieved. Best courses of action can be decided upon, as can the respective responsibilities of each team member and the team as a collective. As a methodology, this serves to ensure that different perspectives are heard and respected, and that the many moral dimensions of the issues are discussed and understood.

Some other approaches use codes of ethics as a foundation to enhance interprofessional discussion and collaboration. Interprofessional teams may focus on their respective codes of ethics in order to understand their various roles and perspectives. In doing so, they have the potential to learn more about both their individual and shared responsibility for patient care.

# Case Scenario

## DO YOU EVER TALK TO EACH OTHER?

Patrick, 65, is being discharged after a total knee replacement. When he was admitted, his nurse did a comprehensive assessment of his home and social situation. She documented that he lives alone, as his wife died six months ago. He lives in a two-storey house that has a bathroom on the main floor, so he plans to sleep on this floor until he is comfortable with stairs. His next-door neighbour has indicated that he will assist him with ambulation and ensure that he has the food he needs during his convalescence.

His surgery went well, and he is now ready for discharge. On his day of discharge, he is visited by his physiotherapist, his dietitian, and finally the home care coordinator. Each of them asks him if he lives alone, whether he has any supports, and whether he has to deal with stairs. By the time the home care coordinator asks these questions, Patrick is extremely abrupt with her and asks whether the team members ever talk to each other. The coordinator asks the nurses if he is always this grumpy!

### Issues

1. A number of professionals are involved in Patrick's care. Are they functioning as a team?
2. How would interprofessional practice change the approach of these caregivers?

Regardless of the methodology chosen to facilitate an approach to interprofessional practice and interprofessional collaboration with respect to addressing challenging issues of ethics and morality, leaders are crucial to ensuring that these processes are in place.

## Patient- and Family-Centred Care

Organizations and leaders play a significant role in ensuring that appropriate models of practices are in place to ensure the delivery of not only the best care but also the most ethical care. One such model and philosophy is that of family- and patient-centred care, which recognizes that the family is essential to the well-being of the patient and that, when possible, the patient should be involved in the planning, delivery, and decisions regarding his or her care. It has been demonstrated that patients have better outcomes and cope better when they are supported by their families, especially during the difficult experiences of illness or injury (Ecenrod & Zwelling, 2000; Shelton, 1999; Van Riper, 2001).

Family- and patient-centred care is an approach to the planning, delivery, and evaluation of health care that ensures collaboration between health care providers, patients, and families with the goal of achieving better health care outcomes and enhanced satisfaction. Family- and patient-centred care applies to patients of all ages and may be practised in any health care setting (Shelton, Jeppson, & Johnson, 1987). It is "a way of caring for children and their families within health services which ensures that care is planned around the whole family, not just the individual child/person, and in which all the family members are recognized as care recipients" (Shields, Pratt, & Hunter, 2006, p. 1318).

It hasn't been that long since families—even the parents of hospitalized children—were restricted from or limited in visiting inpatients. There were concerns regarding infection control, as well as worry that visiting family members would cause the patient distress when they had to leave. Even in children's hospitals this was the case; in some settings, parents were allowed to visit for 2 hours on Sundays. When they left, they invariably left behind crying children. This practice didn't change until the 1950s. Consider the following quotes from *Beyond the Dream: A Legacy of Nursing at SickKids* (The Hospital for Sick Children, 2006).

The thing that's most interesting to me, having nursed for as long as I have, was how little attention was given to the family, really, what this experience meant in having a very ill child. It seemed to me that the children became ours—the institution's. And that was very slow to evolve, I think, to recognize the importance of the family as being central to the child's experience.

Certainly by the time the College Street hospital opened, and after the turn of the century, there was extreme restriction on visiting. Parents were thought to be a nuisance.... They certainly weren't encouraged to participate in any way.

There were stories and descriptions of parents standing outside having to look in on children. The parents weren't allowed in the public wards except for 2 hours on Sunday, 2 to 4. And they barricaded the ward. If the parents brought in candy or food, it was taken from them.

And then after they left, you could hear those children all the way to Bloor Street. Sunday night was bedlam.

Dr. Alan Brown ... wanted to minimize the death rate so the children were not to get any infections. And so there were no visitors.

My superior at Sick Children's was the assistant director of surgical nursing, Lucy Ashton. And Lucy was the one who decided that ... based on some research coming from England—it came out in the '50s actually, but it had to do with separation anxiety. And they realized, in fact, that children did need their parents with them, and it was an important facet to their cure and well-being.

And so that was so much ingrained in my lifestyle that I didn't know whether we could do this or not.... However, we did it. I agreed to it, along with Lucy and Ann. And, of course, then we had to get permission from other powers that be, and so it was opened up for visiting.

One of the things we started doing was liberalizing the visiting hours and, in fact, going the extra mile to establish what we call family-centred care, which involved the parents in the actual care of the children. (The Hospital for Sick Children, 2006)

In contrast, parents now are considered active participants in their children's care and are integral members of the health care team (Ward, 2005). Families and parents help to make the most appropriate decisions regarding care. With their knowledge of the patient, combined with the professional expertise of the health care team, it is hoped that the best interests of the child and family are ensured.

Even though the discussion above focuses on the roles of parents with respect to their children, these same principles apply to the relationships patients of all ages have with family members. There are many views about who represents a person's "family." Today, families may be divorced, blended, adoptive, or gay or lesbian. When a competent adult is the patient, the definition of the family should be made by that person. For example, though one is legally related to parents or siblings, some patients may identify their closest friends as their family and wish their presence. Also, competent patients may designate a substitute decision maker, who might not be a legal relative.

Patients rarely live in isolation but are enmeshed in familial and other relationships and communities that influence their perspectives and provide them with comfort and reassurance. Families share deep, personal connections and commitments and are mutually entitled to receive and obligated to provide support and care (Ward, 2005).

Qualitative studies in neonatal intensive care settings reveal findings that support the need for well established family-centred structures and processes:

- Most parents want to be fully informed and involved in ethical decisions, whereas many providers wanted to protect them from these difficult realities.
- Parents want even more involvement and participation in the care of their child.
- Some caregivers have concerns that parents may not be capable of making competent decisions in these stressful circumstances.
- Many parents did not believe they had received all the necessary information about their infant and had difficulty interpreting information they did receive.
- Parents indicated that when they believe they are getting complete information about their infant, they are more likely to trust the caregivers.

- Patient units with less restrictive visiting reported greater parental involvement in decision making.
- Timing of discussion with parents and effective communication are significant to ensuring a better experience for the parents (Ward, 2005).

The establishment of family- and patient-centred care in all settings has not come without some tension and conflict. Differing understandings, values, perceptions, and expectations may be brought by individuals and constituent groups.

As discussed earlier, whereas in North America, there is a strong focus on the autonomy of the individual, many cultures rely on family involvement in decision making. In circumstances of hospitalization, families may be under stress and in crisis, yet their needs may not always be identified by the health care team. Also, the expertise of families with respect to their unique knowledge of the patient may not always be recognized. Indeed, all families are different. They cope uniquely; for example, some may be information seekers, while others may not be. Some may be highly emotional, while others will be reserved. Some families may challenge the authority of the team, and some families may be perceived by the team to be quietly "watching over them."

Sometimes, teams measure families against each other, potentially resulting in a concerning and pejorative labelling of some families as "difficult." Families become "difficult" when their needs are not being met, when there is a lack of trust, and when they are seriously worried about the care their family members are receiving. A model of family-centred care that respects the family's knowledge and expertise by engaging them both as recipients of care and as commentators of care, results in better relationships and, in the end, better care for the patients.

Recognizing the key role and integral component of family inclusion is crucial to family-centred care. In reality, most health care is delivered in the home by family members. A study of terminally ill patients found that family members, mainly women, provide the bulk of care for dying patients, with little help from paid caregivers or volunteers (Emanuel, Fairclough, Slutsman, Alpert, Baldwin, & Emanuel, 1999). Recognizing families' role in care invites careful attention to supports and resources that facilitate and nurture parents. The Institute for Family-Centered Care has outlined the following elements that together ensure family-centred care (Shelton, Jeppson, & Johnson, 1987):

- Recognize the family as a constant in the child's life.
- Facilitate parent–professional collaboration at all levels of health care.
- Honour the racial, ethnic, cultural, and socioeconomic diversity of families.
- Recognize family strengths and individuality and respect different methods of coping.
- Share complete and unbiased information with families on a continuous basis.
- Encourage and facilitate family-to-family support and networking.
- Respond to child and family developmental needs as part of health care practices.
- Adopt policies and practices that provide families with emotional and financial support.
- Design health care that is flexible, culturally competent, and responsive to family needs.

## Why Is Family-Centred Care Important?

Within the model of family-centred care, patients have a choice regarding family access. In keeping with this philosophy, the right thing to do as a nurse is to partner with patients and families. The health care environment is extremely complex and highly technological; the family's ability to navigate this system is an essential component of keeping patients safe. Key points to consider when advocating for and inviting family involvement are as follows:

- A family member who knows a patient very well can identify even the most subtle signs of discomfort, pain, or change in condition, and alert the team to that.
- A family member may have history that can be of assistance to the health care team. For example, in the hospital setting, the family member will likely know the patient's history and can alert the team to a complication that may have arisen during a previous hospitalization, a reaction to a medication, or treatments that were effective or, conversely, ineffective.
- A family member who is with the patient most of the time can contribute to shift-to-shift reports and to team conferences regarding the patient's progress. Further, parents and other family members can assist nurses and other health care professionals in the monitoring of the patient's condition and his or her response to treatment.
- When the patient is a child, he or she may be developmentally unable to monitor his or her care or appreciate treatment plans. Parents then can take on this role and alert the team when the wrong medication or treatment may be about to be given.
- The health care team can collaborate with families and patients to ensure there is a clear understanding of the discharge plan and transitions (Johnson et al., 1992).

### ROLES THAT FAMILY MEMBERS CAN PLAY

As noted, family members play integral roles in care delivery. In many families, key individuals emerge as primary caregivers and, in this role, provide crucial and diverse care functions. Yet health care professionals may not fully appreciate the costs borne by these individuals or their families in providing this increased level of patient care. For instance, family caregivers might need to quit their jobs, leaving themselves and their family in a precarious financial situation and subject to increased stress. If families lack flexible workplace accommodations, substantial hardship may result. For nurses and other interprofessional team members, supporting the family caregiver and helping families to understand the role they can play in the context of the team may help family members feel more comfortable as team members and, possibly, more able to articulate patient and family needs and challenges.

Clearly, families can play a variety of roles in supporting patients. They play an important role as advocates, by ensuring that the best interests of the patient and the family members are sought and maintained. This is especially important when patients' competency is compromised as a result of illness or hospitalization. Patient safety is enhanced when family members effectively assist in caregiving and ongoing monitoring of care (Burns, 2008; Canadian Patient Safety Institute, 2007; Fleming-Carroll, Matlow, Dooley, McDonald, Meighan, & Streitenberger, 2006; Stevens, Matlow, & Laxer, 2005). In many settings, especially in the home, family caregivers may provide direct care. Whether this care is being provided by family caregivers or alternative care providers such as trusted companions or substitute decision makers (Levine & Zuckerman, 1999), it is for nurses not only to know who is providing care but also to consider ways to provide support and guidance.

STRATEGIES FOR INVOLVING FAMILIES

In some settings, tensions are created with respect to the role of the family and their relationship with the team. Through an ethic of accommodation, health care professionals can better meet the needs of families by gaining greater knowledge and understanding of family needs and dynamics during times of crisis. Through negotiation and accommodation, they can establish partnerships with families and keep avenues of communication and dialogue open. Learning what is important to families, recognizing the various roles that family members play, and sharing with families are important means of supporting them through crisis and uncertainty (Levine & Zuckerman, 1999, 2002).

NEGOTIATION AND ROLES

Family-centred care requires a "process of negotiation between health professionals and the family, which results in shared decision-making" (Corlett & Twycross, 2006, p. 1308). An extensive review of the literature reveals three themes related to negotiation, familial expectations of participation in care, and power and control.

The literature emphasizes the importance of openness and communication regarding mutual understanding of expectations and roles. Though many family members want to participate in care, they differ in the level and extent of their participation. For example, parents who care for a child at home may want respite; when a child's treatment is new, they may or may not want to participate in interventions usually provided by nurses. In the hospital setting, some parents feel they are losing their parental role and are reluctant to hand that role over to others. Some parents perceive nurses (whether the nurses are conscious of this or not) as the "gatekeepers" who decide the extent of parental involvement. They worry about who has control over their child.

The many nuances around family-caregiver inclusion and accommodation in health care provision are complex and multifaceted, inviting careful and critical review of the practice of nurses.

OPPORTUNITIES TO ADVANCE FAMILY-CENTRED CARE

Examples of the benefits of family involvement and hospital presence or visitation abound in the literature. During the SARS outbreaks of 2003, both those with and without SARS in Toronto were isolated from family and friends, as visiting was restricted. Feelings of boredom and anger arose among patients, as did the effect of quarantine on their families. Psychological as well as physical effects appear to emerge when family visits and presence in hospital are withdrawn (Maunder, Hunter, Vincent, Bennett, Peladeau, Leszcz, et al., 2003).

This mounting evidence invites us to consider ways to ensure family presence and, conversely, challenges traditional practices precluding such practices. For instance, traditionally, family members are kept out of the patient's room during emergency or resuscitation procedures even though many studies point to the benefits of their presence (Tsai, 2002). This is a challenging ethical area that is the focus of continued debate among health care professionals, the notion garnering variable support (Sacchetti, Guzzetta, & Harris, 2003). The ethical conflict contrasts the wishes of the family to be present against whether health care professionals can deny them that opportunity (Nibert, 2005). Though it may not always be possible, and though some families may choose not to be present, there are documented positive benefits of family presence. Surviving patients have reported feeling comfort and support from the presence of family members, and in cases in which the patient has died, family members report that their presence at the death helped with the bereavement process.

Studies suggest that when a patient has undergone resuscitation efforts, up to 80% of family members would like to have been offered the opportunity to be present, but only 11% are given the opportunity. All interviewed families present during emergency and resuscitative procedures report that they found it helpful to be present. Most families want to be present if there is a chance their loved one may die. It makes sense that they would want the opportunity to say goodbye while the patient is still alive and that they would want to be present to ensure that all possible efforts are made to save their loved one (Back, 1991).

In advancing family presence in these care situations, a substantial challenge is the attitudes of physicians and nurses (Osuagwu, 1991). These professionals express concern that the family might interfere, detracting from their focus on saving the person's life and causing stress for the team and the family. Yet, the experience of team stress is not uncommon during emergency situations, and this can be balanced by the satisfaction that the patient and family have been helped by having their relational and support needs met.

Some institutions have introduced progressive programs to facilitate family presence in these circumstances. These programs offer an assessment process, education for the team and families, and support for the family during the emergency. This offers families greater opportunity for closure and a chance to say goodbye in the event of death (Nibert, 2005). Studies suggest that family presence does not interfere but can offer great comfort to both the patient and family (Nibert, 2005). Accordingly, nurses have advocated for family presence (Nibert, 2005).

In a recent study of 197 family members present during emergency situations, no incidents of family interference were identified. In only seven cases, a family member was asked to leave for various reasons (e.g., comfort of provider during intubation, needing to discuss potential of child abuse, emotionally overwhelmed). Overall, a low prevalence of negative outcomes appears to indicate negligible negative impacts of family presence on patient care (O'Connell, Farah, Spandorfer, & Zorc, 2007); however, barriers to grapple with include potential negative psychological impacts on family members, family interference in care, and possible increase in staff stress due to families' presence, with a potential influence on performance (O'Connell et al., 2007). At this point, it might be worthwhile for the reader to refer back to "Margaret's Story" (discussed in Chapter 2, page 16) and reflect on that discussion within the context of this additional background information.

## Conclusion

At the crux of family- and patient-centred care is the belief that the family (as defined by the client or patient) is essential to the treatment of illness or injury and is a cornerstone of a thoughtful, philosophical approach to care. Patients cope better when supported by the presence of those they love. The health care environment is extremely complex and highly technological, and families' role in navigating the system is an essential component of keeping patients safe. It invites attention to and innovation in altering processes for partnerships in care; fosters decision making that ensures the best interests of patients and families; and emphasizes the moral responsibility of team members to facilitate family-centred care in an interprofessional health care environment.

## Summary

In any organization, how business is conducted matters, and this is especially true in health care. In the health care sector, there is the added dimension of having responsibility for a vulnerable client population and aiming to provide the best care possible. The continuum of patient care is influenced by organizational and clinical systems and processes that must meet the same ethical standards as does practice.

In this chapter, organizational ethics and leadership ethics were explored as vital to ensuring the engagement of staff through the development of trusting relationships, collaboration, transparency, the provision of opportunities for professional advancement, and the maintenance of a consistent approach to addressing ethical challenges. Leaders also contribute to positive patient, client, and family outcomes by ensuring that important processes and structures are in place to address the many challenges in health care today.

Canada is becoming more culturally diverse; health care is changing; and technology is expanding and influencing the globalization of health care. This is, in turn, affecting the nature of health care and the need for and availability of nurses now and into the future. Nursing leaders must implement a nursing human resources plan that fosters a healthy and ethical work environment and sustains quality patient care.

In a country as diverse as Canada, it is impossible for nurses to be knowledgeable about all cultures. However, in order to provide culturally competent nursing care, assessments should include the exploration of a patient's or family's culture, values, and what is meaningful regarding care and the involvement of family.

There are positive outcomes for patients when health care professionals work and learn together, and this is especially true when interprofessional teams face complex ethical issues and challenges. Collaboration and open discussion among team members are essential to ensuring ethical issues are addressed. Interprofessional practice is strongly aligned to family-centred care, in which the right thing to do is to partner with patients and families. The health care environment is extremely complex and highly technological; the role of the family in navigating this system is an essential component of keeping patients safe. Ethical leaders and ethical organizations ensure all of these processes are in place and, in doing so, ensure a positive, healthy, and ethical culture.

# Critical Thinking

## STAY WITH ME

Gilda is an 80-year-old woman who has just been transferred via ambulance to an emergency department. She is extremely short of breath and experiencing some chest pain. She is accompanied by her daughter, who proceeds to follow her mother but is stopped by the receptionist, who tells her she must stay in the waiting room until she is called. Upset because her daughter cannot stay with her, Gilda starts to cry. Gilda and her daughter are told that the physician must assess her first. The daughter says she has information to share with the team and is told they will interview her later.

### Questions
1. Do you have concerns with this scenario?
2. How can the Emergency Room become more family-centred?
3. Are there patient safety issues here?
4. Do you think Gilda's emotional stress will influence her outcome?
5. If Gilda is admitted, how might this experience influence the role her daughter has with the health care team?

## WHO IS MOST COMPETENT?

Lisa is a 16-year-old girl with cerebral palsy. All her life, she has been cared for at home by her parents with the support of community agencies. She is not ambulatory, needs assistance with feeding, and has trouble being understood by anyone other than her parents.

She has had some trouble recently with a chest infection, and has been admitted to the local hospital with pneumonia. The hospital has relatively open visiting hours, but family members are not allowed to stay during the night unless the patient is palliative.

Lisa's parents are very worried about leaving her alone, especially since she may not be able to communicate effectively with the nurses during the night. They are also concerned that they are not permitted to assist with her care and are asked to leave the room when care is provided. When they ask whether they might hire one of the community nurses to remain with her

continued on following page >>

412

during the night, they are told that it is against hospital policy to have non–hospital-employed nurses providing care.

## Questions

1. Is Lisa at risk in this situation? If so, what are those risks?
2. What might the leaders in this organization do to change practice?

## Discussion Points

1. This chapter discussed leadership, diversity, interprofessional practice, and patient- and family-centred care. How are they related to one another? Are they integrated? Can excellence in any of these domains be achieved in exclusion of another?
2. Consider the clinical environments within which you have had experience, and evaluate them from the perspective of leadership, approaches to diversity, patient-centred care, and interprofessional practice.
3. What strategies should be implemented in the clinical environment to advance leadership, approaches to diversity, patient-centred care, and interprofessional practice?
4. Consider a leader whom you value and look up to, and reflect on why.
5. Do you see yourself as different from others? In what ways are you different? In what ways are you the same?

## References

### Texts and Articles

Andrews, M. M., & Boyle, J. S. (2002). Transcultural concepts in nursing care. *Journal of Transcultural Nursing, 13*(3), 178–180.

Arnold, O. F., & Bruce, A. (2006). Nursing practice with Aboriginal communities: Expanding worldviews. *Nursing Science Quarterly, 18*(3), 259–263.

Back, K. J. (1991). Sudden, unexpected pediatric death: Caring for the parents. *Pediatric Nursing, 17*(6), 571–575.

Barr, H. (2000). Interprofessional education: 1997–2000. *A Review for the UKCC.* London: United Kingdom Central Council for nursing, midwifery and health visiting.

Baumann, A., Blythe, J., Kolotylo, C., Underwood, J. (2004). The international nursing labour market report. In *Building the future: An integrated strategy for nursing human resources in Canada.* Ottawa, ON: The Nursing Sector Study Corporation.

Botes, A. (2000). An integrated approach to ethical decision-making in the health team. *Journal of Advanced Nursing, 32*(5), 1076–1082.

Brodeur, D. (1998). Health care institutional ethics: Broader than clinical ethics. In J. F. Monagle & D. C. Thomasma (Eds.), *Health care ethics: Critical issues for the 21st century* (pp. 497–504). Gaithersburg, MD: Aspen Publishers.

Brown, J. (2003). Women leaders: A catalyst for change. In R. Adlam & P. Villiers (Eds.), *Leadership in the twenty-first century: Philosophy, doctrine and developments* (pp. 174–187). Winchester, UK: Waterside Press.

Burns, K. K. (2008). Canadian patient safety champions: Collaborating on improving patient safety. *Healthcare Quarterly, 11*(Special Issue), 95–100.

Canadian Nursing Advisory Committee. (2002). Our health, our future: Creating quality workplaces for Canadian nurses. Ottawa, ON: Advisory Committee on Health Human Resources.

Canadian Patient Safety Institute. (2007). Ask. Talk. Listen. Be involved in your health care and safety. *Canadian Patient Safety Institute*. Retrieved August 2008 from http://www.patientsafetyinstitute.ca/uploadedFiles/Ask%20Talk%20Listen%20For%20Patients%20and%20Families.pdf

Clegg, S., Kornberger, M., & Rhodes, C. (2007). Organizational ethics, decision making, undecidability. *The Sociological Review, 55*(2), 393–409.

Corlett, J., & Twycross, A. (2006). Negotiation of parental roles within family-centred care: A review of the research. *Journal of Clinical Nursing, 15*(10), 1308–1316.

Cowan, M. J., Shapiro, M., Hays, R.D., Afifi, A., Vazirani, S., Ward, C.R., et al. (2006). The effect of a multidisciplinary hospitalist/physician and advanced practice nurse collaboration on hospital costs. *Journal of Nursing Administration, 36*(2), 79–85.

Coward, H., & Sidhu, T. (2000). Bioethics for clinicians: 19. Hinduism and Sikhism. *CMAJ: Canadian Medical Association Journal, 163*(9), 1167–1170.

Curran, V. (2004). *Interprofessional education for collaborative patient-centred practice research synthesis paper.* Health Canada. Retrieved August 2008 from http://www.hc-sc.gc.ca/hcs-sss/hhr-rhs/strateg/interprof/synth-eng.php

Davis, C. (1988). Philosophical foundations of interdisciplinarity in caring for the elderly, or the willingness to change your mind. *Physiotherapy Practice, 4*, 23–25.

Ecenrod, D., & Zwelling, E. (2000). A journey to family-centered maternity care. *American Journal of Maternal Child Nursing, 25*(4), 178–185; Quiz 186.

Emanuel, E. J., Fairclough, D. L., Slutsman, J., Alpert, H., Baldwin, D., & Emanuel, L. L. (1999). Assistance from family members, friends, paid care givers, and volunteers in the care of terminally ill patients. *New England Journal of Medicine, 341*(13), 956–963.

Fleming-Carroll, B., Matlow, A., Dooley, S., McDonald, V., Meighan, K., & Streitenberger, K. (2006). Patient safety in a pediatric centre: Partnering with families. *Healthcare Quarterly, 9*(Special Issue), 96–101.

Griffith, H. (2001). So long home: Hello Canada. *Nursing BC, 33*(2), 16–19.

Grosenick, L. E. (1994). Governmental ethics and organizational culture. In T. L. Cooper (Ed.), *Handbook of administrative ethics* (pp. 183–197). New York: Marcel Dekker.

Hewison, A., & Sim, J. (1998). Managing interprofessional working: Using codes of ethics as a foundation. *Journal of Interprofessional Care, 12*(3), 309–321.

The Hospital for Sick Children (Producer). (2006). *Beyond the dream: A legacy of nursing at SickKids* [Documentary DVD].

International Council of Nurses. (2001). *Position statement: Ethical nurse recruitment.* Retrieved August 2008 from http://www.icn.ch/psrecruit01.htm

Irvine, R., Kerridge, I., & McPhee, J. (2004 October–December). Towards a dialogical ethics of interprofessionalism. *Journal of Postgraduate Medicine, 50*(4), 278–280.

Irvine, R., Kerridge, I., McPhee, J., & Freeman, S. (2002, August). Interprofessionalism and ethics: Consensus or clash of cultures? *Journal of Interprofessional Care, 16*(3), 199–210.

Johnson, B. H., Seale Jeppson, E., & Redburn, L. (1992). *Caring for children and families: Guidelines for hospitals.* (1st ed.). Bethesda, MD: Association for the Care of Children's Health.

Keatings, M. (2005, February 23). *Values: Shaping organizational culture.* Bioethics Seminar presented at the Joint Centre for Bioethics, University of Toronto.

Kenny, G. (2002). The importance of nursing values in interprofessional collaboration. *British Journal of Nursing, 11*(1), 65–68.

Kingma, M. (2006). *Nurses on the move: Migration and the global health care economy.* New York: Cornell University Press.

Kupperschmidt, B. R. (2004). Making a case for shared accountability. *Journal of Nursing Administration, 34*(3), 114–116.

Laschinger, H. K. S., Finegan, J., Shamian, J., & Casier, S. (2000). Organizational trust and empowerment in restructured health care settings: Effects on staff nurse commitment. *Journal of Nursing Administration, 30*(9), 413–425.

Laschinger, H. K. S., Shamian, J., & Thomson, D. (2001). Impact of magnet hospital characteristics on nurses' perceptions of trust, burnout, quality of care and work satisfaction. *Nursing Economics, 19,* 209–219.

Lessard, L., Morin, D., & Sylvain, H. (2008). Understanding teams and teamwork. *Canadian Nurse, 104*(3), 12–13.

Levine, C., & Zuckerman, C. (1999). The trouble with families: Toward an ethic of accommodation. *Annals of Internal Medicine, 130*(2), 148–152.

Levine, C., & Zuckerman, C. (2000). Hands on/hands off: Why health care professionals depend on families but keep them at arm's length. *Journal of Law, Medicine & Ethics, 28*(1), 5–18.

Lozano, J. M. (2003). An approach to organizational ethics. *Ethical Perspectives, 10*(1), 46–65.

Maunder, R., Hunter, J., Vincent, L., Bennett, J., Peladeau, N., Leszcz, M., et al. (2003). The immediate psychological and occupational impact of the 2003 SARS outbreak in a teaching hospital. *Canadian Medical Association Journal, 168*(10), 1245–1251.

McGillis-Hall, L. M., & Donner, G. J. (1997). The changing role of hospital nurse managers: A literature review. *Canadian Journal of Nursing Administration, 10*(2), 114–139.

McGuire, M., & Murphy, S. (2005). The internationally educated nurse. *Canadian Nurse, 101*(1), 25–29.

Nibert, A. T. (2005). Teaching clinical ethics using a case study: Family presence during cardiopulmonary resuscitation. *Critical Care Nurse, 25*(1), 38–44.

Nicholas, D. B., Fleming-Carroll, B., & Keatings, M. (2007). *Advancing interprofessional practice in a paediatric setting: A framework for change.* Manuscript submitted for publication.

O'Connell, K. J., Farah, M. M., Spandorfer, P., & Zorc, J. J. (2007). Family presence during pediatric trauma team activation: An assessment of a structured program. *Pediatrics, 120*(3), 565–574.

Osuagwu, C. C. (1991). ED codes: Keep the family out. *Journal of Emergency Nursing, 17*(6), 363–364.

Parsons, M. L., Clark, P., Marshal, M., & Cornett, P. A. (2007). Team behavioral norms: A shared vision for a healthy patient care workplace. *Critical Care Nursing Quarterly, 30*(3), 213–218.

Piette, M., Ellis, J. L., St. Denis, P., & Sarauer, J. (2002). Integrating ethics and quality improvement: Practical implementation in the transitional/extended care setting. *Journal of Nursing Care Quality, 17*(1), 35–42.

Racine, L. (2003, June). Implementing a postcolonial feminist perspective in nursing research related to non-Western populations. (Review). *Nursing Inquiry, 10*(2), 91–102.

Renz, D. O., & Eddy, W. B. (1996). Organizations, ethics, and health care: Building an ethics infrastructure for a new era. *Bioethics Forum, 12*(2), 29–39.

Sacchetti, A. D., Guzzetta, C. E., & Harris, R. H. (2003). Family presence during resuscitation attempts and invasive procedures: Is there science behind the emotion? *Clinical Pediatric Emergency Medicine, 4*(4), 292–296.

Sashkin, M, & Williams, R. L. (1990, Spring). Does fairness make a difference? *Organizational Dynamics, 19*(2), 56–71.

Seeger, M. W. (2001). Ethics and communication in organizational contexts: Moving from the fringe to the center. *American Communication Journal, 5*(1).

Shelton, T. L. (1999). Family-centered care in pediatric practice: When and how? *Journal of Developmental and Behavioral Pediatrics, 20*(2), 117–119.

Shelton, T. L., Jeppson, E. S., & Johnson, B. H. (1987). *Family-centered care for children with special health care needs.* Washington, DC: Association for the Care of Children's Health.

Shields, L., Pratt, J., & Hunter, J. (2006). Family centred care: A review of qualitative studies. *Journal of Clinical Nursing, 15*(10), 1317–1323.

Shockley-Zalabak, P., Ellis, K., & Winograd, G. (2000). Organizational trust: What it means, why it matters. *Organizations Development Journal, 18*(4), 35–48.

Sicotte, C., D'Amour, D., & Moreault, M. P. (2002). Interdisciplinary collaboration within Quebec community health care centres. [Evaluation Studies. Journal Article]. *Social Science & Medicine, 55*(6), 991–1003.

Stevens, P., Matlow, A., & Laxer, R. (2005). Building from the blueprint for patient safety at the Hospital for Sick Children. *Healthcare Quarterly, 8*(Special Issue), 132–139.

Tomblin Murphy, G., Maaten, S., Smith, R., Butler, C. (2005). Review of concurrent research on nursing labour market topics. In *Building the Future: An Integrated Strategy for Nursing Human Resources in Canada*. Ottawa, ON: The Nursing Sector Study Corporation.

Tsai, E. (2002). Should family members be present during cardiopulmonary resuscitation? *The New England Journal of Medicine, 346*(13), 1019–1021.

Uys, L. R., & Smit, J. H. (1994). Writing a philosophy of nursing? *Journal of Advanced Nursing, 20*(2), 239–244.

Van Riper, M. (2001). Family-provider relationships and well-being in families with pre-term infants in the NICU. *Heart & Lung, 30*(1), 74–84.

Verkerk, M. A., Lindemann, H., Maeckelberghe, E., Feenstra, E., Hartoungh, R., & de Bree, M. (2004). Enhancing reflection: An interpersonal exercise in ethics education. *Hasting Center Report, 34*, 31–38.

Walsh, M., Brabeck, M., & Howard, K. (1999). Interprofessional collaboration in children's services: Toward a theoretical framework. *Children's Services: Social Policy, Research, and Practice, 2*(4), 183–208.

Ward, F. R. (2005). Parents and professionals in the NICU: Communication within the context of ethical decision making—An integrative review. *Neonatal Network, 24*(3), 25–33.

Williams, L. L. (2006). The fair factor in matters of trust. *Nursing Administration Quarterly, 30*(1), 30–37.

Wong, T. K. S., & Pang, S. M. C. (2000). Holism and caring: Nursing in the Chinese health care culture. *Holistic Nursing Practice, 15*(1), 12–21.

Worthley, J. A. (1999). Compliance in the organizational ethics context. *Frontiers of Health Services Management, 16*(2), 41–44.

Yi, M., & Jezewski, M. A. (2000). Korean nurses' adjustment to hospitals in the United States of America. *Journal of Advanced Nursing, 32*(3), 721–729.

Zwarenstein, M., & Reeves, S. (2000). What's so great about collaboration? *British Medical Journal, 320*, 1022–1023.

# Glossary

**Abortion.** The interruption of a pregnancy either spontaneously or intentionally by means of medical intervention.

**Action.** A *lawsuit* or court proceeding in which an injured party asserts a claim for damages or some other remedial court order against a wrongdoer.

**Actus reus.** The physical element of a criminal offence that results in physical or other harm (e.g., assault causing bodily harm).

**Adjudicate.** In law, the functions of a court or *administrative tribunal* in hearing evidence in a legal controversy between two or more parties, assessing the evidence, making findings of fact and credibility, and rendering a decision (e.g., a verdict of guilty or not guilty in a criminal trial, or a finding of liability and assessment of damages against a defendant in a civil trial).

**Administrative tribunals.** Government boards, agencies, councils, and commissions charged with administration of a particular area (e.g., property taxes, human rights complaints, energy rates, transport licences). These often operate like courts in that they decide claims, grant licences, and so on.

**Advance directive.** A document made and signed by a mentally competent adult detailing specific medical treatments that are to be administered or withheld in the event that the maker later becomes incapable of expressing such wishes owing to mental or physical illness (e.g., Alzheimer's disease, coma).

**Affidavit.** A written statement of facts made under oath or solemn affirmation.

**Appeal.** A legal proceeding in which a superior *appellate court* is asked by one or more parties to the original proceedings to review those proceedings in order to determine whether the inferior court or administrative tribunal committed any errors of law, misconstrued the evidence before it, exceeded its powers, or otherwise acted contrary to law in adjudicating upon the matter. This is not a retrial but a review of the proceedings at trial or at the hearing.

**Appellate court.** A court that hears appeals or reviews decisions of lower or inferior courts.

**Applied ethics.** The application of particular *ethical theories* to actual problems or issues.

**Assault.** Conduct that creates in another person an apprehension or fear of imminent harmful or offensive contact (e.g., a physical or verbal threat).

**Assisted insemination.** A form of *donor insemination*, typically used when the male partner's sperm count is low, in which sperm are extracted and concentrated before being artificially introduced into the recipient's uterus.

**Assisted suicide.** Any aid directed at terminating the life of persons who, due to severe physical limitations or illness, cannot do the act by themselves.

**Autonomy.** An *ethical principle* founded on respect for persons that assumes that a capable and competent person is free to determine a self-chosen plan unless that plan interferes with the rights of others.

**Bargaining agent.** In labour relations, a *union* certified by provincial statute and authorized to negotiate collectively on behalf of a group of employees.

**Bargaining unit.** In labour relations, a group of employees who are members of a *union* and who are bound by the terms of a *collective agreement* (employment contract) negotiated by the union on their behalf with their employer.

**Battery.** Harmful or offensive and nonconsensual contact with the person or clothing of another.

**Beneficence.** A principle that obliges us to act in such a way as to produce some good or benefit for another.

**Bill.** A draft or proposed law that is not yet passed and must be voted upon by Parliament or a legislature; usually introduced by the governing party, but any member of Parliament may introduce a bill.

**Biomedical ethics.** A field of ethics that focuses on issues associated with science, medicine, and health care.

**Burden of proof.** The obligation on a party to litigation (i.e., a criminal or civil lawsuit) to prove a certain fact or facts to a judge or jury.

**Case law.** The law as set forth in decided cases. This is called jurisprudence in civil law systems. (See also *Precedent*.)

**Categorical imperative.** In Kantian ethics, a supreme principle that a law of morality must follow.

**Causation.** In negligence law, a series of related successive events, each of which is dependent upon the previous one, that ultimately result in damage or injury to persons or property.

**Certification.** In labour relations law, the process whereby a particular *union* is legally recognized as the official representative for collective bargaining and labour relations purposes of a certain group of employees in a certain industry.

***Charter of Rights and Freedoms.*** A portion of Canada's *Constitution Act* that sets out the fundamental rights and freedoms of all persons in Canada and limits the rights of the state to infringe upon these rights. Laws or governmental actions that violate these rights without proper justification are null and void.

**Civil code.** A central written and formal source of *civil law* principles and rules.

**Civil law.** A system of law based on Roman law, prevalent in most European countries and in the province of Quebec, in which legal principles and rules are *codified*, or written in an organized fashion into a central statute or code.

**Closed shop.** In labour relations, a place of employment in which, as a condition of employment, a worker is required to belong to the *union* representing the employees.

**Codify.** To formally arrange legal rules and principles into a central written source of law known as a code.

**Collective agreement.** A written contract of employment between an employer and a unionized group of nonmanagerial employees. It binds all employees, lasts for at least one year, and sets out conditions of employment (e.g., wages, hours of work, benefits, sick leave, pension, layoffs, termination, disciplinary action, arbitration of grievances).

**Collective bargaining.** In labour relations, the process by which a *union* (the *bargaining agent*) negotiates the conditions of employment of a group of nonmanagerial employees (the *bargaining unit*) with an employer or group of employers.

**Committee of the person.** One or more persons charged by court appointment with responsibility for the affairs of a person who has been found to be mentally incapable of managing their affairs.

**Common law.** English system of law dating back to the eleventh century, based on unwritten principles derived from judicial *precedents*.

**Complainant.** In professional disciplinary matters, a person who complains, through a formal disciplinary procedure, about the treatment accorded him or her by a member of a self-governing profession (e.g., a physician, nurse, dentist, lawyer).

**Conciliator.** In labour relations, a person usually appointed by the provincial Minister of Labour to intervene in a strike or other labour dispute in an attempt to work out a settlement agreeable to both sides, to narrow the issues under dispute, and to canvass possible solutions.

**Consent.** The permission given by a person to allow someone else to perform an act upon the person giving such permission. Consent can be explicit (expressed verbally or in writing) or implicit (implied by the circumstances or the conduct of the person giving it).

**Constitution.** A written law that sets forth the fundamental rules and principles defining how a country is organized, how its laws are passed, and the extent of the power of its government and its courts.

**Constitutional convention.** In British, Canadian, and Commonwealth constitutional law, a practice that is not a part of the legal written *Constitution* yet is followed by tradition. For example, it is a convention that the Queen (or the Governor General, the Queen's representative in Canada) always follow and accept the advice of her ministers and give royal assent to all legislation submitted to her (or the Governor General). Although the Queen can legally decline to give such assent, to do so would create a constitutional crisis and political impasse.

**Contract.** An oral or written agreement between two or more parties that creates legally binding, mutual obligations and rights.

**Contributory negligence.** A situation in which a *plaintiff* is held partly responsible for the damage or injury sustained because he or she is partly at fault.

**Controlled act.** In Ontario (under the *Regulated Health Professions Act, 1991,* S.O. 1991, c. 18, s. 27), a specific medical act or procedure that may be performed only by a person who is a member of a health care profession (e.g., a nurse, doctor, dentist) and who is authorized by a health profession act (e.g., the *Nursing Act, 1991,* S.O. 1991, c. 32) to perform such an act. (See Chapter 5.) Also called *restricted act* in Manitoba.

**Cooling-off period.** In labour relations, the period between the breakdown in negotiations and the time in which unionized employees may legally commence a strike against the employer or after which the employer may legally lock out the employees. Its purpose is to attempt to settle tensions between labour and management and assist in the resumption of negotiations.

**Coroner's inquest.** An inquiry convened under the authority of a coroner to investigate the circumstances of a death under suspicious circumstances, as a result of wrongdoing, possible negligence, or accident (i.e., not through natural causes). The inquest is presided over by a deputy coroner, and determinations of fact and recommendations are made by a jury.

**Costs.** In legal proceedings, the lawyers' fees and other expenditures associated with the conduct of the proceeding from beginning to end.

**Court of first instance.** See *Original jurisdiction.*

**Criminal Code of Canada.** An act of Parliament that lists and defines all criminal offences and sets out procedural rules for trying such offences and punishing convicted persons.

**Criminal law.** The body of law that prohibits certain specified conduct or acts set out in a criminal code or other statute and includes sanctions (punishment), such as imprisonment or fines, for breach. It includes all rules of criminal procedure used in trying accused persons charged with offences; regulates relationships between the state (society) and the individual; and aims to keep and maintain order.

**Criminal negligence.** Conduct in which the actor (the accused) has acted intentionally in a reckless or wanton manner, showing disregard for the rights or safety of others who might reasonably be expected to suffer harm or damage as a result of such conduct, and in which damage or harm ensues.

**Cryopreservation.** The freezing of tissue for later use. For example, sperm or embryos may be preserved for use in *assisted insemination.*

**Cultural relativism.** The view that individual and group responses to morality are relative to the norms and values of that particular culture or society, or to the specific situation. Also called *normative relativism.*

**Custom.** In law, practice or rules of a particular trade or industry given force of law by the courts in the absence of specific statute law, case law, or doctrine governing the particular area.

**Damages.** A sum of money awarded by a court to a plaintiff at the end of a civil trial as compensation for an injury to person or property caused by the defendant.

**Decertification.** In labour law, the process by which a union loses its right to represent a group of employees and to bargain collectively on employees' behalf, either through its failure to take steps to negotiate a collective agreement or through a vote of the members themselves.

**Defendant.** A person or party against whom a lawsuit is brought; the party sought to be made responsible for the plaintiff's damages.

**Delegation.** In health care, the assignment by a health care professional to another person of a certain act or procedure that the professional is authorized by law and by his or her professional regulatory body to perform. Delegation is lawful if the person to whom the task is delegated is adequately trained to perform the act and properly supervised.

**Delict.** In the *civil law* system of Quebec, a civil wrong, such as an assault. *Delict* corresponds to the word *tort* in common law.

**Democratic rights.** Rights enshrined in the *Charter of Rights and Freedoms*, which provide for democratic participation of citizens in government. These include the right to vote; a maximum five-year-term limit on the life of Parliament or a provincial legislature (i.e., an election at least every five years); and the requirement that Parliament or a legislative assembly sit at least once per year (i.e., no rule by decree or dispensing with legislative approval of laws).

**Descriptive ethics.** A systematic explanation of moral behaviour or beliefs.

**Detain.** To hold in police custody or control without freedom to leave.

**Directive.** See *Advance directive*.

**Disclosure.** The obligation of each party to a lawsuit under the rules of civil procedure to reveal to the other party or parties all evidence, documents, reports, records, and so on that will be relied upon at trial.

**Distributive justice.** A process for deciding how resources are allocated.

**Doctrine.** Texts, journal articles, treatises, restatements of the law, and other learned writings of legal scholars on any legal subject; used by lawyers and judges as an aid in interpreting or developing the law.

**Documentary discovery.** The right of each party in a lawsuit to obtain copies of all relevant documents possessed by or in the control of the opponent(s) and upon which the opponent(s) will rely at trial.

**Donor insemination.** A therapeutic procedure in which sperm from a healthy donor (who may or may not be the woman's partner) are artificially introduced into a fertile woman's uterus.

**Double effect.** A morally correct action intended for good purposes resulting in a negative, unintended outcome (e.g., the provision of appropriate pain relief with the good intention to eliminate pain, and a subsequent effect of that good intention is the hastening of the person's death).

**Dual procedure offence.** In criminal law, an offence that may be tried either as a *summary conviction offence* or an *indictable offence* at the option of the Crown attorney. The choice usually depends on the seriousness of the facts surrounding the laying of charges.

**Due process.** The right of every citizen, regardless of race, sex, colour, creed, or religion, to receive fair treatment according to established procedures and rules of natural justice.

**Duty of care.** A legal obligation imposed on an individual to act or refrain from acting in a way such as to avoid causing harm to the person or property of another who might reasonably be affected and whose rights and well-being ought to be considered by the actor.

**Ectogenesis.** The maintenance of an embryo in an artificial womb.

**Embryo donation.** The making available of surplus cryopreserved embryos that are no longer needed or wanted by the couple who originated them (i.e., by in vitro fertilization). The alternatives are to destroy the embryos or to use them for research purposes.

**Equality rights.** The right to be treated equally by and before the law regardless of one's race, gender, sexual orientation, religion, ethnic origin, physical or mental disability, age, or skin colour. These rights are specifically enshrined in the *Canadian Charter of Rights and Freedoms*.

**Ethical dilemma.** A situation in which the most ethical course of action is unclear, in which there is a strong moral reason to support each of several positions, or in which a decision must be made based on the most right or the least wrong choice of action.

**Ethical principles.** A set of values based on ethical theory and intended to guide right action.

**Ethical theory.** A framework of assumptions and principles intended to guide decisions about morality.

**Ethics.** The philosophical study of questions regarding what is morally right and wrong.

**Euthanasia.** Based on the Greek language, *eu* for good, and *thanatos* for death, in its strictest sense euthanasia is defined as a painless death. The term is used in a number of situations including active voluntary or involuntary euthanasia, in which steps are taken with consent to actively end the life of a dying patient, and situations of passive euthanasia, in which the person is allowed to die; that is, no active steps are taken to preserve the life of a dying person.

**Evidence.** The material with which a party builds its case against another and proves a fact or set of facts. It may take the form of oral testimony given under oath by witnesses, documentary or real physical evidence such as DNA, blood samples, hair and clothing fibres, photographs, and so on.

**Examination for discovery.** A preliminary oral examination at which the lawyer for each party in a trial has the opportunity to ask relevant questions of the other party or parties, under oath, to obtain full disclosure of all evidence and facts that will be relied upon at trial.

**Fidelity.** A guiding principle of relationships based on loyalty, promise keeping, and truth telling.

**Findings of fact.** In law, conclusions drawn by a trier of fact (i.e., a judge or jury) as to what actually occurred, and in what sequence, in a given case. These are based upon an examination and assessment of the evidence adduced at trial by the parties to the litigation (whether criminal or civil). For example, in a civil action in a motor vehicle accident case, one witness may testify that A. drove his vehicle through the intersection against a red light, while another witness may say that the light was green. The trier of fact will assess the evidence given by these two witnesses, determine which is more credible, and make a finding of fact as to which colour the light was when the accident occurred.

**Fundamental rights.** Specific rights enshrined the *Charter of Rights and Freedoms* that are considered to be basic and necessary in every democratic society (e.g., the freedoms of religion, conscience, thought and expression, press, peaceful assembly, association).

**Garnishment.** A court-ordered procedure by which individuals or corporations owing money to a defendant debtor are required to pay a portion or all of it to the sheriff for distribution among the defendant's creditors, including the plaintiff.

**Grantor.** A person of sound mind and usually (in most provinces) over the age of majority who signs a document giving another power to make medical treatment decisions on his or her behalf or decisions respecting his or her property or finances. (See also Power of attorney for personal care.)

**Harm.** Negative consequences to persons, usually as a result of action or nonaction, related to their physical, emotional, and psychological well-being.

**Health disciplines board.** A provincial regulatory body that governs a health care profession with respect to licensing members and that ensures appropriate educational and professional qualifications, standards of practice, and ethical conduct by members. This body's name varies among provinces.

**Homicide.** The death of a human being caused by the actions or omissions of another.

**Hybrid offence.** In criminal law, an offence that can be tried either by indictment or summarily at the option of the Crown. (See also Dual procedure offence.)

**Indictable offence.** The most serious of criminal offences; usually triable by a jury but only after a preliminary hearing at which the accused is ordered to stand trial. Punishment ranges from heavy fines and/or several years' to life imprisonment.

**Inferior court.** A level of court that is judicially subordinate to a superior one; usually a trial court, which is bound by previous decisions of an appeal court.

**Informed consent.** In health care, a legally capable person's consent to a specific medical treatment, the nature and purpose of which, material risks and benefits of which, and material risks of not proceeding with which the person is informed by the health care practitioner. A material risk is one that a person would reasonably wish to know prior to making the decision of whether to undergo or forgo the proposed treatment.

**Injunction.** A court order obtained by one party against one or more other parties that directs those others to refrain from a specific conduct or to perform a specific act.

**Interdisciplinarity.** When more than one discipline is involved with the client, but planning and implementation are undertaken collaboratively.

**Interprofessional practice.** The continuous interaction of two or more health care professionals, organized with a common goal of solving or exploring mutual issues and achieving the best outcomes, with the best possible inclusion of the patient and family.

**Intradisciplinarity.** Individuals or teams within a specific discipline collaborating toward the achievement of positive client outcomes (e.g., a team of nurses planning the patient's care together).

**In vitro fertilization.** A process whereby fertilization occurs outside the body and without intimate human contact.

**Judgement debtor.** A person who has been sued and against whom a court has issued a judgement finding him or her liable to pay a sum of money to the *plaintiff*.

**Judgement debtor examination.** An oral examination at which the *defendant* gives answers under oath to questions by the plaintiff's lawyer concerning his or her finances, sources of income, and ability to pay the judgement against him or her.

**Jurisdiction.** The authority of a court to hear and decide a legal dispute (e.g., civil or criminal) in a particular territory, as well as the types of orders and judgements it may make.

**Jurisprudence.** Judges' written decisions in past court cases, which serve as *precedents* for future decisions in civil law systems; not binding, but seen as evidence of how past courts have interpreted a civil code provision or legal principle. (See also *Case law*.)

**Juror.** Member of a jury.

**Jury.** A group of 12 (in criminal juries) or six (in civil juries) citizens over the age of majority who are convened to hear evidence, make findings of fact, and ultimately deliver a verdict in a criminal or civil trial.

**Justice.** A principle that focuses on the fair treatment of individuals and groups within society.

**Lawsuit.** See *Action*.

**Legal rights.** Rights of all persons residing in Canada that are invoked upon arrest or detention or when such persons are charged with a criminal offence. These are enshrined in the *Charter of Rights and Freedoms* and include the right to life, liberty, and security of the person (e,g., the right not to be compelled to give evidence against oneself in a police investigation and the right to remain silent); the right to be secure against unreasonable search and seizure (e.g., having one's home searched by the police without permission, without good reason, and without a warrant issued by a justice of the peace); the right not to be arbitrarily detained or imprisoned; the right to be informed of the reason for one's arrest and to be informed of the charge; the right to speak to a lawyer in private and to be informed of this right; the right to have the legality of one's detention determined by an impartial court and to be immediately released if that detention is judged to be unlawful; and the right to be tried within a reasonable time by an impartial court, to be presumed innocent until proven guilty, to reasonable bail, and to a jury trial if the punishment for the offence with which one is charged is five or more years' imprisonment. If acquitted or convicted of a criminal offence, a resident of Canada has the right not to be tried again for the same offence (the "double jeopardy" rule). Residents have the right, when punished for an offence of which they have been convicted, not to be subjected to cruel or unusual punishment (e.g., torture or degrading punishment and treatment, inhumane treatment or living conditions while in prison, and, arguably, capital punishment).

**Legislative assembly.** A provincial parliament consisting of only one house. Also called *the legislature.*

**Liability.** The legal responsibility owed by a party at fault to another for *damages* incurred or injury suffered by that other.

**Licensing.** The granting by a nursing regulatory body, such as a college of nurses or provincial nursing association, to an otherwise qualified nurse, of the right to practise within the province in accordance with recognized standards of care and ethics and subject to any restrictions specified in the licence.

**Litigant.** A person or corporation who is a party to a *lawsuit.*

**Living will.** A written document signed by a mentally competent person setting forth specific instructions regarding medical treatments to be applied or withheld in the event that the maker later becomes incapable of expressing those wishes. For example, the document might indicate whether resuscitation should be attempted in the event of a cardiac arrest.

**Lockout.** In labour relations, the employer's equivalent of the strike, in which the employer locks out its unionized employees from the workplace or refuses to continue to employ them, in an effort to pressure them to concede during contract negotiations or in labour disputes. In most provinces, a lockout, like a strike, may occur only after the expiry of a *collective agreement* and only after a *cooling-off period* under the applicable provincial labour statute.

**Malfeasance.** In law, doing an act that is one's duty, but doing it poorly, incorrectly, or negligently.

**Malpractice.** The failure of a health care professional or other specialist to observe and adhere to the appropriate *standards of care* for a given act or procedure; the negligent performance of a procedure or act requiring a reasonable degree of professional skill and ability. (See also *Negligence.*)

**Mens rea.** The mental element of a criminal offence (i.e., the accused's state of mind when he or she is alleged to have committed a crime); the requirement that the accused was aware and willfully intended to commit the act, knew that the act was wrong, or was reckless as to the consequences of the act.

**Metaethics.** A philosophical focus on the meaning and nature of morality and ethics.

**Misconduct.** See *Professional misconduct.*

**Mobility rights.** The rights of all persons legally resident in Canada to move in and out of Canada and between various provinces and cities, to take up residence anywhere in the country in order to pursue employment or educational and other opportunities. These rights are enshrined in the *Charter of Rights and Freedoms.*

**Moral distress.** Stress caused by situations in which one is convinced of what is morally right but is unable to act; results when moral issues are unresolved and when supportive processes are not in place.

**Multidisciplinarity.** The involvement of professionals from more than one discipline (e.g., a nurse, physician, and physiotherapist) in the care of a patient.

**Narrative.** The examination of stories for the purpose of revealing notions of morality and helping to clarify one's moral perspectives.

**Negligence.** The nonintentional category of *tort* law wherein one person has, through carelessness, failed in a *duty of care* toward another such that that other has sustained injury to person or property as a result of the person's act or failure to act.

**New reproductive technologies.** Techniques to promote pregnancy by overcoming or bypassing infertility, including *donor insemination, assisted insemination, in vitro fertilization, cryopreservation,* ovum and *embryo donation,* and *surrogacy.* Advanced genetic technologies have also been developed that include sex selection, embryo research, prenatal diagnosis, and human embryo cloning.

**Nightingale pledge.** Composed by a committee chaired by Lystra Gretter, a nursing instructor at the old Harper Hospital in Detroit, Michigan. Adapted from the Hippocratic Oath, it was first used by its graduating class in the spring of 1893.

> *I solemnly pledge myself before God and in the presence of this assembly, to pass my life in purity and to practice my profession faithfully. I will abstain from whatever is deleterious and mischievous, and will not take or knowingly administer any harmful drug. I will do all in my power to maintain and elevate the standard of my profession, and will hold in confidence all personal matters committed to my keeping and all family affairs coming to my knowledge in the practice of my calling. With loyalty will I endeavor to aid the physician, in his work, and devote myself to the welfare of those committed to my care.*

**Nonfeasance.** Failing to do that which is one's legal duty or obligation to do.

**Non-heart-beating organ donation (NHBOD).** This alternative to brain death allows for the retrieval of organs for donation once the heart has stopped and death is declared after five minutes.

**Nonmaleficence.** A principle that obliges us to act in such a way as to prevent causing harm to others.

**Normative relativism.** See *Cultural relativism.*

**Nursing ethics.** The study of moral questions that fall within the sphere of nursing practice and nursing science.

**Objective standard.** The standard of the reasonable or "average" person against which someone's particular conduct in a given situation is judged. For example, a nurse performing a given task in a particular manner will have his or her methods of doing such task measured against the manner in which one would expect a reasonably competent and skilled nurse to perform it.

**Obligation.** In civil law (as opposed to common law), some act or course of conduct that the law requires an individual or individuals to perform, either for the benefit of another party or parties or for that of society in general. (See also *Duty.*)

**Open shop.** A place of employment in which *union* membership is not mandatory. (See also *Closed shop.*)

**Organizational ethics.** Those values and standards that influence how an organization functions; the methods an organization uses to undertake its business (in hospitals, patient care); and how ethical standards are met in leadership, structures, and processes (e.g., recruitment).

**Original jurisdiction.** The first court to hear a criminal or civil case (i.e., the court in which the litigation process begins).

**Originating process.** A document issued out of a court that begins a legal proceeding and must be formally served upon (delivered to) a *defendant* or responding party or parties. (See also *Statement of claim* and *Writ of summons.*)

**Palliative care.** Care intended to ensure that, through emotional and psychological support and effective symptom management, the patient experiences a quality dying process and a dignified death.

**Parliament.** A body of elected lawmakers (members of Parliament, or MPs) entrusted with the power to make laws for the country or a province. The Canadian Parliament consists of two houses (the Senate and the House of Commons) and the Queen (the Head of State).

**Plaintiff.** The party who brings a lawsuit and seeks *damages* against another for breach of contract or other wrong done.

**Pleadings.** The court documents filed by each party to the lawsuit outlining the nature of the claim, the defence to the claim, and the issues to be tried in the action.

**Power of attorney.** Generally, in Canada, a document in which a legally capable person appoints another to manage the maker's financial affairs and make decisions on the maker's behalf in the maker's absence or unavailability. In Ontario, for example, under the *Substitute Decisions Act, 1992,* S.O. 1992, c. 30, two types of powers of attorney are recognized in law: a power of attorney for property and a power of attorney for personal care (see below).

**Power of attorney for personal care.** In Ontario, a legal document in which the maker appoints someone to make decisions on his or her behalf regarding medical treatment, care, feeding, clothing, shelter, hygiene, and so on, in the event that he or she becomes incapable owing to physical or mental illness. This document takes legal effect only on the maker's becoming incapable of making treatment decisions and giving consent for himself or herself. (See also *Grantor.*)

**Precedent.** A judge's previous decision that serves as a guide or basis for deciding future cases having similar facts or legal issues. A higher-court precedent is usually binding on an inferior court. (See also *Case law.*)

**Preliminary inquiry.** In criminal law, a hearing held before a provincial court judge at which the Crown prosecutor is required to show that the evidence presented is such that a reasonable jury properly instructed could convict the accused. If the evidence is found insufficient in this regard, the accused must be discharged.

**Presumption of innocence.** The principal of law that holds that a person charged with a criminal offence is not guilty until and unless proven guilty of the offence at trial. The Crown (i.e., the prosecution) is obliged to prove beyond a reasonable doubt that the accused committed the offence; the accused need not prove that he or she did not commit the offence.

**Pretrial conference.** A conference of all parties and their lawyers held a few weeks before trial in the presence of a judge other than the one who will hear the trial. The judge reviews the facts of the case and the positions of each party, as well as the strengths and weaknesses of each party's case. Then the judge advises the litigants how the case might be decided. This is a last attempt to reach a settlement without a lengthy and expensive trial.

**Prima facie duties.** Those duties that one must always act upon unless they conflict with those of equal or stronger obligation.

**Principles.** See *Ethical principles.*

**Procedural law.** Law that regulates how individual rights are asserted and enforced in the judicial system, such as which court hears the matter, what documents must be filed and when, and so on.

**Procedural justice.** The perception that processes (e.g., how decisions are made, who is involved, and what process is undertaken) have been fair and inclusive regardless of the outcome.

**Professional misconduct.** In the regulation of the nursing profession, any conduct by a licensed or certified nurse that specifically contravenes the ethical and professional standards or rules of conduct set out by the provincial regulatory body.

**Professions Tribunal.** In Quebec, an administrative tribunal that hears appeals (with leave) of disciplinary decisions involving members of the Ordre des infirmières et infirmiers du Québec and other professional regulatory bodies in the province.

**Proximate cause.** A concept of causation wherein damage, injury, or other resulting event must not be too remote or unforeseeable a consequence of a particular act or omission.

**Proxy.** In health care, a person appointed or otherwise authorized by law to give consent to a specified medical treatment or procedure on behalf of another if the patient is unable to give such consent owing to physical or mental incapacity.

**Proxy consent.** In health care, the consent given by a patient via another person authorized by the patient to give consent to medical treatment.

**Rationality.** The notion of thinking and reasoning, associated with comprehension, intelligence, or inference. Rationality requires explanations, or justifications, particularly for the purpose of supporting an opinion or conclusion. For example, a rational person would have reasons or arguments to support an ethical opinion.

**Reasonable doubt.** The standard of proof in a criminal case. This means that the Crown (the prosecution) must satisfy the trier of fact (either a judge or a jury) that the accused committed the offence with which he or she is charged, giving sufficient *evidence* such that no real or logically compelling reason exists in the trier's mind that the accused did not commit such act.

**Recertification.** Further training and further examination undertaken by a health care professional to demonstrate proficiency in certain professional skills or to maintain such proficiency as a condition of being licensed or certified to practise.

**Registration.** In the regulation of nursing practice, the recording of a nurse's name and other particulars and enrolment of that person as a member of a provincial nursing *regulatory body*.

**Regulations.** Detailed secondary laws passed by a federal or provincial cabinet pursuant to a specific statute. The statute usually gives the cabinet the power to make detailed rules to carry out the intent and purpose of the act but are too detailed and time-consuming for Parliament to enact.

**Regulatory body.** A provincially created professional organization, such as a provincial nursing association or college, charged with licensing and regulating entry into a given health care profession.

**Reprimand.** In nursing disciplinary matters, a penalty administered against a member of the profession by the provincial nursing regulatory body for contravention of the body's *regulations* or for *professional misconduct*, in which the member is admonished before the body orally or in writing (in public or private).

**Restricted act.** See *Controlled act*.

**Revocation.** In nursing disciplinary matters, the cancellation of a nurse's licence or certificate to practise nursing in the province, usually administered against the nurse for violating the regulatory body's professional or ethical standards and rules of conduct.

**Right.** A claim or privilege to which one is justly entitled or may do, either legally or morally.

**Rule of law.** A fundamental principle of Canada's constitution, which demands that all persons, including the state, be subject to the same rules and laws, free from any exercise of arbitrary power. This includes the principle that all persons are equal before the law regardless of wealth, social status, race, gender, etc., and that no one is above the law.

**Rules of civil procedure.** Detailed rules and regulations that govern procedure in the commencement and conduct of court actions, trials, the gathering of evidence, documentation, and the enforcement of court orders and judgements.

**Sanctity of life.** A principle that respects life and emphasizes the continuation of life at all costs.

**Sexual harassment.** Any unwanted conduct, language, or behaviour of a sexist or sexual nature directed by one person toward another.

**Sheriff.** An officer of the court in a particular county or judicial district who is responsible for enforcing court orders, carrying out judicial sales of real estate or other property, and serving court documents on witnesses.

**Slippery slope**. An argument that suggests that when an exception to the rule is made, exceptions will continue to be made until the rule no longer exists. For example, consider the notion of sanctity of life. If we were to allow physician-assisted suicide, soon, euthanasia in all circumstances may become the norm.

**Standard of care.** Legal yardstick against which a person's conduct is measured to determine whether that person has been *negligent* and whether the person's conduct or actions in a given situation have met those expected of a competent health care professional.

**Stare decisis.** Rule of English common law whereby courts are legally bound to follow previous court decisions, which have the force of law. Usually, courts will follow *precedents* whose facts and legal issues are similar or identical to the case they are deciding unless there is good reason to depart from following the precedent (e.g., clear evidence that the court that issued the precedent decision failed to consider relevant facts or another clearly applicable previous precedent). (See also *Precedent* and *Case law.*)

**Statement of claim.** A document prepared and filed by a *plaintiff* in a lawsuit initiating the court *action*. It sets out the *damages* and other relief sought from the court and the bare facts (but not the evidence) upon which the plaintiff relies to support a claim against a *defendant*.

**Statement of defence.** A document prepared and filed by the *defendant* in a lawsuit. It sets forth the defendant's version of the facts (but not the evidence) giving rise to the *action* and the legal grounds or reasons that the defendant is not liable for the *plaintiff*'s damages.

**Statute law.** A formal written law passed by *Parliament* or a provincial legislature that takes precedence over and supersedes common law case law. Also found in *civil law* systems.

**Stem cells.** Cells that are able to renew themselves through cell division. Stem cells exist in the human embryo, where they differentiate to become a fetus and then a human being. Current research induces stem cells to differentiate to replace, for example, brain cells that have been damaged and can be stimulated to become cells with special functions, such as heart muscle and insulin-producing cells.

**Substantive law.** Law that sets out detailed rights and obligations of citizens in private dealings with one another and with society in general.

**Summary conviction offences.** In criminal law, offences of a less serious nature that are tried without a jury in a fairly rapid, straightforward way and for which the maximum punishment is six months' imprisonment or a fine of up to $2000, or both.

**Superior court.** A higher trial court of a province or territory.

**Surrogacy.** An arrangement whereby a woman bears a child for another couple or individual. The gestational mother may be the biological mother (through sperm donation of either the male partner or a donor) or may carry the embryo of the couple, an embryo donated by another couple, or one created from a donor egg and donor sperm.

**Tort.** An intentional or nonintentional (i.e., negligent) wrongful act that causes damage or injury to another's person, reputation, or property.

**Transdisciplinarity.** Disciplines crossing traditional boundaries to share roles with other professionals in the areas of education and practice (e.g., recognizing that more than one discipline may function in a particular role).

**Trial court.** See *Original jurisdiction*.

**Unidisciplinarity.** A focus on the self as a practitioner, not necessarily as a contributor to the broader team. When an individual first enters the profession, his or her focus as a novice is on learning and becoming confident in the knowledge and competencies required of that discipline.

**Union.** In labour law, a group of nonmanagerial employees in a common trade or industry organized in association with a constitution and membership for the purpose of advancing the common interests of its members respecting employment relations with a common employer or group of employers.

**Utilitarian theory.** An ethical theory that considers an action to be right when it leads to the greatest possible number of good consequences or to the least possible number of bad consequences.

**Utility.** A term that considers the value of an outcome or consequence from many perspectives.

**Value.** An ideal that has significant meaning or importance to an individual, a group, or a society.

**Veracity.** A moral principle that emphasizes truth telling.

**Vicarious liability.** In negligence law, the liability of a principal (an employer) for the *negligent* or tortious acts of the principal's agent (an employee) done within the scope of the agent's authority or employment.

**Virtue.** A characteristic of the person that promotes good or high ethical standards.

**Voluntary assumption of risk.** In negligence law, a situation in which an injured *plaintiff* is in possession of sufficient information or has knowledge of dangerous conditions or a state of affairs but assumes the risk that he or she may be injured as a result of such conditions despite this knowledge. For example, a participant in a hockey game assumes the risk that he or she may be injured during the game. This may reduce the liability of a defendant in a subsequent negligence suit.

**Whistle-blowing.** The bringing forward, to an employer or regulator, of allegations that may be related to *misconduct* (e.g., a legal issue, the breach of a regulation, or a direct threat to public interest). Such misconduct may involve fraud, health and safety violations, or corruption. The person bringing forward the concern (the whistle-blower) may fear reprisal.

**Workplace violence.** Violence that occurs in the course of work (e.g., bullying, disrespectful and threatening behaviour, verbal or physical abuse). It may occur between peers, from a manager to staff, from clients, patients, or families to health care professionals. Workplace violence may result in psychological or physical harm.

**Worldview.** The way different cultures and societies view the world and the reality within which they exist. For example, one culture may view society as being made up of individuals who have individual choice and autonomy; others may view society as an interdependent community.

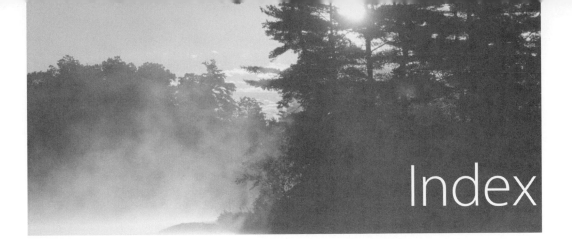

# Index